THE
HERBAL
APOTHECARY

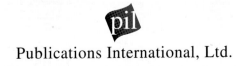

Publications International, Ltd.

Contributing writer: Lisa Brooks

Photography: Alamy Stock Photo, Andrew Massyn, Shutterstock.com

Louis Weber, CEO
Publications International, Ltd.
8140 Lehigh Avenue
Morton Grove, IL 60053

ISBN: 978-1-64030-105-4

Manufactured in China.

8 7 6 5 4 3 2 1

CONTENTS

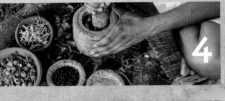
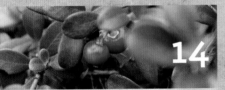
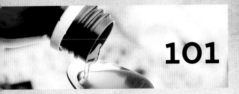
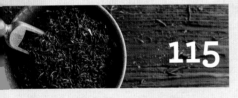
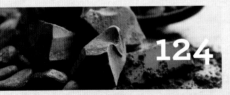
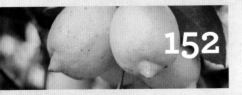
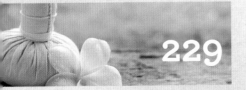

INTRODUCTION

Herbs have long intrigued us—and for good reason. Because of their potential as food and as medicine, they have enjoyed a special relationship with humans throughout the ages.

To our ancestors, knowledge of herbs meant survival. But the passage of time did not diminish human beings' respect for the herb. Druids revered the oak and mistletoe, both rich in medicinal attributes. In the Eastern world, physicians wrote tomes on herbal remedies, some prized to this day as authoritative medical sources. Later, the Greeks and Romans cultivated herbs for medicinal as well as culinary uses. Hippocrates, considered the father of Western medicine, prescribed scores of curative herbs and taught his students how to use them. The search for precious herbs and spices led Europeans to the New World. There they found scores of new plants which they brought back with them to the courts of England, Spain, and France.

The development of pharmaceutical drugs some 100 years ago changed our focus from herbs and natural healing to the new "wonder drugs." Medical practice turned away from botanicals and embraced these new chemical-based medicines. In addition, the Industrial Revolution meant urbanization, and city dwellers, who now had limited access to gardens, welcomed the convenience of shopping for—instead of growing—their medicines and foods.

But there was a renewed interest in herbs in the latter half of the 20th century. Though lifesavers in countless cases, pharmaceutical drugs proved not to be the magic bullets we'd hoped for. Seeking ways to feel better without the side effects of pharmaceutical drugs, countless people began rediscovering herbs as natural remedies.

What exactly is an herb? No group of plants is more difficult to define. In general, an herb is a seed-producing plant that dies down at the end of the growing season and is noted for its aromatic and/or medicinal qualities. Among the most utilitarian of plants, herbs lend themselves to a seemingly endless array of medicinal preparations. And you don't have to be a pharmacist—or a shaman—to make them.

Like other healing traditions, herbal medicine recognizes and respects the forces of nature: Health is seen as the proper balance or rhythm of natural forces while disease is an imbalance of these forces. Because the forces of nature are not easily grasped and manipulated, herbal traditions turn to the earth's masters of natural balance and symmetry— plants.

Indeed, plants are ideal biochemical medicines. We have built-in systems for metabolizing plants and using their energies. But our bodies have difficulty metabolizing and excreting synthetic chemical medicines. And think about the negative terms used to describe the actions of synthetic pharmaceuticals: they suppress, they fight, they inhibit. They do little to support overall health. Medicines made from plants, on the other hand, tend to nourish the body without taxing it, to support the body system rather than suppressing it.

Some pharmacists and pharmacologists argue that synthetic drugs derived from plants have an action identical to the active constituents in the plants. (Constituents are the elements of the plant; active constituents are the elements that produce an effect.) While this is true in some cases (digoxin and ephedrine, to name just two), most synthetic drugs are not identical to their natural counterparts.

Most plants contain a dozen or more different constituents. The idea that we can entirely duplicate the action of a plant by simply synthesizing a single active constituent is somewhat misguided. Part of a plant's healing effect is due to the sum total of all the constituents. To isolate certain constituents is to rob a plant of its deeper healing potential. This concept of a healing vitality or life force in the whole plant is central to the tradition of herbal medicine and is recognized in all the ancient medical systems.

There's no doubt that pharmaceuticals have their place. They enable dramatic alterations of biochemical processes—they can halt severe inflammation, slow the rate of the heart or respiration, or stimulate the bowels to move. These medicines are often necessary in emergencies, acute conditions, and cases of severe illness. But plants offer us nourishment and healing actions that synthetic medications cannot. Many herbs have shown profound healing effects when used as tonics over long periods. Furthermore, synthetic drugs are combined with waxes, stabilizers, tableting agents, and coatings. Plants, on the other hand, are complex collections of naturally occurring and nourishing substances that may have vital roles in health, including vitamins, minerals, amino acids, fatty acids, fiber, and bioflavonoids. Synthetic drugs can also cause side effects and long-term toxicities that are rare in plants. Botanical medications restore the body's processes to normal function; synthetic drugs can push these processes to unnecessary extremes.

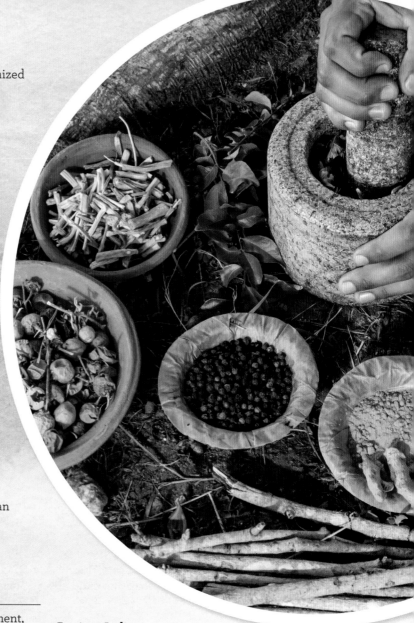

HERBAL MEDICINE YESTERDAY AND TODAY

It was our ancestors, in their search for nourishment, who uncovered the roots of medicine. The Neanderthal and Paleolithic peoples were hunters and gatherers who lived intimately with nature, using plants as food, clothing, shelter, tools, weapons, and medicine. They discovered certain plants could optimize their health while others reduced fertility or made them ill. As they learned which plants were not poisonous, which were nourishing, and which were palatable, they also noted which could calm a nauseous stomach, ease the pains of childbirth, and heal wounds. Some Stone Age artifacts appear to be tools that could grind grains, roots, seeds, and bark—precursors of the mortar and pestle we use today.

Ancient India and Ayurvedic medicine (about 10,000 BC to present). Some of the oldest known writings are clay tablets unearthed in what is now the Middle East. Many of these ancient clay tablets mention healing plants. Within these early writings are four books of classic wisdom, called the *Vedas*, from which the system of Ayurvedic medicine, as well as the Hindu religion, arose. Believed to have been recanted orally since at least 10,000 BC, the information within the *Rig Veda*—the oldest of the four books—describes this ancient medical system.

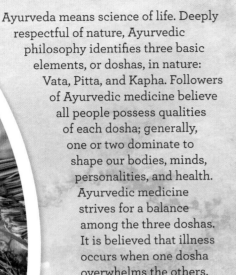

Ayurveda means science of life. Deeply respectful of nature, Ayurvedic philosophy identifies three basic elements, or doshas, in nature: Vata, Pitta, and Kapha. Followers of Ayurvedic medicine believe all people possess qualities of each dosha; generally, one or two dominate to shape our bodies, minds, personalities, and health. Ayurvedic medicine strives for a balance among the three doshas. It is believed that illness occurs when one dosha overwhelms the others.

Ayurvedic medicine looks to nature as the source of wellness, thus its use of healing plants. An Ayurvedic doctor or herbalist begins by identifying which dosha type(s) an individual is; this allows him or her to use an herb with a corresponding physiologic action. A person who tends to have dominant Vata energies, for example, will benefit from plants that decrease excess Vata and/or increase Kapha and Pitta. The effective use of herbs in Ayurvedic medicine requires an intimate understanding of the natural forces within a plant.

Ancient China and Taoism (5000 BC to present). Ancient Asian cultures also embraced the idea that one should seek a balance with the natural forces within all life forms. Chinese Taoism embraces a bipolar medical system rather than the tripolar system of the Ayurvedic doshas. The life force is seen as the ever-churning circular motion of two opposing actions, yin and yang. All diseases are understood as an imbalance of yin and yang. The Chinese believe that *qi* (pronounced chee and sometimes written as chi), or vital energy, is responsible for health. An imbalance of qi results in illness.

All matter, including plants and animals, is yin and yang (although one usually dominates); therefore, plant qi can be used to balance animal qi. A disturbance in a person's qi may affect the balance of yin and yang. For example, if qi is blocked, yang may predominate. Some herbs are predominantly yin tonics, some are yang tonics, and most are a complex combination of yin and yang. Chinese herbalists must be familiar with each plant's energy to prescribe the herbal remedies with the most healing potential.

Ancient Chinese healers were quite sophisticated in their use of plant medicines. One surviving materia medica (Latin for "on medicine"; the term refers to a list of medicinal substances) of more than 365 plants is the *Pen-ts'ao Ching (The Classic of Herbs)*. This oldest-known Chinese pharmacopoeia is said to be the work of the Emperor Shen Nung who ruled in the 28th century BC. The *Pen-ts'ao Ching* lists plants still in use today, including ma huang, ginger, and cinnamon.

Other written records of Chinese herbalism include the *Huang ti Nei Ching*, written in 2500 BC by Huang ti, the "Yellow Emperor." This work is a comprehensive review of Chinese medical arts. A classic on internal medicine, it is still used today in acupuncture schools in the United States. The *Li Shih-Chen* is another ancient Chinese herbal materia medica written by a Chinese scholar by the same name. It was translated into English and published in Britain in 1596 after centuries of use in China. This compendium, which lists more than 2,000 drugs and 8,000 prescriptions, is still studied by traditional Chinese physicians.

Ancient Egypt (4000 BC to 1000 BC). The Eber's papyrus is one of Egypt's most important surviving medical writings. Dating from approximately 1550 BC, this 65-foot papyrus scroll was discovered in 1873 by Georg Ebers, a German Egyptologist. The document includes both herbal and medical therapies, including numerous substances still thought to be medicinally active, such as garlic and moldy bread. The Egyptians had a sophisticated knowledge of plants, as their practice of using myrrh in embalming attests.

Ancient Greece (1000 BC to AD 1). In Greek mythology Asclepias, the Greek god of healing and medicine, carried a caduceus. In ancient Greece, the caduceus, a snake wrapped around the staff of knowledge, symbolized knowledge and healing. Today, the caduceus remains the symbol of medical science.

formed, foreign lands were explored, and goods were traded. The spice trade was particularly strong; ultimately, it stimulated transoceanic explorations by the Europeans. Many kings and emperors hoped to lay claim to new lands and the resources these lands offered. Poisons were frequently used to deal with enemies and achieve these goals.

One of the medical schools founded in Alexandria emphasized the study of poisonous plants. Crateuas, who lived about 100 BC, was a plant collector and herbalist for King Mithradates VI, known as The King of Poisons. (Mithradates is said to have taken various poisons prepared by Crateuas, increasing the doses over time so his body would develop a tolerance for them. He hoped to make himself immune to the threat of poisoning.) The drawings by Crateuas are the earliest known botanical illustrations. His was the first illustrated pharmacopoeia, which classified the plants and explained their medicinal uses.

Pendanius Dioscorides, a Greek who lived around AD 100, served as a physician to the Roman army. He traveled extensively throughout Europe and published the five books commonly referred to as *De Materia Medica*. A compendium of nearly 600 plants, it was the leading pharmacologic text for 16 centuries. This thorough work included most of the previously existing herbal literature.

Greek healers and physicians came to be known as Asclepiads. Aristotle, who lived approximately 384–322 BC, was believed to be a descendant of Asclepias. Perhaps best known for his school of philosophy, founded about 335 BC, Aristotle also wrote hundreds of books on numerous subjects, including one work that described 500 plants, called *De Plants*.

The Iron Age witnessed the flourishing of civilizations. During that time, the first medical schools were

A review of classical Greek medicine would not be complete without mention of Hippocrates. Born about 460 BC, Hippocrates was the son of the Asclepiad physician Heraklides, but he eschewed the Asclepiads for their many superstitious practices. Considered the father of modern medicine, Hippocrates believed in gathering data and employing observation and experiments in his practice and study of medicine. Hippocrates banished magic, superstition, and incantations. Instead, he embraced the life force, the laws of nature, the body's innate ability to heal itself, and the healing power of nature—all principles that relate to herbalism. He stated, "Nature heals, the physician is only Nature's assistant." Out of the school of medicine named after Hippocrates came the Hippocratic Oath, a code of medical ethics taken by physicians, which remains in use today.

Galen was a Roman physician during the period that Rome was the hub of the world (around AD 130–200). As a result of his thorough medical research on cadavers, he is sometimes referred to as the father of anatomy. (During the era of gladiators, vicious battles were common, and Galen gained some of his knowledge of anatomy by attending to injured warriors.) Galen authored an astounding 400 books, half of them on medical subjects, including *De Simplicus,* an herbal. He created potent medicines by combining plant, animal, and mineral substances. One well-known recipe, Galen's Theriac, had an opium base and more than 70 ingredients, including animal flesh, herbs, minerals, honey, and wine. It remained in use for several centuries.

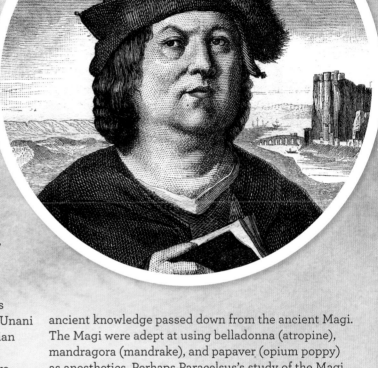

Arabia (AD 800 to present). Arabic medicine was derived from classical Greek medicine—its name, Unani Tibb, means Greek medicine. The Arabian physician Avicenna is credited as the first to distill essential oils from aromatic plants. One of his books, the five-volume *Canon of Medicine,* an authoritative and monumental compendium of all medical knowledge at the time, remained in use in Europe for more than 700 years from its publication about AD 1020. Unani Tibb remains the primary medical system for about 200 million people in the Middle East and southern Asia.

Europe in the Elizabethan era (late 1500s to early 1600s). The Swiss physician Paracelsus lived from 1493 to 1541. Paracelsus traveled throughout Europe studying chemistry, alchemy, and metallurgy and their application to medicine. He reasoned that plants had some sort of active chemicals that were responsible for their actions. Because Paracelsus wrote in the common language of the people rather than in Latin, he was lauded by folk healers, and, likewise, Paracelsus respected them. He believed these healers possessed

ancient knowledge passed down from the ancient Magi. The Magi were adept at using belladonna (atropine), mandragora (mandrake), and papaver (opium poppy) as anesthetics. Perhaps Paracelsus's study of the Magi led to his thoughts on homeopathy (the use of extreme dilutions of plant, animal, and mineral products to promote healing), which closely approximate modern homeopathic philosophy.

An English apothecary, Nicolas Culpeper sought to remove power from medical doctors and put it in the hands of the apothecary profession. He supported educating people to care for themselves—especially those who could not afford doctor visits. He disturbed the entire medical profession by translating the *London Pharmacopoeia* from Latin to English in 1649, putting it in the hands of the common people. Culpeper is also known for his association with the Doctrine of Signatures, an ancient concept that held that the physiologic action of a particular plant on the human body can be learned or inferred from observing the plant and getting to know its character and appearance. John Gerard, an Englishman who lived around the same time as Culpeper, was a barber-surgeon. In those days, many physicians dispensed medicine only. Barber-surgeons filled the gap by offering minor surgical procedures. The red and blue striped barber pole is a remnant of the old symbol used by the barber-surgeons—the blue stripe represents venous blood and the red stripe represents arterial blood. And yes, you could also get your hair cut while you were undergoing surgery. Gerard published the *General History of Plants,* more commonly known as *Gerard's Herbal,* in 1597.

Early American Medicine. The medicine of the early Americans was a pragmatic blend of Native American remedies and numerous European traditions. The early settlers brought valued seeds and plants with them from Europe to the new land; some indigenous American plants, such as plantain, dandelion, and red clover, were already familiar to them. Many households had a family herbal—held in nearly equal esteem with the family Bible—to which they often referred during times of illness. As the colonies grew, the new Americans learned from each other and the Native Americans, incorporating the practices of the different cultures into their medical knowledge. This broad knowledge base gave rise to the early American Eclectic physicians.

The Eclectics, whose philosophy was popular from the end of the 1800s through the early 1900s, were licensed physicians, but they opposed some of the current medical trends such as bloodletting and the use of arsenic as a medicine. The Eclectics espoused tailoring the medicine very closely to each individual and defined very specifically the herbs that best treated a particular condition. The temperature of the patient; the appearance of the skin, tongue, and eyes; the gait; and the pulse were all carefully noted. Their skill in noting which plant was most specific for which symptom or collection of symptoms made their system of prescribing known as "specific medication."

Modern Times. Herbal medicine and other alternative therapies, such as homeopathy and hydrotherapy, flourished in early America. In fact, at the beginning of the 20th century, 25 percent of all doctors practiced

some form of homeopathy, and a homeopath could be found on the staff of nearly every major hospital. So prominent and popular, in fact, were all types of healing arts that there is reported to have been a glut of doctors—all types of physicians competed for business.

The American Medical Association (AMA) was formed in the 1840s at a time when allopathic (conventional, Western) medicine was in decline, and homeopathy and herbal medicine were the dominant medical systems. The decline of traditional allopathic medicine followed the success of the homeopaths and herbal physicians in treating people during epidemic diseases in the cities in the 1830s—diseases the allopathic physicians were not equipped to handle. The AMA was organized to protect the interests of this declining profession; the organization chose its weapons of protection well.

In 1910, the Carnegie Foundation for the Advancement of Teaching published a report by educator Abraham Flexner. The Flexner Report examined American medical schools and education programs and recommended approval only to allopathic-oriented schools. Foundation grants and state regulators, in general, followed the Flexner Report's recommendations, with prompting by the emerging drug companies and the political lobbying of the AMA. This economic and political trend effectively killed the Eclectic and homeopathic medical professions, which formerly had been on an equal footing with the allopaths. It also eliminated the semi-professional herbalists. Formal medical-level herbalism was kept alive into the 1930s by a few remaining Eclectic physicians as well as by an emerging naturopathic medical profession.

When pharmaceutical science emerged around the early 1900s, the allopathic practitioners in the United States relied solely on pharmaceuticals at the expense of herbal medicines. Penicillin and other drugs saved millions of lives; indeed, it seemed that pharmaceuticals were long-awaited miracles.

But pharmaceuticals cannot nourish or strengthen the health and vitality of the entire body. They usually address only a single symptom and force certain pharmacologic effects. Many pharmaceuticals achieve

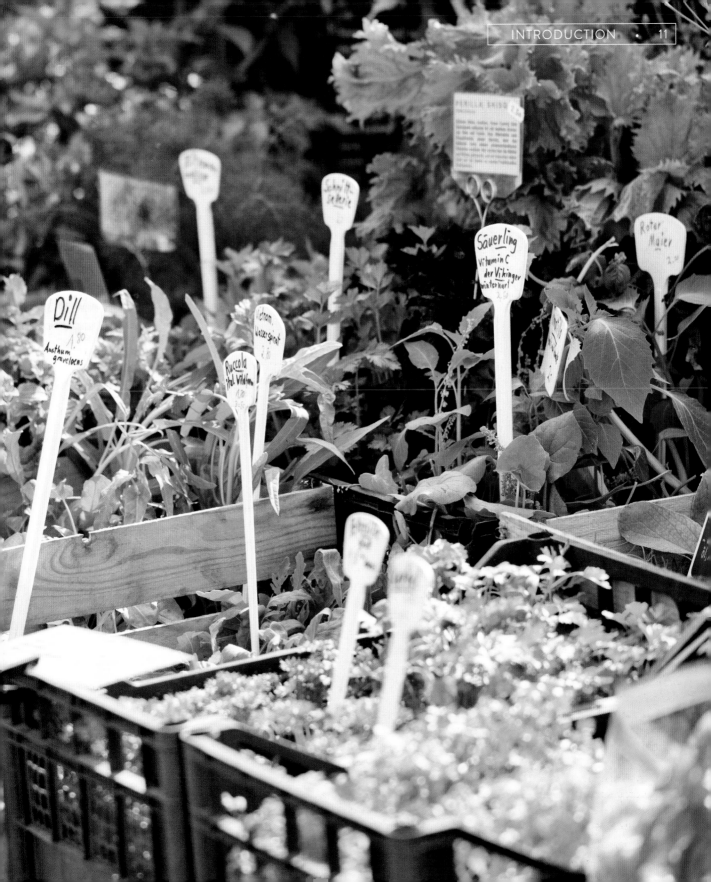

these effects at a cost, which we refer to as side effects. For example, while antibiotics kill bacteria, they don't address the underlying cause of infection. And at the same time they kill harmful bacteria, they also destroy beneficial bacteria (such as *Lactobacillus acidophilus*) within the intestines and vagina, making it easier for yeast and other pathogens to move in. More troubling is that many types of infection are becoming resistant to pharmaceuticals. Widespread use of antibiotics in medicines—as well as their use in animals whose meat is intended for human consumption—may be responsible for the evolution of super bacteria that are resistant to most pharmaceuticals.

Armed with the realization that pharmaceuticals are not the panacea once imagined, many people are returning to natural therapies. Herbalism in the United States has been undergoing a renaissance since the early 1970s, with the reemergence of the naturopathic medical profession after its decline in the 1950s and 1960s. Many new schools of herbal medicine have emerged in North America, and are now graduating several hundred clinically trained herbalists a year. Research dollars are increasingly becoming available to investigate botanical therapies. Nurseries stock a wide assortment of culinary and medicinal herbs. Public seminars and symposia on herbal medicine are often filled to capacity. Numerous books, journals, and community programs have emerged to help the public gain a working knowledge of this important field of medicine.

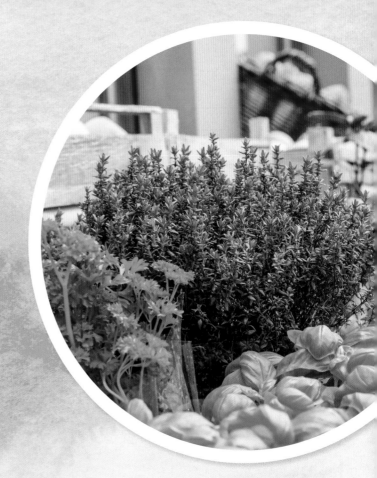

SHOPPING FOR HERBS

The interest in herbs and herbal medicines continues to boom. A whole gamut of herb types and strengths is now available, and there's a variety of ways to use and consume them. With so many herb products available, you may not know where to start. But don't despair: Anyone can learn how to use the most common herbs—safely and easily.

You can purchase herbal medicines at your local health food store or natural-product pharmacy. You can also make herbal remedies yourself, which is a less expensive—and more satisfying—alternative. Whichever route you choose to take, you need to know a few herb basics before you head to the store.

When buying a bulk herb for use as a cooking spice or tea, or for making your own homemade herbal products, choose herbs with a strong aroma, color, and flavor. Selection is fairly easy once you become familiar with an herb's characteristic odor, taste, and appearance. Compare an herb's characteristics in preparations, too. If an herbal tea imparts a strong color to the water, with a good aroma and strong flavor, its quality is probably good. Teas and tinctures with pale colors and weak flavors are of poor quality. If possible, select teas that have been harvested less than one year ago. Look for tinctures made from fresh plants.

Herbal teas and essential oils from an herbalist are likely to be much stronger than their grocery store counterparts. Even the common spices an herbalist dispenses, such as cinnamon or ginger, are likely to be of stronger color, flavor, and smell than the cinnamon or ginger in your kitchen spice rack. But as interest in herbs grows, fresh herbs and specialty teas of good, strong quality are becoming more accessible to the general consumer.

In general, an herb's potency as a flavoring is intimately linked to its potency as a medicine, and the two actions are likely to diminish equally with time. This is because much of an herb's medicinal actions are due to essential (volatile) oils—the oils in herbs we cherish as aromatic and flavoring substances. As the name "volatile" suggests, these are fairly unstable compounds; they are one of the first constituents in any herb to decompose and become less potent. So if an herb or spice has a strong smell and flavor, it is probably still strong as a medicine. As the flavor and aroma wane, the medicinal activity wanes concurrently.

Dried and powdered herbs remain at full potency for about a year. Most tinctures and essential oils maintain a good, strong potency for three to five years.

Be aware that "safe" and "nontoxic" do not mean 100 percent reaction-free; they do mean nonlethal and almost always harmless. Individual reactions can occur from any substance, including mint, garlic, or alfalfa. Always use caution when using an herbal medicine for the first time—don't take handfuls of capsules or drink pots of tea. Begin with 2 to 3 capsules or 1 to 2 cups of tea daily for a few days to see how your body reacts. People who have a history of reacting to prescription drugs or people who are very sensitive to perfumes or soaps should be cautious. For any serious or persistent health complaints, you should consult a naturopathic or other type of physician.

PURCHASING HERBAL PREPARATIONS

When buying herbs in capsule or tablet form, it's often impossible to assess the quality of the herbs. Naturopathic physicians, herbalists, or individuals who have used the product are good sources of information. It's a good idea to do some careful study about the herbs you are considering. Make sure they are indicated for the condition you wish to treat or prevent, and make sure you understand the appropriate therapeutic dosage.

Increasingly, herb suppliers are "standardizing" the botanical extracts they sell to consumers. This means these herbal preparations have been tested to determine the type and amount of at least one chemical constituent contained in the plant. Standardization sounds like a good idea. But the practice has its pros and cons.

The good news is that standardization ensures the potency of some components of an herbal product. Many of the healing properties of ginkgo, for example, are thought to reside in chemicals called heterosides. Thus, if you buy a standardized ginkgo preparation, you can be fairly certain you're getting a sufficient amount of heterosides. The problem is, ginkgo also contains flavonoids and super oxide dismutase. Should we standardize for these chemicals? If we discover five more active constituents in the next decade, will they all need to be standardized? If so, we can expect to be paying plenty for the herbs we buy.

Another problem with standardization is that as we study the medicinal effects of herbs, we're learning that healing may result not from a single element contained in a plant, but from a complex combination of constituents. Standardization implies that an herb is good only for the standardized constituent. But herbs contain many nourishing substances, and, unlike drugs, herbs are not administered to produce a single chemical effect. If we begin to value plants for their standardized chemicals only, it won't be long before pharmaceutical companies are isolating extracts and packaging them as drugs. And that's not what herbal medicine is about.

Herbal healing is a holistic process. Forgoing traditional Western thinking, herbalists do not use drugs to suppress symptoms of an illness. Herbs are meant to spur our bodies to heal naturally. So next time you get a headache, cold, or minor cut or scrape, pay a visit to nature's pharmacy. Of course, you should never attempt to diagnose a serious illness and treat it yourself. In such cases, seek advice from a physician.

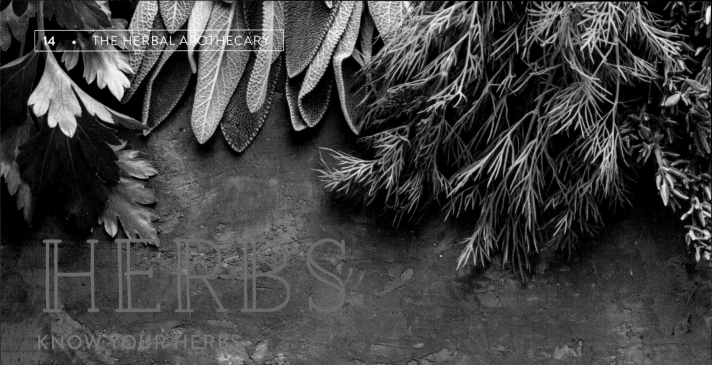

HERBS

KNOW YOUR HERBS

From earliest times, human beings have been captivated by the mystical, seemingly magical ability of herbs to heal and nurture us. The Bible is rife with references to herbal healing: "Go up into Gilead and take Balm . . . ." (Jeremiah 46:11); "And Isaiah said, 'Take a lump of figs.' And they took it and laid it on the boil, and he recovered . . . ." (2 Kings 20:7).

Those who had knowledge of herbal healing were revered by their neighbors. In an age before science, these simple healers meant the difference between life and death. After the Industrial Revolution, as the population became urbanized and science evolved, interest in herbs waned.

But in the last 50 years, as those of us who live in industrialized nations have grown more health-conscious and less willing to turn to synthetic drugs, herbal medicine has enjoyed a resurgence in popularity. Pharmaceuticals, though lifesavers in countless cases, are not without side effects. As more people strive to lead more natural lives, they are looking in increasing numbers to herbs as natural remedies. In doing so, they are participating in an ancient healing tradition.

USING MEDICINAL HERBS SAFELY

Most herbs are safe to use in moderate amounts. But unless your ailment is minor—a common headache, for example—never attempt to diagnose yourself. If you do use herbs medicinally, be sure you know what you're taking and the effect it is intended to have on you. And don't take herbs—or any medicine—without making sure the herb is appropriate for your condition. In other words, do your homework. This is especially important if you're pregnant or nursing because anything you ingest affects your child.

If you use prescription medications regularly, you should seek advice from a naturopathic physician or herbalist before using herbs medicinally. Blood thinning medications, in particular, may interact with herbs, other drugs, and even some foods and are the drug class most often responsible for hospitalization due to adverse side effects. Also note that children and the elderly sometimes require lower doses of herbs.

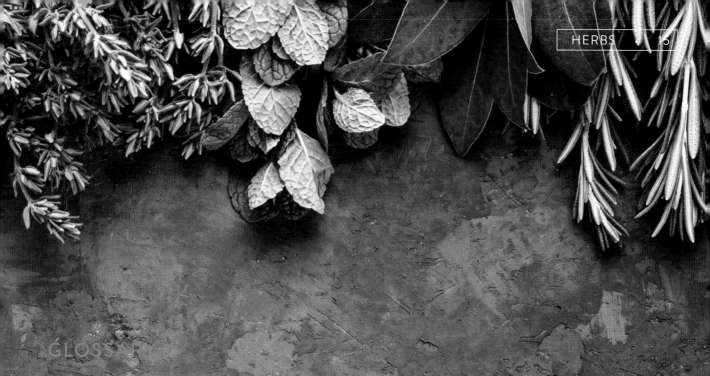

GLOSSARY

Alterative: Gradually and favorably alters a medical condition

Analgesic: Relieves pain

Antacid: Neutralizes excess stomach acids

Antipyretic: Reduces fever

Antiseptic: Prevents growth of bacteria

Antispasmodic: Prevents or relaxes muscle spasms

Astringent: Dries, constricts, and binds inflamed or draining tissues

Bitter: Plant with a sharp, sometimes unpalatable taste that stimulates appetite and enhances digestion

Carminative: Relieves gas and pain in the bowels

Compress: Cloth soaked in an herbal tea and applied externally

Decoction: Tea made by boiling the tough, woody parts of a plant

Demulcent: Protects damaged or inflamed tissues

Diaphoretic: Induces sweating

Diuretic: Increases urine flow

Evergreen: Bears foliage throughout the year

Expectorant: Assists in expelling mucus from lungs and throat

Genus: Botanical name for a group of closely related plants

Herbaceous: Perennials with non-woody stems, which die down at the end of the growing season

Infusion: Tea made by steeping an herb's leaves or flowers in hot water

Laxative: Promotes bowel movements

Mucilage: Gelatinous substance found in some herbs

Nervine: Calms tension and nourishes the nervous system

Perennial: Lives from year to year

Poultice: Plant matter applied to injured or inflamed skin

Salve: Healing ointment

Sedative: Quiets the nervous system and promotes sleep

Shrub: Perennial with branched, woody stems

Species: Classification applied to a plant within a genus

Stimulant: Increases circulation

Tincture: Herbal extraction of a plant, usually with alcohol

Tonic: Improves overall function of a particular organ or tissue

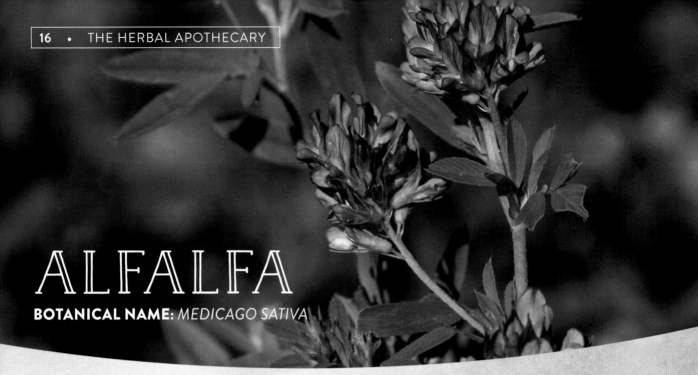

ALFALFA

BOTANICAL NAME: *MEDICAGO SATIVA*

You've probably encountered alfalfa as sprouts in the produce section of your grocery store, on a sandwich, or at salad bars, but did you know the entire plant is valuable? The sprouts are a tasty addition to many dishes, and the leaves and tiny blossoms of this tall, bushy, leafy plant are used for medications. Herbalists often recommend alfalfa in cases of malnutrition, debility, and prolonged illness. Alfalfa tea and capsules are taken for several months build up the body. Alfalfa contains substances that bind to estrogen receptors in the body. Estrogen binds to these receptors like a key in a lock. If the estrogen level is low, and many of these "locks" are empty, the constituents of alfalfa bind to them instead and increase estrogenic activity. These keys, although similar to estrogen, are not nearly as strong. If estrogen levels in the body are too high, the alfalfa keys fill some of the locks, denying the space to estrogen, thereby reducing estrogenic activity. Because alfalfa may provide some estrogenic activity when the body's hormone levels are low and compete for estrogen binding sites when hormone levels are high, alfalfa is said to be hormone balancing.

Both alfalfa sprouts and leaf preparations may help lower blood cholesterol levels. The saponins in alfalfa seem to bind to cholesterol and prevent its absorption. Alfalfa is high in vitamins A and C, niacin, riboflavin, folic acid, and the minerals calcium, magnesium, iron, and potassium. Alfalfa also contains bioflavonoids.

PREPARATIONS

Alfalfa is available in capsules, which you may take daily as a nutritional supplement. You can also find bulk alfalfa leaves, which you can infuse to make a nourishing tea. Infuse 1 tablespoon per cup of boiling water and steep for 15 minutes.

PRECAUTIONS

Excessive consumption of alfalfa may cause the breakdown of red blood cells. Also, a constituent in alfalfa, canavanine, may aggravate the disease lupus. Canavanine is an unusual amino acid found in the seeds and sprouts but not in the mature leaves. Thus, alfalfa tea and capsules made from leaves would not contain canavanine. Avoid alfalfa during pregnancy because of its canavanine content and hormonally active saponins. If you are pregnant, you may put a few sprouts on a sandwich now and then, but avoid daily consumption of alfalfa.

ALOE

BOTANICAL NAME: *ALOE VERA* or *A. BARBADENSIS*

Aloe vera is the most common of the more than 300 species of aloe. Resistant to salt and drought, this hardy herb can be found on rocky shorelines or dunes or intermingled with other vegetation. A common houseplant, aloe is characterized by pointed, fleshy leaves that exude a mucilaginous sap when broken.

This common plant has many uncommon virtues. Modern clinical studies show that aloe is one of the best herbs for soothing skin and healing burns, rashes, frostbite, and severe wounds. It is also used to treat eczema, dandruff, acne, ringworm, gum disease, and poison oak and ivy. Aloe is found commercially in a number of creams and lotions for softening and moisturizing skin. It works by inhibiting formation of tissue-injuring compounds that gather at the site of a skin injury. The plant contains chrysophanic acid, which is effective in healing abrasions. Some compounds from aloe show promise as potential cancer fighters.

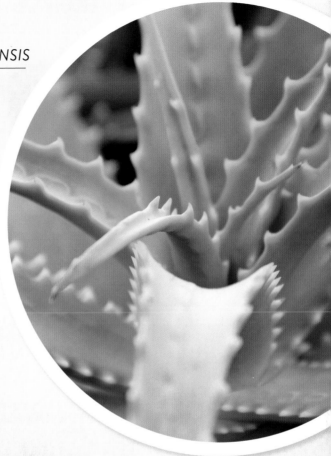

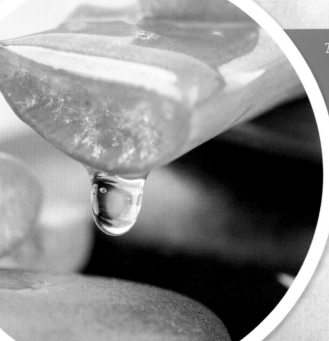

The fleshy leaves produce a skin-healing sap. Aloe produces new leaves from its center, so if you are obtaining sap from your own plant, cut the outermost (oldest) leaves first.

PRECAUTIONS

Aloin, the yellow portion of aloe just under the leaf's peel, is a strong laxative that may cause severe cramping and diarrhea, so use aloe cautiously internally and always with a carminative such as ginger, fennel, or coriander. Commercial aloe juice has this property removed, so it is safe to drink as recommended on the bottle. People with diabetes should be careful using aloe—studies have shown it can reduce blood sugar levels.

ANGELICA

BOTANICAL NAME: *ANGELICA ARCHANGELICA*

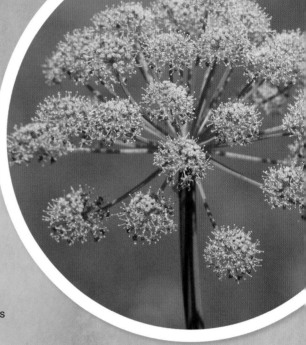

For centuries, peasants gathered angelica because it was purported to ward off evil spirits. Early physicians prescribed angelica for a number of illnesses. Angelica syrup was taken as a digestive aid, and American Indians used angelica to treat lung congestion and tuberculosis. Today angelica is used primarily to treat digestive and bronchial conditions and as an expectorant and cough suppressant. It has antibacterial, antifungal, and diaphoretic (induces sweating) properties. It also increases menstrual flow. Japanese studies have shown that a related species of angelica has anti-inflammatory properties that may be useful in an arthritis treatment. In China, the Asian species is prescribed to improve liver function in people with cirrhosis and chronic hepatitis, to regulate menstruation, and to relieve menopausal symptoms. Studies have shown that compounds from Chinese angelica may also have cancer-fighting properties.

Commercially, angelica roots and seeds are used to flavor Benedictine and Chartreuse liqueurs, gin, vermouth, and some brands of tobacco. The herb's distinctive flavor is also found in fresh or dried leaves and stems. Add very small amounts of fresh leaves to salads, fruits, soups, stews, desserts, and pastries.

This large, boldly attractive plant produces lush growth, making it a striking focal point for your garden. Angelica looks much like a very large celery or parsnip plant. This herb produces large white umbel flower heads and decorative yellow-green seedpods.

PRECAUTIONS

Don't attempt to gather wild species of angelica; they look a lot like water hemlock, which is extremely toxic. Angelica increases menstrual flow, so avoid it if you're pregnant. It contains chemicals called psoralens, which can cause some sensitive people to develop a rash when exposed to sunlight; some people get dermatitis when handling the leaves. Use small amounts of the herb since it can act strongly on the nervous system. If angelica causes you any problems, discontinue use.

Also known as dong quai, the dried root of the related species Angelica sinensis is revered in traditional Chinese medicine. It is used to treat a variety of gynecological conditions, including premenstrual syndrome, fibroids, endometriosis, and menopause. It is generally considered useful for conditions related the blood and may be prescribed for headaches, high blood pressure, infections, and inflammation.

ANISE

BOTANICAL NAME: *PIMPINELLA ANISUM*

Anise has been considered a valuable herb since at least the 6th century BC. The Romans cultivated the plant for its distinctive fragrance and flavor, which is similar to licorice. They also used anise extensively as a medicine. For centuries, anise was used to induce a mother's milk to flow, to ease childbirth, and as an aphrodisiac. Today herbalists recommend anise to aid digestion and prevent gas. Because it loosens bronchial secretions and reduces coughing, anise is often found in cough syrups and lozenges. The herb has some antimicrobial properties.

Anise is a prime ingredient in many ethnic cuisines, including Scandinavian, Greek, East Indian, Arabic, and Hispanic foods. The herb intensifies the flavor of pastries, cakes, and cookies, and it complements eggs, stewed fruit, cheese, spinach, and carrots. Use leaves whole in salads or as a garnish. Anise cookies are a traditional Christmas treat in Europe. Dried leaves make a pleasant-tasting tea, and the herb has been used to flavor liqueurs, including the well-known Greek ouzo. With its licorice-like taste, it is used to flavor most of the "licorice" candy in the United States and other candies as well.

PRECAUTIONS

Although anise has been recommended to treat morning sickness, the herb has an estrogen-like property. Pregnant women should avoid any herbs or drugs that might have an estrogenic effect.

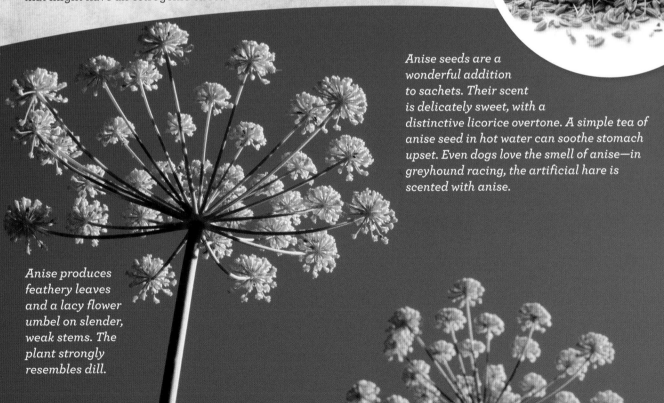

Anise seeds are a wonderful addition to sachets. Their scent is delicately sweet, with a distinctive licorice overtone. A simple tea of anise seed in hot water can soothe stomach upset. Even dogs love the smell of anise—in greyhound racing, the artificial hare is scented with anise.

Anise produces feathery leaves and a lacy flower umbel on slender, weak stems. The plant strongly resembles dill.

ARNICA

BOTANICAL NAME: *ARNICA MONTANA*

The next time your calves ache after a strenuous morning run, try massaging them with an arnica liniment. European herbalists and American Indians have long recognized arnica's abilities to soothe and relax sore, stiff muscles. More than 100 commercial drug preparations in Germany contain arnica. The herb is also used to make homeopathic remedies. The flower is the most potent part of the plant, but sometimes the leaves are also used.

Arnica's healing powers have been attributed to two chemicals, helenalin and arnicin, which have anti-inflammatory, antiseptic, and pain-relieving properties. Arnica also increases blood circulation.

Arnica is available in tinctures, salves, and ointments to treat minor wounds, sprains, and bruises. You can lay a compress made with arnica tea or the diluted tincture on such injuries, or place a compress on the stomach to relieve abdominal pain. To make an arnica oil, heat 1 ounce of flowers in 10 ounces of any vegetable oil for several hours on low heat. Strain and let the oil cool before applying it to bruises or sore muscles.

The plant is best used fresh. Gather flowers in midsummer, just as they reach their blooming peak. Preserve them in alcohol to make a liniment.

PRECAUTIONS

The helenalin in arnica causes dermatitis in a few people after repeated applications. Discontinue use if you develop any skin problems. Otherwise, arnica is safe for topical use. But do not ingest arnica. Taken internally, the herb can irritate the kidneys and the digestive tract, cause dizziness, and elevate blood pressure.

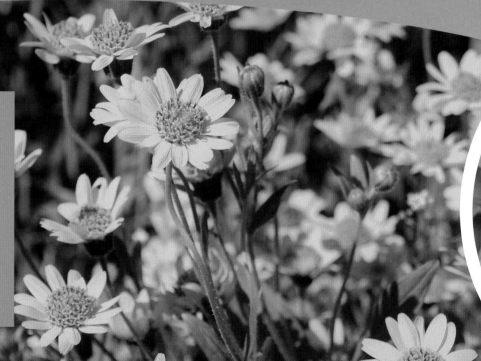

Arnica is also known as leopardsbane, mountain tobacco, and wolfsbane. The plant grows from a horizontal, dark brown root and produces round and hairy stems. These send up as many as three flower stalks with blossoms that resemble daisies. Lance-shaped, bright green, and toothed, arnica's leaves appear somewhat hairy on their upper surfaces.

ASTRAGALUS

BOTANICAL NAME: *ASTRAGALUS MEMBRANACEUS*

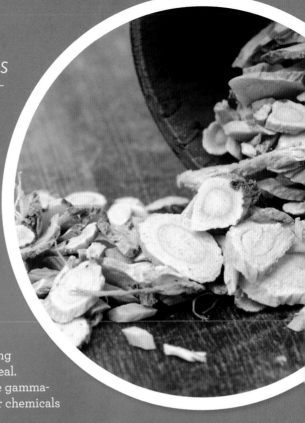

Here in the West we're just beginning to appreciate the healing properties of astragalus. Compiled by Chinese physicians in the first century AD, *The Divine Husbandman's Classic of the Materia Medica* lists astragalus as its number-one health-giving plant. Because of its immune-system–enhancing properties, astragalus is often prescribed for people with "wasting" diseases such as fatigue or loss of appetite due to chronic illness, or for people who need to strengthen their body's systems. It is not uncommon in China to use astragalus extracts to fight several kinds of cancer. It is used in Chinese hospitals to lessen the side effects of chemotherapy and radiation.

Astragalus lowers fevers and has a beneficial effect on the digestive system. Other illnesses for which herbalists use astragalus include arthritis; diabetes; inflammation in the urinary tract; prolapsed uterus, stomach, or anus; uterine bleeding and weakness; water retention; and skin wounds that refuse to heal. Astragalus' ability to lower blood pressure is probably due to the gamma-aminobutyric acid it contains, which dilates blood vessels. Other chemicals in the root have been found to strengthen the lungs.

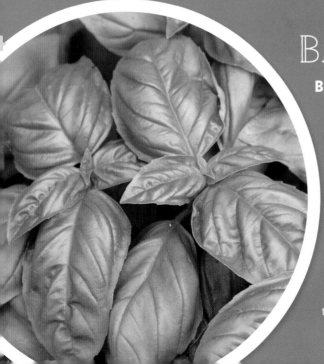

BASIL

BOTANICAL NAME: *OCIMUM BASILICUM*

Basil is recommended to aid digestion and expel gas. It's also good for treating stomach cramps, vomiting, and constipation. It has been found to be more effective than drugs to relieve nausea from chemotherapy and radiation.

Studies show that extracts of basil seeds have antibacterial properties. Basil contains vitamins A and C as well as antioxidants, which prevent cell damage. One study found that basil increases production of disease-fighting antibodies up to 20 percent. It also combats the herpesvirus. Strongly fragrant, basil is used in sachets and potpourri. A basil infusion used as a hair rinse adds luster to the hair and helps treat acne and itching skin.

BILBERRY

BOTANICAL NAME: *VACCINIUM MYRTILLUS*

Bilberry contains vitamins A and C and was a folk remedy in Scandinavia to prevent scurvy and treat nausea and indigestion. The berries were once steeped in gin and taken as a digestive tonic. They are a popular Russian remedy for colitis and stomach ulcers because they decrease inflammation in the intestines and protect the lining of the digestive tract. The herb has astringent, antiseptic, and tonic properties, making it useful as a treatment for diarrhea.

Berries contain flavonoid anthocyanidins, which have a potent antioxidant action and protect body tissues, particularly blood vessels. Several studies have shown that bilberry extracts stimulate blood vessels to release a substance that helps dilate (open) veins and arteries. Bilberries may keep platelets from clumping, thus preventing clotting and improving circulation. The berry may help prevent many diabetes-related conditions caused by poor circulation.

Because they contain a substance that slightly lowers blood sugar, the leaves are a folk remedy to manage diabetes. However, you should not use the leaves to self-treat diabetes. German researchers are investigating the leaves as a treatment for gout and rheumatism.

Bilberry preparations may be particularly useful for treating eye conditions and have been prescribed for diabetic retinopathy, cataracts, night blindness, and macular degeneration. Modern European prescription medications that contain bilberry are used to improve eyesight and circulation.

Bilberry is a deciduous shrub with thin, creeping stems. Leaves are bright green, alternate, and oval. One of more than 100 members of the genus Vaccinium, bilberry is related to blueberries and huckleberries.

In England, World War II pilots were given bilberry jam to improve their eyesight. You can obtain the berries' benefits this way, eat the tart fruit raw, or make it into a syrup. You can also use bilberry capsules, tea, or tincture.

BLACK COHOSH

BOTANICAL NAME: *CIMICIFUGA RACEMOSA*

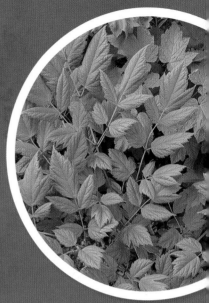

North American Indians used black cohosh to treat fatigue, sore throat, arthritis, and rattlesnake bite, but the herb's primary use historically was as a medicine to ease childbirth. Nineteenth-century American herbalists also recommended black cohosh for fever and menstrual cramps. Black cohosh is a diuretic, expectorant, astringent, and sedative, but today it is most often recommended for treating symptoms of menopause. The herb seems to have an estrogenic effect by binding to estrogen receptors in the body. Black cohosh contains the anti-inflammatory salicylic acid (the main ingredient of aspirin) and has been used for a variety of muscular, pelvic, and rheumatic pains, especially those caused by nervous tension. Herbalists in China use a related species, *C. foetida,* to treat headache, measles, and gynecologic problems.

PRECAUTIONS

An overdose of black cohosh may cause dizziness, diarrhea, abdominal pain, vomiting, visual dimness, headache, tremors, and a depressed heart rate. Don't use it if you have a heart condition. Because the herb seems to affect hormones, don't use it if you're pregnant.

BLUE COHOSH

BOTANICAL NAME: *CAULOPHYLLUM THALICTROIDES*

American Indians considered blue cohosh a panacea for women's ailments. Over the centuries and up to the present time, the herb has been used to treat uterine abnormalities and relieve menstrual cramps. Before the introduction of forceps, American obstetricians used blue cohosh to help induce labor.

In the past, herbalists also used blue cohosh to treat bronchitis, rheumatism, and irregular menstruation. They also combined it with other herbs, including motherwort and partridge berry, for women in the last few weeks of pregnancy to promote smooth labor. It was listed as an "official" medicine in the *U.S. Pharmacopoeia* until 1936.

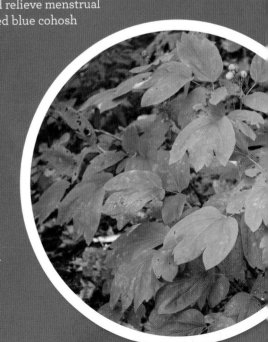

PRECAUTIONS

Blue cohosh contains several strong compounds. It can constrict coronary blood vessels, so do not use it if you have a history of stroke or have high blood pressure, heart disease, or diabetes. The powdered rhizome irritates mucous membranes, so handle it with care; don't inhale it or get it in your eyes. And don't take blue cohosh during labor unless you are working with an herbalist or midwife knowledgeable about herbs. Above all, do not eat the berries: They are poisonous!

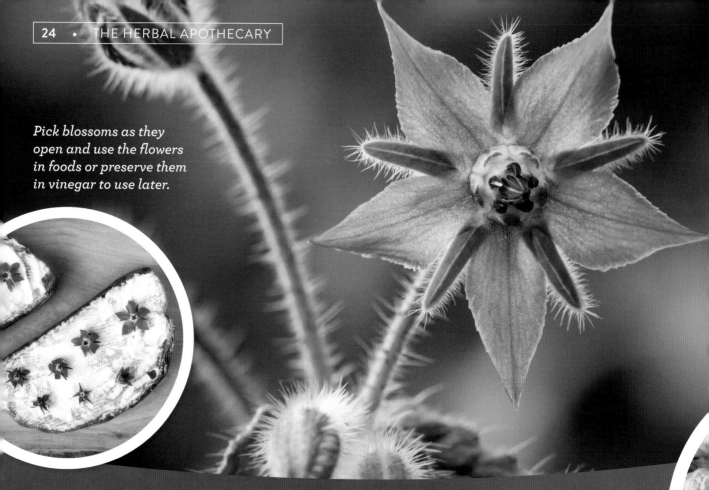

Pick blossoms as they open and use the flowers in foods or preserve them in vinegar to use later.

BORAGE

BOTANICAL NAME: *BORAGO OFFICINALIS*

Celtic warriors drank borage wine because they believed it gave them courage. Romans thought borage produced a sense of elation and well-being. The Greeks turned to the herb when their spirits sagged. Today, herbalists consider borage a diuretic, demulcent, and emollient, and prescribe the plant to treat depression, fevers, bronchitis, and diarrhea. The malic acid and potassium nitrate it contains may be responsible for its diuretic effects. Poultices of leaves may be useful in cooling and soothing skin and reducing inflammation and swelling. The plant also has expectorant properties.

The crisp flavor of borage flowers complements cheese, fish, poultry, most vegetables, salads, iced beverages, pickles, and salad dressings. You can eat small amounts of young leaves: Steam well or sauté as you would spinach so the leaves are no longer prickly. You can also candy the flowers.

PRECAUTIONS

Borage is safe to use in moderation. Claims that it may harm the liver have not been substantiated, but you may want to limit how much you use; the herb contains the same type of alkaloids as comfrey. Some researchers strongly suggest not eating the leaves, which contain higher amounts of pyrrolizidine alkaloids than the flowers do.

BURDOCK

BOTANICAL NAME: *ARCTIUM LAPPA, A. MINUS*

If you've ever returned from an outdoor romp with your pet and discovered burrs clinging tenaciously to the cuffs of your trousers and your pet's fur, you've encountered burdock, an herb whose primary use is as a blood purifier. The root is also considered a diuretic, diaphoretic, and laxative. It has also been used to treat psoriasis, acne, and other skin conditions. Research has found that several compounds in burdock root inhibit growth of bacteria and fungi. A poultice of leaves is effective in healing bruises, burns, and swellings. The Chinese also use burdock root to treat colds, flu, measles, and constipation and burdock seeds to treat skin problems. Herbalists use burdock to treat liver disorders.

Burdock also contains a substance called inulin, a starch that is easily digested. Burdock root tastes like a marriage of potato and celery; eat it fresh, steamed, or sautéed. Eat young stalks raw or steam them as you would asparagus. Burdock root is a staple of Japanese cuisine and sold in Japanese grocery stores, often under the name gobo root.

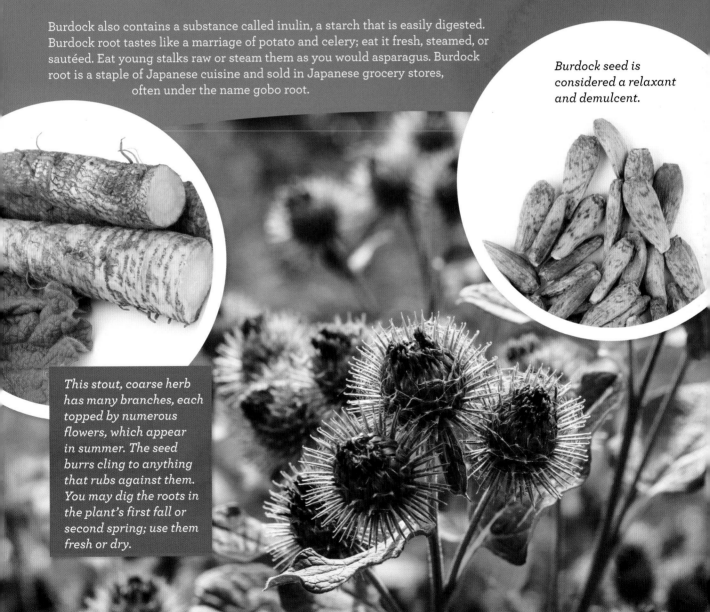

Burdock seed is considered a relaxant and demulcent.

This stout, coarse herb has many branches, each topped by numerous flowers, which appear in summer. The seed burrs cling to anything that rubs against them. You may dig the roots in the plant's first fall or second spring; use them fresh or dry.

BURNET

BOTANICAL NAME: *POTERIUM SANGUISORBA*

Useful to control bleeding, burnet's name, in fact, means "to drink up blood." The herb is considered helpful in treating vaginal discharges and diarrhea. Burnet leaves contain vitamin C and tannins; the latter gives it astringent properties. Practitioners of traditional Chinese medicine use the root topically on wounds and burns to reduce inflammation and the risk of infection. It is also used to treat gum disease. While burnet is rarely used medicinally in North America, Europeans and Russians still use it in their folk medicine. It is used to heal ulcerative colitis as a folk remedy in Northern Europe and Russia. Apparently, its medicinal properties are due to more than simply the astringent tannins it contains. Russian research shows that the leaves improve circulation to the uterus, especially in pregnant women. The leaves also have immune-enhancing properties that may help correct some abnormalities during pregnancy.

In the kitchen, use tender, young, well-chopped leaves in salads, vinegars, butters, and iced beverages. Add leaves to vinegars, marinades, and cheese spreads. And flowers make attractive garnishes.

BUTCHER'S BROOM

BOTANICAL NAME: *RUSCUS ACULEATUS*

Butcher's broom enjoys a venerable history as a medicinal herb. The ancient Greeks recommended butcher's broom for treating kidney stones, gout, and jaundice.

Today, butcher's broom is experiencing a comeback. There is scientific evidence it may have value in treating circulatory problems, such as varicose veins and hemorrhoids. In German studies, it decreased the inflammation of varicose veins, helped to tighten them, and encouraged the blood to flow up the legs. In addition to strengthening blood vessels, the plant reduces fever and increases urine flow.

For 300 years—from the 16th to 19th centuries—butcher's broom was associated with the meat industry. Butchers used the leaves to repel vermin and animals. Later, they made "brooms" from the plant to scrub chopping blocks. With its waxy green leaves and scarlet berries, butcher's broom has been used to decorate meats at Christmas; indeed, another name for the herb is box holly.

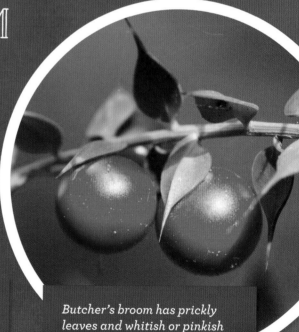

Butcher's broom has prickly leaves and whitish or pinkish flowers that appear from mid-autumn to late spring. Its round berries are scarlet or yellow.

CALENDULA

BOTANICAL NAME: *CALENDULA OFFICINALIS*

The Romans grew these plants to treat scorpion bites. Calendula's yellow flowers were once believed to be an effective treatment for jaundice.

The herb is used today to treat wounds, skin conditions, and peptic and duodenal ulcers. Calendula's primary use is to heal the skin and reduce swelling. Apply calendula to sores, cuts, bruises, burns, and rashes. It even soothes the discomfort of measles and chicken pox—simply make a double strength tea and wash over the skin eruptions. It also helps prevent and relieve diaper rash. Calendula induces sweating, increases urination, and aids digestion. Researchers have found that compounds in calendula may be useful in treating cancer. It has traditionally been used to treat tonsillitis and any condition related to swollen lymph glands, including breast cancer. It is also an excellent treatment for infection due to *Candida albicans*. Calendula tincture is used topically on varicose veins, bruises, and sprains.

In the kitchen, add a few calendula flowers to salads and sandwiches. Powdered yellow flowers may substitute for saffron's color (they once were used to color butter, custards, and liqueurs), although go easy—they have a bitter taste. The flowers produce a bright yellow dye and are commercially grown. Dry flowers for potpourri. A calendula rinse brings out highlights in hair. It is a popular ingredient in skin cream and lotions, baby oils, and salves.

To treat thrush, an infection with the *Candida* organism that appears in the mouth, swab the area with a tincture diluted in an equal amount of distilled water. Calendula is rarely drunk as a tea. A strong infusion, however, makes a good compress. For a poultice, mash fresh flowers and apply to the skin. To make calendula oil, crush dried or wilted flowers, then heat in olive oil for a few hours on low heat. Strain.

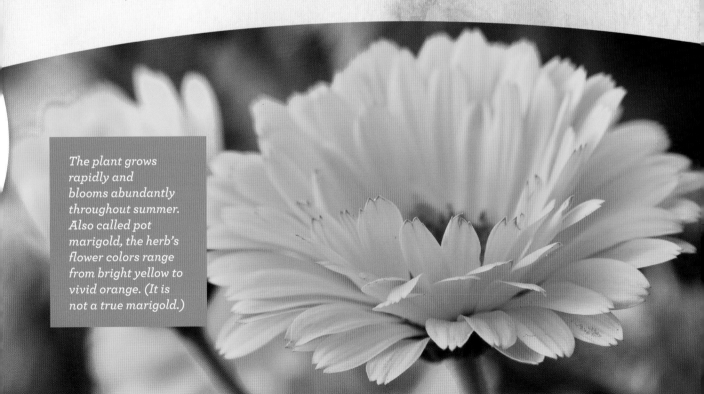

The plant grows rapidly and blooms abundantly throughout summer. Also called pot marigold, the herb's flower colors range from bright yellow to vivid orange. (It is not a true marigold.)

CARAWAY

BOTANICAL NAME: *CARUM CARVI*

Caraway seeds were found in ancient tombs, indicating the plant was used at least 5,000 years ago. As a medicine, caraway is used—most often as a cordial—to relieve an upset stomach and dispel gas. Caraway water has long been given to babies with colic. A compress soaked in a strong infusion or the powdered and moistened seed relieves swelling and bruising. But you may be most familiar with caraway from eating sauerkraut, rye crackers, and rye bread—foods that rely heavily on its strong aroma and taste. Add caraway seeds to beef dishes, stews, and breads. Add leaves to salads and soups. The herb complements eggs, cheese, sauces, barley, oats, pork, and fish, as well as cabbage, beets, spinach, potatoes, peas, cauliflower, turnips, and zucchini. Cooking it a long time can make it bitter, so add caraway no more than 30 minutes before a dish is done. It also makes children's medicines more tasty.

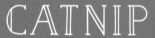

The most popular way to use caraway medicinally is in food. It is rare to find anyone using it by itself as a tincture or tea, but sometimes it flavors tinctures or syrups.

CATNIP

BOTANICAL NAME: *NEPETA CATARIA*

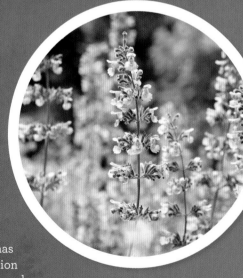

Your cat may go crazy over catnip, but the herb has actually been used as a mild sedative for about 2,000 years. The Romans harvested catnip, and colonists carried the herb to America, where it quickly became naturalized. Catnip tea aids digestion, promotes sleep, and treats colds, nervousness, and headaches. Its most important use is as a sedative that is safe enough even for children and the elderly. Catnip contains sedative constituents similar to valerian, another popular herbal relaxant. One of catnip's most famous uses is to treat colic in babies—a condition for which it has been used for hundreds of years. It also makes a good tea for treating indigestion associated with anxiety or nervousness. The tea treats measles and chicken pox when used both internally and topically. An infusion applied to the skin relieves hives and other rashes. The herb increases perspiration, reduces fevers, and increases menstrual flow. But catnip finds its greatest commercial value in the pet industry, as filling for cat toys. Cats react differently than humans do to the herb; they find it very stimulating, not sedating at all. The herb's fragrance also repels many insects.

CAYENNE PEPPER

BOTANICAL NAME: *CAPSICUM ANNUUM*

Cayenne has many medicinal uses. The main ingredient in cayenne is capsaicin, a powerful stimulant responsible for the pepper's heat. Although it can set your mouth on fire, cayenne, ironically, is good for your digestive system and is now known to help heal ulcers! It reduces substance P, a chemical that carries pain messages from the skin's nerve endings, so it reduces pain when applied topically. A cayenne cream is now in use to treat psoriasis, postsurgical pain, shingles, and nerve damage from diabetes. It may even help you burn off extra pounds. Researchers in England have found that about ¼ ounce of cayenne burns from 45 to 76 calories by increasing metabolism.

Taking cayenne internally stabilizes blood pressure. You can apply powdered, dry cayenne as a poultice over wounds to stop bleeding. And in the kitchen, cayenne spices up any food it touches. Cayenne is also the source for the infamous "pepper spray," used by both the public and many police forces.

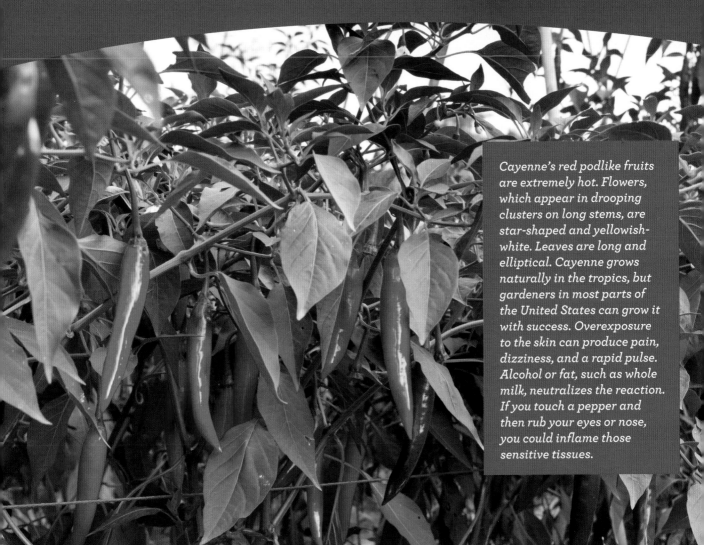

Cayenne's red podlike fruits are extremely hot. Flowers, which appear in drooping clusters on long stems, are star-shaped and yellowish-white. Leaves are long and elliptical. Cayenne grows naturally in the tropics, but gardeners in most parts of the United States can grow it with success. Overexposure to the skin can produce pain, dizziness, and a rapid pulse. Alcohol or fat, such as whole milk, neutralizes the reaction. If you touch a pepper and then rub your eyes or nose, you could inflame those sensitive tissues.

CHAMOMILE, GERMAN

BOTANICAL NAME: *MATRICARIA RECUTITA*

Chamomile is one of the world's best-loved herbs. The herb produces a pleasant-tasting tea, which has a strong aroma of apples. The early Egyptians valued chamomile and used it to cure malaria and bring down fevers. The ancient Greeks called on chamomile to relieve headaches and treat illnesses of the kidney, liver, and bladder. Today herbalists prescribe the herb to calm nerves and settle upset stomachs, among its other uses.

Chamomile's medicinal properties derive from its essential oils. The herb has three primary medicinal uses: an anti-inflammatory to reduce swelling and infection; an antispasmodic to relieve digestive upsets, headaches, and menstrual cramps; and an anti-infective for cleansing wounds. Chamomile is often found in creams and lotions to soothe sensitive or irritated skin and treat rashes and skin allergies. Cosmetics employ it to reduce puffiness, especially around the eyes. It reduces the swelling that results from allergies or colds. It is used on bruises, sprains, and varicose veins and almost any time the skin becomes inflamed. Chamomile infusions make excellent skin cleansers. Use chamomile both internally and topically to relieve muscle pain. Its calming action not only relieves pain but also induces sleep and relieves nervous indigestion—it has been used to calm children and babies for hundreds of years. Chamomile reduces gastric acid, which helps prevent or speed healing of ulcers. It even shows immune-system activity. Chamomile's fragrant aroma makes it a good addition to potpourri and flower arrangements.

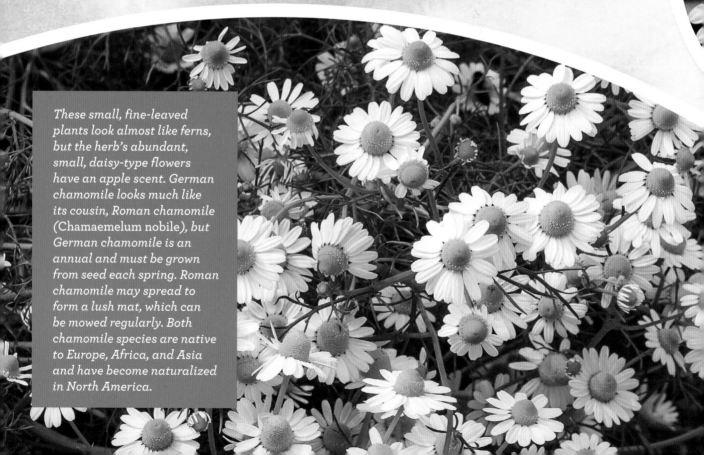

These small, fine-leaved plants look almost like ferns, but the herb's abundant, small, daisy-type flowers have an apple scent. German chamomile looks much like its cousin, Roman chamomile (Chamaemelum nobile), but German chamomile is an annual and must be grown from seed each spring. Roman chamomile may spread to form a lush mat, which can be mowed regularly. Both chamomile species are native to Europe, Africa, and Asia and have become naturalized in North America.

Although the plant contains not a hint of blue, chamomile contains a potent volatile oil that is a brilliant blue when isolated. This oil, called chamazulene after its dark azure color, has strong anti-inflammatory actions. Apply a preparation made from its volatile oil to skin infections, or apply cloths soaked in strong chamomile tea to eczema patches and other inflamed skin surfaces.

PRECAUTIONS

Chamomile flowers may cause symptoms of allergies in some people allergic to ragweed and related plants, although the risk of this is quite low.

Roman chamomile

TEETHING BABY TEA

You may give chamomile to teething infants to calm them and reduce gum inflammation. If a child will not drink chamomile tea from a bottle or take it from a spoon, soak a cloth in ½ cup of strong chamomile tea to which you've added 2 drops of clove oil. Place the cloth-tea mixture in the freezer for 20 minutes, then give to the baby to chomp on.

Steep 1 tablespoon of chamomile flowers per cup of water for 15 minutes. Drink a half cup up to five times a day for digestive problems. For nervous conditions, combine chamomile with equal parts of passion flower, skullcap, oats, or hops.

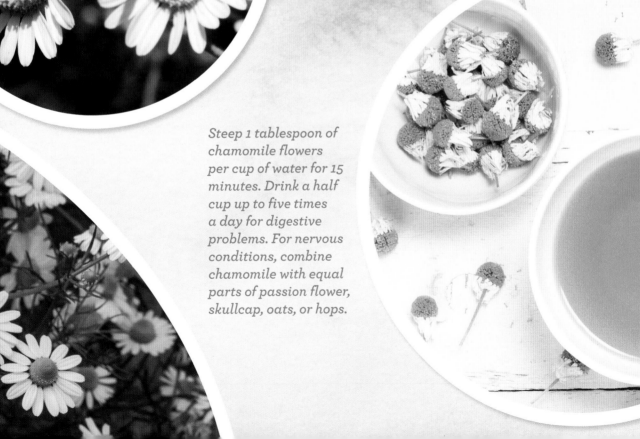

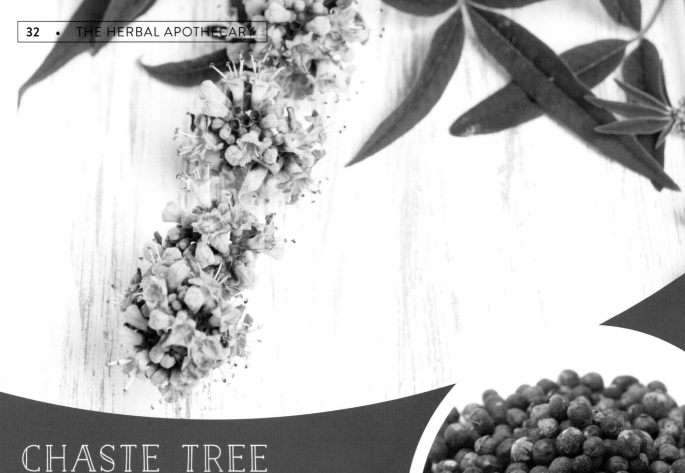

CHASTE TREE

BOTANICAL NAME: *VITEX AGNUS CASTUS*

During the Middle Ages, monks used chaste tree to diminish their sexual drive, hence the herb's common name, monk's pepper. Today chaste tree, which is often referred to as vitex, is used primarily to treat women's discomforts. The flavonoids in chaste tree produce a progesterone-like effect. The herb may raise progesterone levels by acting on the brain. Chaste tree helps to normalize and regulate menstrual cycles, reduce premenstrual fluid retention, reduce some cases of acne that may flare up during PMS or menstruation, reduce hot flashes, and treat menopausal bleeding irregularities and other menopausal symptoms. It is also useful in helping dissolve fibroids and cysts in the reproductive system and may be used for treating some types of infertility.

Chaste tree may be used after childbirth to promote milk production. It is a slow-acting herb and may take months to take effect.

PRECAUTIONS

Because of chaste tree's complex hormonal actions, be cautious using it during pregnancy. It may also interfere with hormonal drugs. Little information is available about the physiologic activity of chaste tree in men.

The berries are the only part of chaste tree typically used. Because of their unpleasant taste, they are usually taken in capsule form or as a tincture.

CHIVES

BOTANICAL NAME: *ALLIUM SCHOENOPRASUM*

Archaeologists tell us that this herb has been in use for at least 5,000 years. By the 16th century, it was a popular European garden herb. Chives' few medicinal properties derive from the sulfur-rich oil found in all members of the onion family. The oil is antiseptic and may help lower blood pressure, but it must be consumed in fairly large quantities.

Chives' pleasant taste—like that of mild, sweet onions—complements the flavor of most foods. Use fresh minced leaves in dishes containing potatoes, artichokes, asparagus, cauliflower, corn, tomatoes, peas, carrots, spinach, poultry, fish, veal, cheese, eggs, and, of course, in cream cheese atop your bagel or in sour cream on a baked potato. Add chives at the last minute for best flavor. Flowers are good additions to salads and may be preserved in vinegars.

Chives produces tight clumps of long, thin, grasslike leaves that resemble those of onion in appearance and taste. The herb produces abundant, small, rose-purple, globe-shaped flower heads in early summer. Chives may be planted as edging, grown alone, or grown with other plants in containers. The herb is native to Greece, Sweden, the Alps, and parts of northern Great Britain.

COMFREY

BOTANICAL NAME: *SYMPHYTUM OFFICINALE*

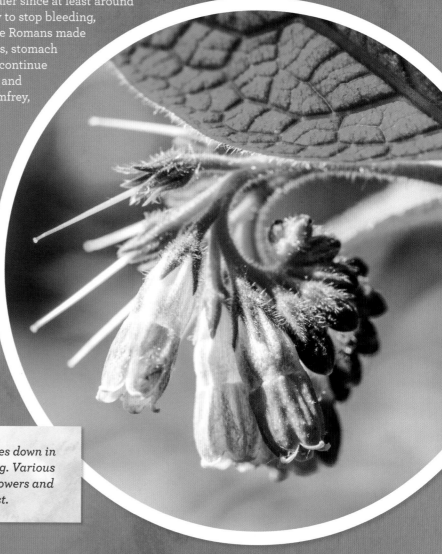

Comfrey has been regarded as a great healer since at least around 400 BC, when the Greeks used it topically to stop bleeding, heal wounds, and mend broken bones. The Romans made comfrey poultices and teas to treat bruises, stomach disorders, and diarrhea. Today herbalists continue to prescribe comfrey for bruises, wounds, and sores. Allantoin, a compound found in comfrey, causes cells to divide and grow, spurring wounds to heal faster. It also inhibits inflammation of the stomach's lining. Comfrey has been recommended for treating bronchitis, asthma, respiratory irritation, peptic ulcers, and stomach and intestinal inflammation. Studies show it inhibits prostaglandins, substances that cause inflammation. It was once promoted as a salad green and potherb; however, internal use of comfrey has become a much-debated topic.

In cosmetic use, comfrey soothes and softens skin and promotes growth of new cells. Comfrey is found in creams, lotions, and bath preparations. It dyes wool brown.

Comfrey is a hardy, leafy plant that dies down in winter and comes back strong in spring. Various species of comfrey have purple-pink flowers and appear from May through the first frost.

PRECAUTIONS

There is some evidence that excessive consumption of comfrey root, especially *Symphytum uplandicum*, contributes to liver damage, though this has not been confirmed. Several people who consumed comfrey have experienced liver damage. It has been suggested that other substances they took simultaneously may have interacted adversely with the comfrey. Do not use comfrey root topically until it receives a clear bill of health. Comfrey contains pyrrolizidine alkaloids, which are responsible for its harmful effects. The dried leaf contains no pyrrolizidine alkaloids; it is considered relatively safe to use as tea and does contain some of the healing allantoin. The fresh leaves contain very little pyrrolizidine, especially the large, mature leaves.

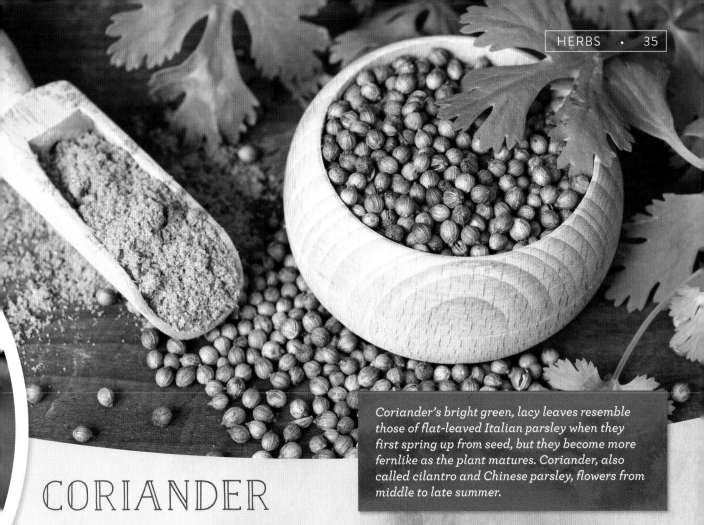

CORIANDER

BOTANICAL NAME: *CORIANDRUM SATIVUM*

Coriander's bright green, lacy leaves resemble those of flat-leaved Italian parsley when they first spring up from seed, but they become more fernlike as the plant matures. Coriander, also called cilantro and Chinese parsley, flowers from middle to late summer.

Coriander has been cultivated for 3,000 years. The Hebrews, who used coriander seed as one of their Passover herbs, probably learned about it from the ancient Egyptians, who revered the plant. The Romans and Greeks used coriander for medicinal purposes and as a spice and preservative. The Chinese believed coriander could make a human immortal. Throughout northern Europe, people would suck on candy-coated coriander seeds when they had indigestion; chewing the seeds soothes an upset stomach, relieves flatulence, aids digestion, and improves appetite. Poultices of coriander seeds have been used to relieve the pain of rheumatism. The Chinese prescribe the tea to treat dysentery and measles. Coriander relieves inflammation and headaches. But its most popular medicinal use has been to flavor strong-tasting medicines and to prevent intestinal gripping common with some laxative formulas.

Coriander's leaf flavor is a cross between sage and citrus. The herb's bold flavor is common to several ethnic cuisines, notably those of China, southeast Asia, Mexico, East India, Spain, Central Africa, and Central and South America. Add young leaves to beets, onions, salads, sausage, clams, oysters, and potatoes. Add seeds to marinades, salad dressings, cheese, eggs, and pickling brines. Coriander seed is used commercially to flavor sugared confections, liqueurs such as Benedictine and Chartreuse, and gin. Its essential oil is found in perfumes, aftershaves, and cosmetics because of its delightfully spicy scent. It is no longer as popular a cosmetic as it was from the 14th to 17th centuries, but coriander "refines" the complexion and was in the famous Eau de Carnes and Carmelite water. It is still used in soaps and deodorants.

COSTMARY

BOTANICAL NAME: *CHRYSANTHEMUM BALSAMITA*

Costmary flourished in English gardens and was used to spice ale. The herb is antiseptic and slightly astringent and has been used in salves to heal dry, itchy skin. It promotes urine flow and brings down fevers. Although rarely used for this purpose today, its principle medicinal use was as a digestive aid and to treat dysentery, for which it was included in the British Pharmacopoeia. The cosmetic water was commonly used to improve the complexion and as a hair rinse. Costmary is good for acne and oily skin and hair.

Costmary's flavor complements beverages, chilled soups, and fruit salads. You can add dried leaves to potpourri, sachets, and baths, or slip them in books to deter bugs that eat paper—this was once a common practice. Dried branches have been used to make herbal baskets.

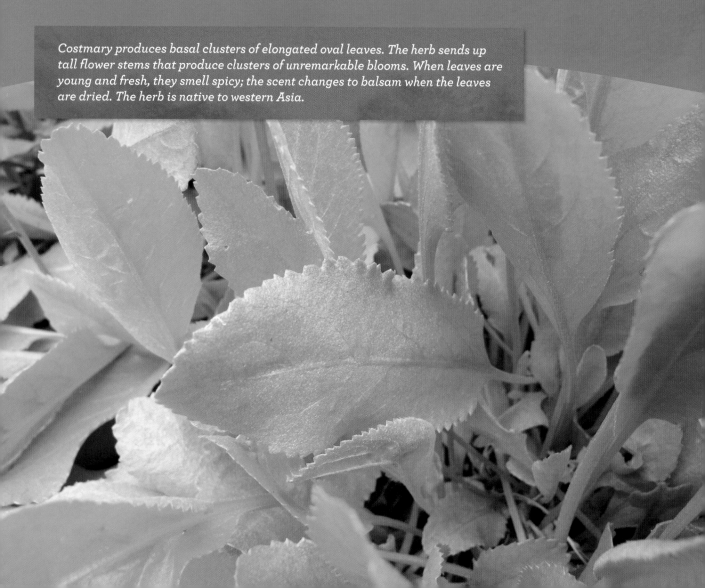

Costmary produces basal clusters of elongated oval leaves. The herb sends up tall flower stems that produce clusters of unremarkable blooms. When leaves are young and fresh, they smell spicy; the scent changes to balsam when the leaves are dried. The herb is native to western Asia.

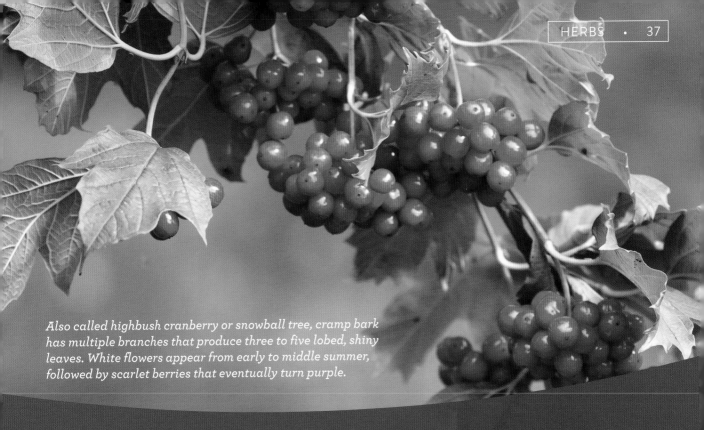

Also called highbush cranberry or snowball tree, cramp bark has multiple branches that produce three to five lobed, shiny leaves. White flowers appear from early to middle summer, followed by scarlet berries that eventually turn purple.

CRAMP BARK

BOTANICAL NAME: *VIBURNUM OPULUS*

Cramp bark's name tells you how the tree is used. American Indian women relied extensively on cramp bark to ease the pain of menstrual cramps and childbirth. An early American formula known as Mother's Cordial was given to women in childbirth. Cramp bark is used to halt contractions during premature labor and prevent miscarriage. It has also been used to prevent uterine hemorrhaging.

An antispasmodic, cramp bark may reduce leg cramps, muscle spasms, and pain from a stiff neck. Nineteenth-century herbalists often prescribed cramp bark as a sedative and muscle relaxant. The herb's medicinal actions may be attributed in part to a bitter called viburnin, as well as valerianic acid (also found in valerian), salicosides (also found in willow bark), and an antispasmodic constituent. Clinical studies indicate cramp bark may be useful in treating cardiovascular problems, reducing blood pressure and heart palpitations, and fighting influenza viruses. Cramp bark is considered an astringent as well.

The tree's cooked berries taste somewhat like cranberries, which is why it is often called cranberry tree or bush. In Scandinavia, liquor is distilled from the fruit. A Russian brandy made with the berries is used as a stomach ulcer remedy. From a species that grows in Japan, the Japanese make a vinegar to treat cirrhosis of the liver.

PRECAUTIONS

Do not eat fresh berries, which contain viburnin and may cause indigestion. The toxicity dissipates when berries are cooked.

DANDELION

BOTANICAL NAME: *TARAXACUM OFFICINALE*

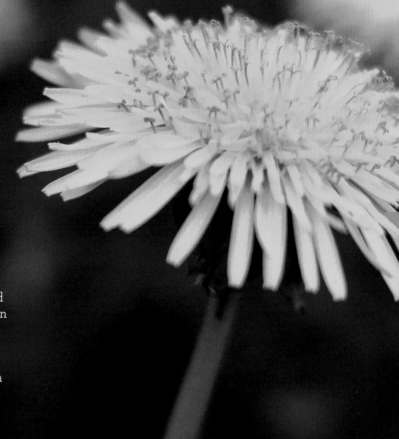

The Arabs were the first to introduce dandelion's healing and nutritive abilities to the Europeans through their writing. By the 16th century, dandelion was considered an important culinary and blood-purifying herb in Europe. The root is used to treat liver diseases, such as jaundice and cirrhosis. It also is considered beneficial for building up blood and curing anemia.

Dandelion root's diuretic properties may help lower blood pressure and relieve premenstrual fluid retention. Unlike most diuretics, it retains potassium rather than flushing it from the body. Clinical studies have favorably compared dandelion's actions with the frequently prescribed diuretic drug Furosemide. Dandelion roots contain inulin and levulin, starchlike substances that are easy to digest, as well as a bitter substance (taraxacin) that stimulates digestion. Dandelion roots, stems, and leaves exude a white sticky resin that dissolves warts, if applied repeatedly.

Wine made from dandelion flowers tastes like sherry. An Arabian dish, *yublo*, contains the flower buds and oil, flour, honey, and roses. The roasted ground root makes a good coffee substitute. Dandelion leaves are rich in minerals and vitamins, particularly vitamins A, B2, C, and K and calcium. Add young leaves to salads, or sauté them as you would spinach. The English sometimes put the flowers in sandwiches. Dandelion makes a tonic bath and facial steam. Its flowers produce a

Long considered a lawn pest, dandelion produces a taproot that is white on the inside and dark brown on the outside. You're probably familiar with the bright yellow flowers that top dandelion's hollow stems. Flowers appear in late spring and close at night. Dark green leaves are jagged and grow close to the ground.

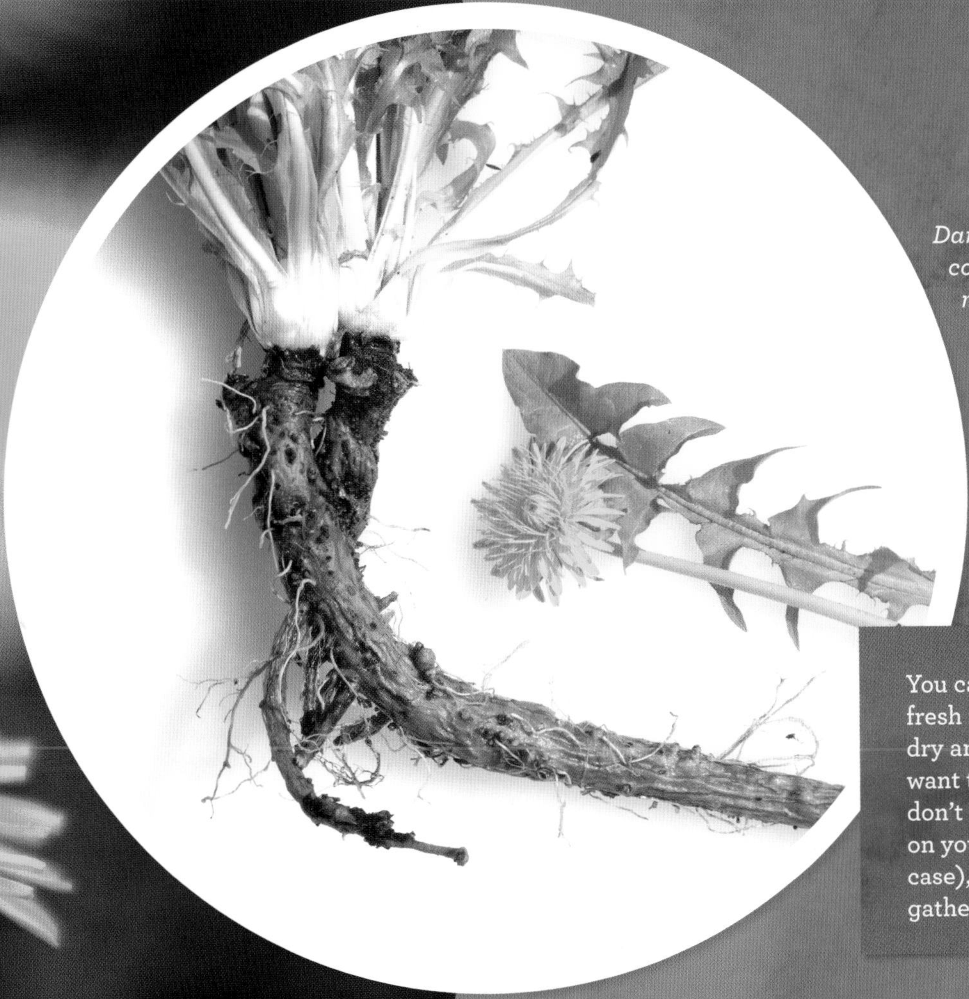

Dandelion roots make wonderful colon cleansing and detoxifying medications because any time digestion is improved, the absorption of nutrients and the removal of wastes from the body improves as well.

You can eat dandelions prepared fresh from your yard or you can dry and tincture them. If you want to use your own dandelions, don't use any chemical sprays on your lawn (a good idea in any case), and be wary where you gather dandelions.

DANDELION JUICE SPRING TONIC

Make a cleansing, nourishing juice from the dandelions you weed out of your lawn. The sweetness of the apples and carrots improves the bitter taste of the dandelion. Consume this preparation in small quantities as a spring tonic.

- **3 cups dandelion roots**
- **10 organic carrots**
- **6 organic apples**

In a home juicer, juice the dandelion roots, carrots, and apples separately. Combine the juices in a blender and chill 30 minutes to allow flavors to blend. Blend with any of the following: 1 tsp vitamin C crystals, 1 tsp spirulina powder, ¼ tsp liquid multiminerals.

To treat colds and congestion, add garlic, cayenne, or horseradish, and sip the tonic throughout the day.

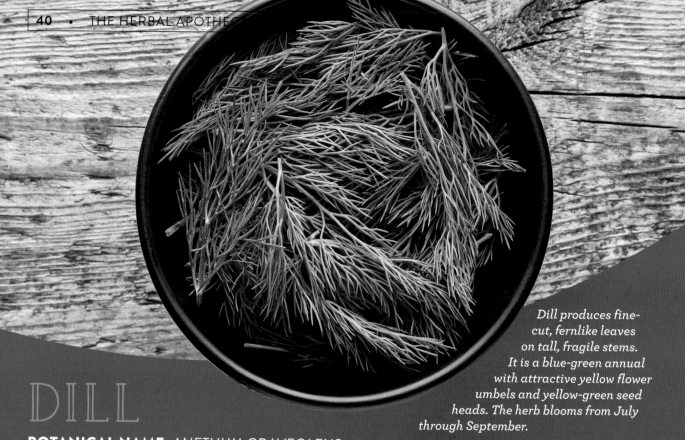

DILL

Dill produces fine-cut, fernlike leaves on tall, fragile stems. It is a blue-green annual with attractive yellow flower umbels and yellow-green seed heads. The herb blooms from July through September.

BOTANICAL NAME: *ANETHUM GRAVEOLENS*

Dill derives from an old Norse word meaning "to lull," and, indeed, the herb once was used to induce sleep in babies with colic. Herbalists also use dill to relieve gas and to stimulate flow of mother's milk. Dill stimulates the appetite and settles the stomach, but the seeds have also been chewed to lessen the appetite and stop the stomach from rumbling—something that parishioners found useful during all-day church services. In India, it is used to treat ulcers, fevers, uterine pain, and problems with the eyes and kidneys, usually in a formula with other herbs. In Ethiopia, the seeds are chewed to relieve a headache.

Add minced dill leaves to salads and use as a garnish. Seeds go well with fish, lamb, pork, poultry, cheese, cream, eggs, and an array of vegetables, including cabbage, onions, cauliflower, squash, spinach, potatoes, and broccoli. Of course, dill pickles would not be the same without dill seed and weed. The herb is particularly popular in Russia and Scandinavia. Its taste somewhat resembles caraway, which shares a similar chemistry.

HARVESTING

Flavor is best retained for later use if frozen; pick leaves just as flowers begin to open. For seeds, harvest entire plants when seed heads begin to turn brown. Hang-dry upside down in paper bags to catch seeds.

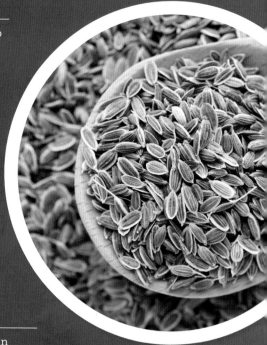

Dill seeds

ECHINACEA

BOTANICAL NAME:
ECHINACEA PURPUREA

American Indians used echinacea extensively to treat the bites of snakes and poisonous insects, burns, and wounds. The root facilitates wound healing. (Sometimes the seeds are combined with the roots for medicinal use.) Echinacea is prescribed to treat various infections, mumps, measles, and eczema. A compound in echinacea prevents damage to collagen in the skin and connective tissues when taken internally. Recent studies suggest that, applied topically, echinacea may treat sunburn.

Today, echinacea root is used primarily to boost the immune system and help the body fight disease. Besides bolstering several chemical substances that direct immune response, echinacea increases the number and activity of white blood cells (the body's disease-fighting agents), raises the level of interferon (a substance that enhances immune function), increases production of substances the body produces to fight cancers, and helps remove pollutants from the lungs. Many studies support echinacea's ability to fend off disease.

Another species, *E. angustifolia*, is used interchangeably with *E. purpurea* although the chemistry of the two species is slightly different.

Also known as purple coneflower, echinacea resembles the black-eyed Susan. The herb produces long black roots and stout, sturdy stems covered with bristly hairs. Cone-shaped flower heads, which appear from middle to late summer, are composed of numerous tiny purple florets surrounded by deep pink petals.

PRECAUTIONS

Echinacea has been shown to be very nontoxic and safe even for children. Some herbalists believe echinacea should not be used by people with auto-immune disorders such as lupus or rheumatoid arthritis because their immune systems are already overstimulated.

ELDERBERRY

BOTANICAL NAME: *SAMBUCUS NIGRA*

Elderberry has probably been used medicinally and nutritively for as long as human beings have gathered plants. Evidence of elderberry plants has been uncovered in Stone Age sites. Ancient people used elderberries to dye their hair black. The wood of old stems is still used to make musical instruments by Native Americans and Europeans.

In the kitchen, the berries are used to make jams, jellies, chutneys, preserves, wines, and teas. For decades, elder flower water was on the dressing tables of proper young ladies who used it to treat sunburn and eradicate freckles. It is still sometimes used in Europe for these purposes. Yellow and violet dyes are made from the leaves and berries, respectively.

Medicinally, elderberry has been used as a mild digestive stimulant and diaphoretic. Elder flowers decrease inflammation so are often included in preparations to treat burns and swellings and in cosmetics that reduce puffiness. The berries have been used traditionally in Europe to treat flu, gout, and rheumatism as well as to improve general health. Several tales attribute longevity to the elderberry.

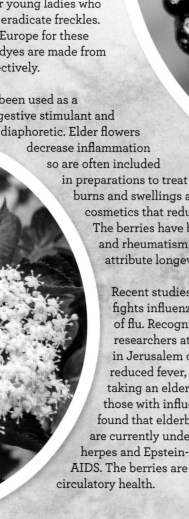

Recent studies in Israel found the berry is a potent antiviral that fights influenza virus B, the cause of one of the common forms of flu. Recognizing that it has long been used as a flu remedy, researchers at the Hebrew University Hadasah Medical Centre in Jerusalem conducted clinical studies and found the berry reduced fever, coughs, and muscle pain within 24 hours. After taking an elderberry syrup only two days, almost two-thirds of those with influenza reported complete recovery. The Centre also found that elderberry stimulates the immune system. The berries are currently under investigation for their ability to inhibit the herpes and Epstein-Barr viruses as well as HIV, the virus that causes AIDS. The berries are also rich in compounds that improve heart and circulatory health.

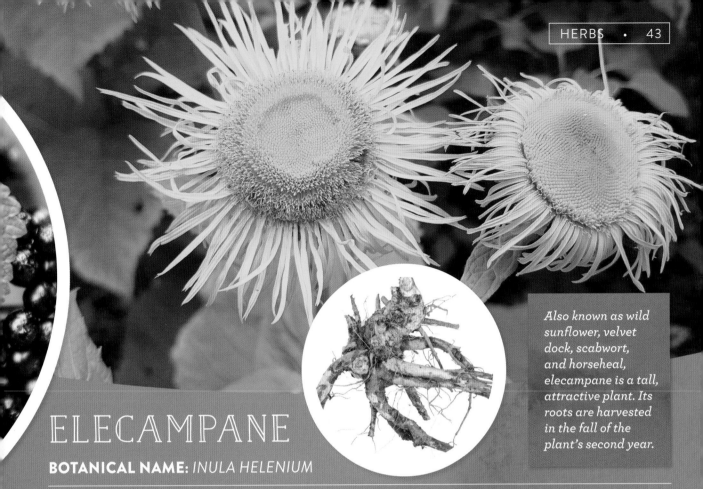

ELECAMPANE

Also known as wild sunflower, velvet dock, scabwort, and horseheal, elecampane is a tall, attractive plant. Its roots are harvested in the fall of the plant's second year.

BOTANICAL NAME: *INULA HELENIUM*

Elecampane's Latin name, *helenium*, refers to the legend that Helen of Troy carried a handful of elecampane on the day Paris abducted her, sparking the Trojan War. Perhaps she carried it because she had worms: Elecampane has been used for centuries to expel parasites in the digestive system, and today we know it contains a compound that expels intestinal worms.

But elecampane has been used most often for treating respiratory diseases. It is especially good for shortness of breath and bronchial problems. Early American colonists grew it for use as an expectorant; in Europe, people with asthma chewed on the root. Indian Ayurvedic physicians prescribe elecampane for chest conditions. In China, the plant is used to make syrup, lozenges, and candy to treat bronchitis and asthma.

European studies show that elecampane promotes menstruation and may be useful in reducing blood pressure. The herb also has been shown to have some sedative effect. The root is added to many medicines and used as a flavoring for sweets. Cordials and sugar cakes are still made from it in parts of Europe. You'll find the flower heads in dried craft arrangements.

PRECAUTIONS

Avoid elecampane if you're pregnant, as the herb has been used traditionally to promote menstruation. Studies have shown that a small dose of elecampane lowers blood sugar levels in animals, but higher doses raise them. Thus, people with diabetes should be careful when using the herb. People occasionally develop a rash from skin contact with the herb.

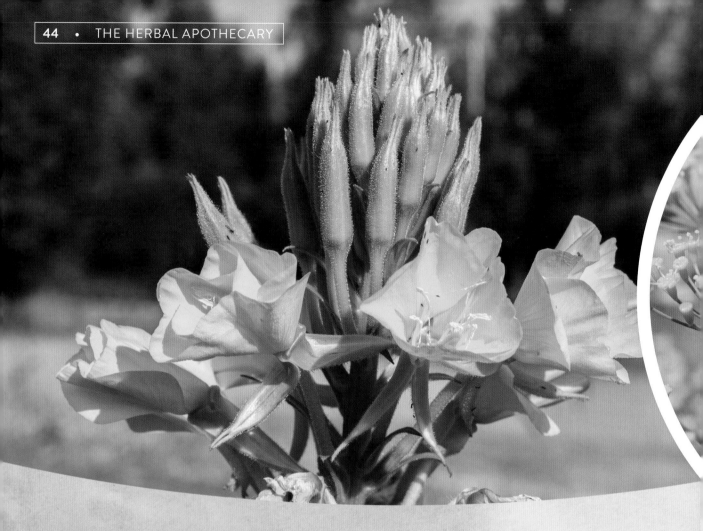

EVENING PRIMROSE

BOTANICAL NAME: *OENOTHERA BIENNIS*

The boiled root of evening primrose, which tastes something like a sweet parsnip, may be pickled or tossed raw in salads. The plant once was grown in monasteries; more recently scientists have found that the seeds contain a rare substance called gamma-linoleic acid (better known as GLA), which may have value in treating multiple sclerosis, thrombosis, premenstrual symptoms, menopausal discomfort, alcohol withdrawal, hyperactivity, and psoriasis. In one study, more than half the study participants found that their PMS symptoms completely disappeared when they used evening primrose. In another study, more than half the arthritis patients who took evening primrose oil also found relief. The oil, when combined with zinc supplements, improves dry eyes and brittle nails, although it often takes two to three months to notice improvement in these conditions. Leaves and bark have been used to ease cough spasms.

The Highland Psychiatric Research Group in Scotland discovered evening primrose helps regenerate damaged liver cells. It is also thought to prevent liver damage, stop alcohol from impairing brain cells, and lessen the symptoms of a hangover. Research is underway to determine if it can protect cells against HIV, the virus that causes AIDS.

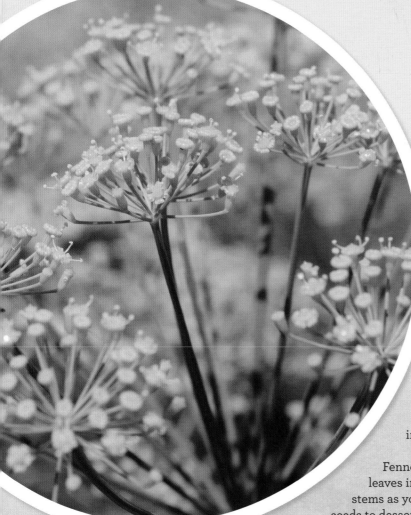

FENNEL

BOTANICAL NAME:
FOENICULUM VULGARE

The Greeks gave fennel to nursing mothers to increase milk flow. Early physicians also considered fennel a remedy for poor eyesight, weight loss, hiccups, nausea, gout, and many other illnesses. Fennel is a carminative, weak diuretic, and mild digestive stimulant. Herbalists often recommend fennel tea to soothe an upset stomach and dispel gas. It aids digestion, especially of fat. In Europe, a popular children's carminative is still made with fennel, chamomile, caraway, coriander, and bitter orange peel. Fennel is also a urinary tract tonic that lessens inflammation and helps eliminate kidney stones.

Fennel tastes like a more bitter version of anise. Use leaves in salads and as garnishes. You can eat tender stems as you would celery, and add seeds to desserts, breads, cakes, cookies, and beverages. Mince bulbs of sweet fennel and eat raw or braise. Fennel complements fish, sausage, duck, barley, rice, cabbage, beets, pickles, potatoes, lentils, breads, and eggs. Add it to butters, cheese spreads, and salad dressings. A fennel infusion acts as a skin cleanser and antiseptic. It reduces bruising when applied topically. The herb dyes wool shades of yellow and brown.

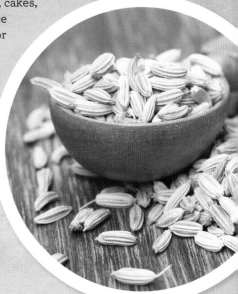

PRECAUTIONS

Fennel has mild estrogenic properties, so avoid it if you're pregnant. Very large amounts can overstimulate the nervous system.

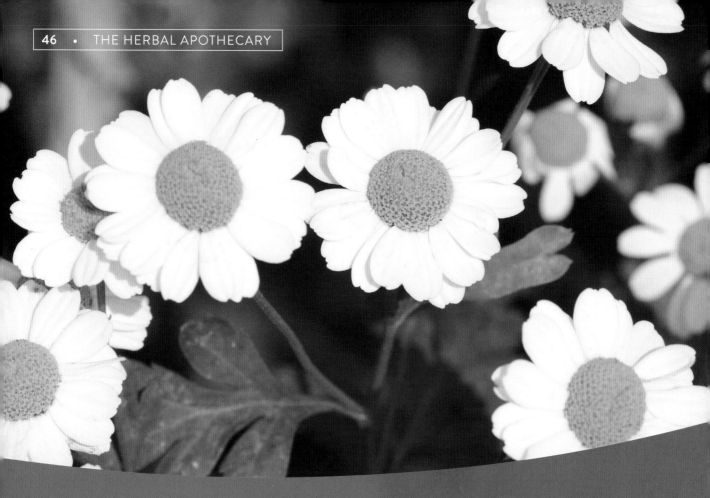

FEVERFEW

BOTANICAL NAME: *TANACETUM PARTHENIUM*

Feverfew's common name derives from the Latin *febrifugia*, which means "driver out of fevers." The Romans used the herb extensively for this purpose, and the Greeks employed it to normalize irregular contractions in childbirth. Today feverfew leaves are best known for their ability to fight headaches, particularly migraines. The herb's constituents relax blood vessels in the brain and inhibit secretion of substances that cause pain. Feverfew is most effective when used long-term to prevent chronic migraines, but some people find it helpful when taken at the onset of a headache. When patients at the Department of Medicine and Haemotology in Nottingham, England, ate fresh feverfew leaves for three months, they had fewer migraines and less nausea when they did experience one. Their blood pressure was reduced, and they reported feelings of well-being. Feverfew also is reported to reduce inflammation in joints and tissues. It has been prescribed for treating menstrual cramps. Pyrethrin, an active ingredient, is a potent insect repellent. Feverfew's leaves and stems produce a dye that is greenish-yellow.

PRECAUTIONS

Feverfew may cause stomach upset. Chewing raw leaves regularly may irritate the mouth. Tinctures and capsules do not cause such irritation. Because feverfew relaxes blood vessels, it may increase blood flow during menstruation.

GENTIAN

BOTANICAL NAME:
GENTIANA LUTEA

Gentian root has been prized as a digestive bitter for more than 3,000 years—the Egyptians, Arabs, Greeks, and Romans used it. In India, Ayurvedic doctors used gentian to treat fevers, venereal disease, jaundice, and other illnesses of the liver. Colonists in Virginia and the Carolinas discovered Indians using a gentian decoction to treat back pain. Chinese physicians use it to treat digestive disorders, sore throat, headache, and arthritis. Gentian, moreover, has been used to increase menstruation, thus easing painful periods.

Today, gentian is used commercially to make liqueurs, vermouth, digestive bitters, and aperitifs. Gentian is also a primary ingredient of Moxie, a patent medicine popular in the late 19th century that is still sold in New England as a soft drink. The herb's bitterness increases gastric secretions and helps a sluggish appetite or poor digestion. It is especially useful for problems digesting fat or protein. Researchers in Germany found that it cures heartburn, intestinal inflammation, and general indigestion. It also destroys several types of intestinal worms.

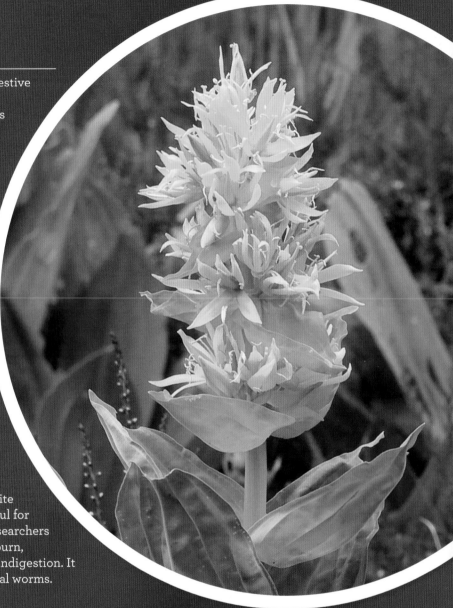

PRECAUTIONS

Don't take gentian if you are pregnant. Although no studies have shown it is dangerous, gentian has been used to promote menstruation. Gentian also contains constituents that may elevate blood pressure. Although the Food and Drug Administration has approved gentian for use in foods and alcoholic beverages, large doses may cause nausea and vomiting. The gentian violet sold in pharmacies is not made from gentian: It is a very potent chemical used to treat skin infection.

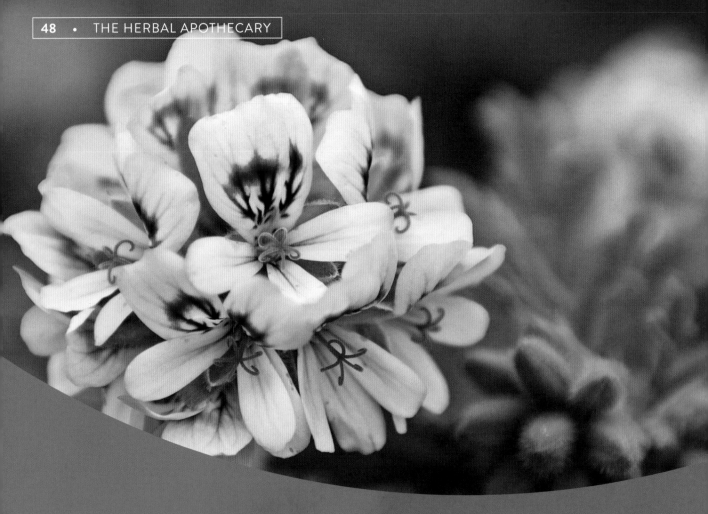

GERANIUM, SCENTED

BOTANICAL NAME: *PELARGONIUM GRAVEOLENS*

You could call the scented geranium the potpourri plant. The herb comes in a wide variety of fragrances, including rose, apple, lemon, lime, apricot, strawberry, coconut, and peppermint, making it an ideal addition to potpourri and sachets. The plant was considered fashionable in Victorian times.

Herbalists sometimes recommend the astringent herb for treating diarrhea and ulcers and to stop bleeding. The essential oil is used to treat ringworm, lice, shingles, and herpes. The pharmaceutical industry uses one of the antiseptic compounds in geranium called geraniol. The leaves of some varieties, including rose, may be used to flavor cookies and jelly. Add other leaves, such as peppermint, to herbal teas. Added to facial steams and baths, they are cleansing and healing to the skin. The scent is popular in men's products—it blends well with woodsy and citrus fragrances. Rose geranium is used in many aromatherapy products for its relaxing and emotional balancing properties. This species is also added to cosmetics to improve the complexion.

The fresh leaves of scented geranium can be added to jellies and fruit dishes or placed on desserts. For a unique herbal treat, place the leaves in the bottom of a buttered cake pan before pouring in the batter. When you turn the finished cake over, it will be decorated with the herb leaves.

GINGER

BOTANICAL NAME: *ZINGIBER OFFICINALE*

Most every child knows the taste of ginger. It's the prime ingredient in ginger ale, gingerbread, and gingersnaps. But the popular kitchen spice enjoys a rich history as a medicinal herb as well. Ginger is a potent anti-nausea medication, useful for treating morning sickness, motion sickness, and nausea accompanying gastroenteritis (stomach "flu"). As a stomach calming aid, ginger reduces gas, bloating, and indigestion and aids in the body's absorption of nutrients and other herbs. Ginger is also a valuable deterrent to several types of intestinal worms. And the herb may work as a therapy and preventive treatment for some migraine headaches and rheumatoid arthritis.

Ginger promotes perspiration if ingested in large amounts. Use internally or topically. The herb stimulates circulation, so if you are cold, you can use warm ginger tea to help raise your body heat. Ginger may occasionally promote menstrual flow. It also prevents platelets from clumping and thins the blood, which reduces the risk of atherosclerosis and blood clots. Grated ginger poultices or compresses ease lung congestion when placed on the chest and alleviate gas, nausea, and menstrual cramps when laid on the abdomen.

Ginger is a staple of many cuisines, including those of southeast Asia, India, Japan, the Caribbean, and North Africa. Add the spicy chopped root to beverages, fruits, meats, fish, preserves, pickles, and a variety of vegetables. Use ground ginger in breads, cookies, and other deserts.

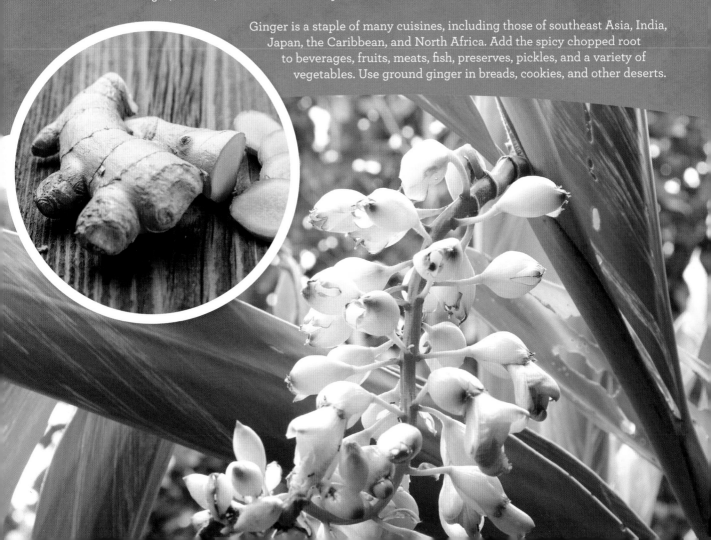

GINGKO

BOTANICAL NAME: *GINKGO BILOBA*

This stately deciduous tree produces male and female flowers on separate plants. Female plants produce orange-yellow fruits the size of large olives. In the fall its leaves turn gold. Found throughout the temperate world, ginkgo may be grown in many parts of the United States.

Ginkgo is one of the oldest species of tree on earth. It is used to treat conditions associated with aging, including stroke, heart disease, impotence, deafness, ringing in the ears, blindness, and memory loss. In many studies, it helped people improve their concentration and memory. Ginkgo promotes the action of certain neurotransmitters, chemical compounds responsible for relaying nerve impulses in the brain.

Ginkgo increases circulation, including blood flow to the brain, which may help improve memory. Several studies show it reduces the risk of heart attack and improves pain from blood clots (phlebitis) in the legs. Additional studies show that, in a large percentage of people, ginkgo helps impotence caused by narrowing of arteries that supply blood to the penis; macular degeneration of the eyes, a deterioration in vision that may be caused by narrowing of the blood vessels to the eye; and cochlear deafness, which is caused by decreased blood flow to the nerves involved in hearing.

Constituents in ginkgo are potent antioxidants with anti-inflammatory effects. A current scientific theory attributes many of the signs of aging and chronic disease to oxidation of cell membranes by substances called free radicals, which may arise from pollutants or from normal internal production of metabolic substances. Ginkgo counters destruction of cells due to oxidation. Researchers also found it can help children with asthma.

The herb produces chemicals that interfere with a substance called platelet activation factor, PAF, which is involved in organ graft rejection, asthma attacks, and blood clots that lead to heart attacks and some strokes.

PRECAUTIONS

Ginkgo may cause problems for people with clotting disorders or those who take blood-thinning medications. Extremely large quantities of ginkgo sometimes cause irritability, restlessness, diarrhea, nausea, and vomiting.

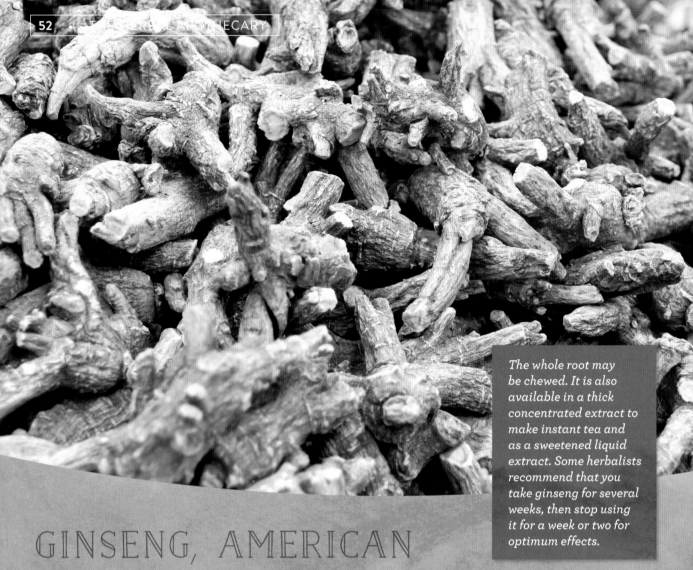

The whole root may be chewed. It is also available in a thick concentrated extract to make instant tea and as a sweetened liquid extract. Some herbalists recommend that you take ginseng for several weeks, then stop using it for a week or two for optimum effects.

GINSENG, AMERICAN

BOTANICAL NAME: *PANAX QUINQUEFOLIUS*

The Chinese have used a close relative of American ginseng since prehistoric times. In the United States, colonists grew rich collecting American ginseng and exporting it to China, where the herb enjoys a strong reputation as an aphrodisiac and prolonger of life. Ginseng is an adaptogen, capable of protecting the body from physical and mental stress and helping bodily functions return to normal.

Clinical studies indicate that ginseng may slow the effects of aging, protect cells from free radical damage, prevent heart disease, and help treat anemia, atherosclerosis, depression, diabetes, edema (excess fluid buildup), ulcers, and hypertension. Its complex saponins, ginsenosides, are responsible for most of its actions. They stimulate bone marrow production and immune-system functions, inhibit tumor growth, and detoxify the liver. Ginseng has many dual roles, for example, raising or lowering blood pressure or blood sugar, according to the body's needs.

Ginseng gently stimulates and strengthens the central nervous system, making it useful for treating fatigue and weakness caused by disease and injury. It reduces mental confusion and headaches.

GOLDENSEAL

BOTANICAL NAME:
HYDRASTIS CANADENSIS

The Cherokee Indians mixed powdered goldenseal root with bear grease and slathered their bodies to protect themselves from mosquitoes and other insects. Pioneers adopted the herb and used it to treat wounds, rashes, mouth sores, morning sickness, liver and stomach complaints, internal hemorrhaging, depressed appetite, constipation, and urinary and uterine problems.

One of goldenseal's active ingredients is hydrastine, which affects circulation, muscle tone, and uterine contractions. The herb is also an antiseptic, astringent, and antibiotic, making it effective for treating eye and other types of infections. Berberine and related alkaloids have been credited with goldenseal's antimicrobial effects. Goldenseal makes a good antiseptic skin wash for wounds and for internal skin surfaces, such as in the vagina and ear; it also treats canker sores and infected gums. The herb has been found to fight a number of disease-causing microbes, including *Staphylococcus* and *Streptococcus* organisms.

It takes about five years for the root to get large enough to harvest.

Berberine may be responsible for increasing white blood cell activity and promoting blood flow in the liver and spleen. Berberine has been used in China to combat the reduction of white blood cells that commonly follows chemotherapy and radiation treatment for cancer. Studies suggest it may have potential in the treatment of brain and skin cancers.

PRECAUTIONS

Hydrastine accumulates in the system and is toxic in large doses. Berberine may lower blood pressure, but hydrastine raises it, so avoid the herb if you have high blood pressure, heart disease, or glaucoma, except under professional guidance.

GOTU KOLA

BOTANICAL NAME: *CENTELLA ASIATICA*

Gotu kola is considered a relaxant, nerve tonic, diuretic, anti-inflammatory, and wound healer. The herb has long been regarded as a life extender. Shepherds in Sri Lanka noticed that elephants ate it and lived a long time. Thus, a later proverb reasoned, "Two leaves a day will keep old age away." Indian Ayurvedic physicians have used the plant extensively to treat the problems of aging. There is no evidence to support the theory that gotu kola prolongs life, but some tests have shown that the plant is a sedative and tonic for the nervous system and could help in treating many neurologic and mental disturbances, especially debility stemming from stress. Ayurvedics also use gotu kola to treat asthma, anemia, and other blood disorders.

In India gotu kola has been called brahmi, in honor of the god Brahma. It is reputed to improve memory, and East Indians again note that elephants, which supposedly never forget, consider gotu kola a delicacy.

The plant also has been used internally to treat rheumatism and other inflammatory diseases. In the Orient, physicians employ gotu kola leaves and roots to treat wounds, ulcers, and lesions that don't heal properly, including leprosy lesions. Gotu kola contains a chemical called asiaticoside, which aids in the treatment of leprosy. It also helps prevent scarring, and it has been used successfully in Germany to heal the skin after surgery.

Gotu kola is thought to stimulate the body's immune system. It improves circulation throughout the body—one reason it may improve memory and brain function. It also improves varicose veins and other circulation disorders.

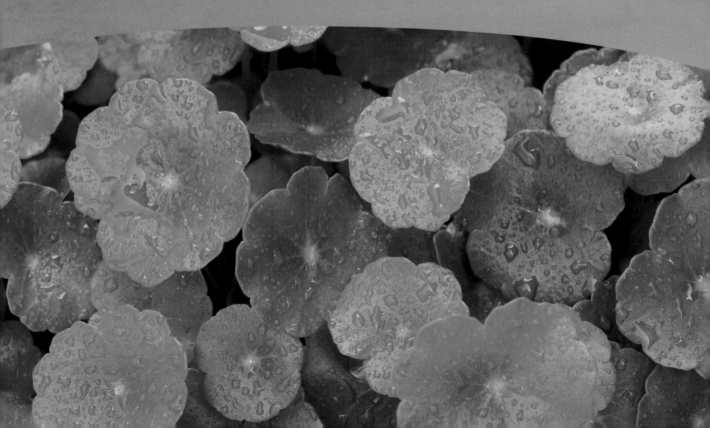

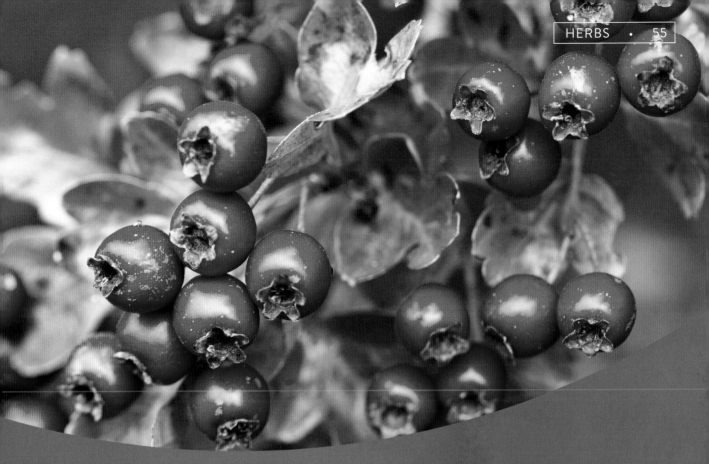

HAWTHORN

BOTANICAL NAME: *CRATAEGUS LAEVIGATA*

Hawthorn has been cherished for centuries. The Druids considered hawthorn a sacred tree. The Pilgrims brought it to America: Mayflower is, in fact, another name for hawthorn.

Hawthorn is an important herb for treating heart conditions. The berries and flowers contain several complex chemical constituents, including flavonoids such as anthocyanidins, which improve the strength of capillaries and reduce damage to blood vessels from oxidizing agents. Hawthorn's ability to dilate blood vessels, enhancing circulation, makes it useful for treating angina, atherosclerosis, high and low blood pressure, and elevated cholesterol levels. Many clinical studies have demonstrated its effectiveness for such conditions—with the use of hawthorn, the heart requires less oxygen when under stress. Heart action is normalized and becomes stronger and more efficient. Hawthorn also helps balance the heart's rhythm and is prescribed for arrhythmias and heart palpitations by European physicians. Although it affects the heart somewhat like the medication digitalis, hawthorn does not have a cumulative effect on the heart.

PRECAUTIONS

Hawthorn is considered safe and may be used for long periods. Do not self-medicate with hawthorn. Consult a physician or herbalist before taking it, especially if you take prescription heart medication: Hawthorn may intensify the effects of these drugs.

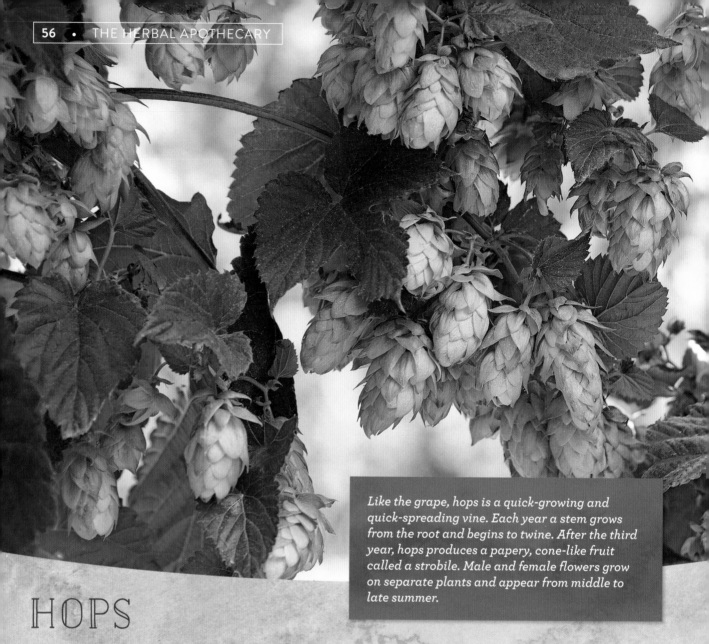

Like the grape, hops is a quick-growing and quick-spreading vine. Each year a stem grows from the root and begins to twine. After the third year, hops produces a papery, cone-like fruit called a strobile. Male and female flowers grow on separate plants and appear from middle to late summer.

HOPS

BOTANICAL NAME: *HUMULUS LUPULUS*

If you worked in a hopyard, you might find yourself falling asleep on the job. Hops contains chemicals that depress the central nervous system, making it a useful sedative herb. Abraham Lincoln and England's King George III, notorious insomniacs, reportedly lay their heads on hops-filled pillows to ensure a good night's sleep. Hops' other constituents are antiseptic, antibacterial, and anti-inflammatory, and they slightly increase activity of the female hormone estrogen. Hops has also been used as a pain reliever, fever cure, expectorant, and diuretic. It has been prescribed to treat nervous heart conditions, PMS, menstrual pain, and nervous symptoms of menopause. The Greeks and Romans used hops as a digestive aid. If you have drunk beer, you will be familiar with hops' pleasantly bitter taste. This bitterness makes hops an excellent digestive aid. Since the 9th century AD, brewers have used hops to flavor and preserve beer. In some Scandinavian countries, weavers make a coarse cloth from hops vine. Dried hops also makes an interesting addition to dried floral arrangements.

HOREHOUND

BOTANICAL NAME: *MARRUBIUM VULGARE*

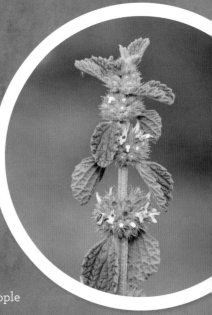

Your recent ancestors may have sucked on horehound lozenges to open clogged nasal passages and alleviate other symptoms associated with the sniffles. One of the Hebrews' ritual bitter herbs, horehound was also prized by the Greeks and Egyptians. Herbalists have employed it to treat hepatitis and jaundice. But horehound's most reliable uses are to soothe sore throats, help the lungs expel mucus, and treat bronchitis. A weak sedative, it also helps normalize an irregular heartbeat. It induces sweating and will lower a fever, especially when infused and drunk as a hot tea.

The herb's primary constituents include an essential oil, tannin, and a bitter chemical called marrubiin. The plant also contains vitamin C, which adds to its ability to fight colds. Horehound has a taste similar to sage and hyssop but more bitter. At one time it was used in England as a bitter to flavor ale. Today some people use the leaves to make an old-fashioned candy called horehound drops.

PRECAUTIONS

In very large doses, horehound may cause cardiac arrhythmias.

HORSERADISH

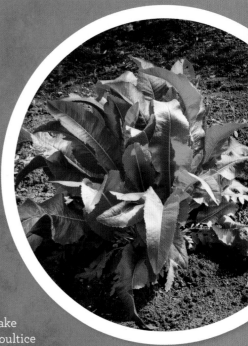

BOTANICAL NAME: *ARMORIACIA RUSTICANA*

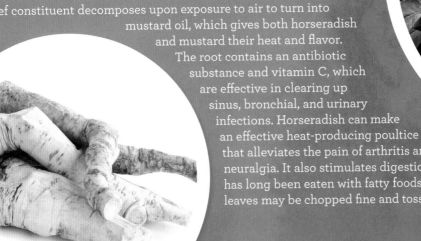

Horseradish has been used as a medicine for centuries. Its chief constituent decomposes upon exposure to air to turn into mustard oil, which gives both horseradish and mustard their heat and flavor. The root contains an antibiotic substance and vitamin C, which are effective in clearing up sinus, bronchial, and urinary infections. Horseradish can make an effective heat-producing poultice that alleviates the pain of arthritis and neuralgia. It also stimulates digestion and has long been eaten with fatty foods to help digest them. Tender new leaves may be chopped fine and tossed in salads.

HORSETAIL

BOTANICAL NAME: *EQUISETUM ARVENSE*

Horsetail is high in minerals, particularly silica. The herb contains so much silica, in fact, that you can use it to polish metal. Early Americans used horsetail to scour pots and pans. Horsetail treats water retention, bed-wetting, and other bladder problems, including kidney stones. It is also used to decrease an enlarged prostate. Used externally, it stops bleeding and helps wounds to heal. It was once used to prevent the lungs from scarring in people with tuberculosis.

Because it contains minerals, horsetail strengthens bone, hair, and fingernails. Horsetail infusions—often combined with nettles—are drunk to help broken bones mend. The silica in it encourages the absorption of calcium by the body and helps prevent build-up of fatty deposits in the arteries.

PRECAUTIONS

Make sure your horsetail was not gathered near an industrial site. Horsetail tends to pick up large amounts of nitrates and selenium from the soil. Equisetene, a chemical found in the plant, is a nerve toxin in large doses. It increases in amount as the plant matures, so pick horsetail only in the spring when it is in its second stage. Long-term use of horsetail could result in kidney damage. Do not use horsetail if you have high blood pressure or are pregnant.

The young shoots can be gathered and cooked like asparagus.

One of the earth's oldest plant species, horsetail has been around for 200 million years. The herb's name refers to the resemblance of its needle-like leaves to a horse's tail.

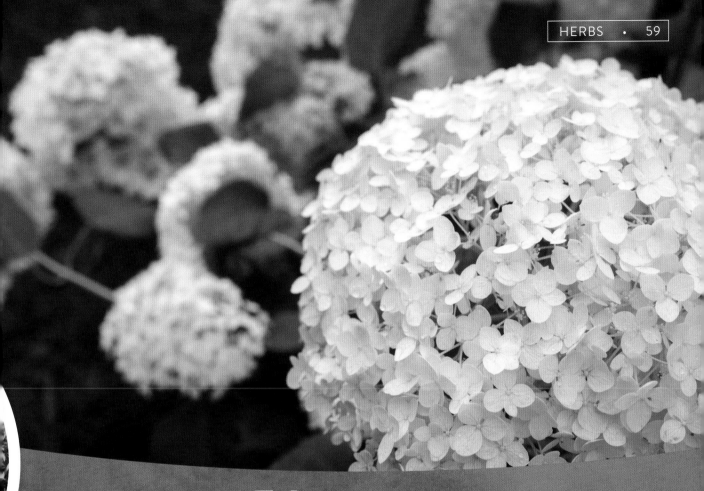

HYDRANGEA

BOTANICAL NAME: *HYDRANGEA ARBORESCENS*

Hydrangea root, which contains a number of glycosides, saponins, and resins, is used most often for treating enlarged prostate glands. The herb is employed to treat urinary stones and cystitis, and it can help prevent the recurrence of kidney stones. But you should not self-medicate for urinary or kidney stones, as these conditions require professional medical treatment.

The root is a laxative and diuretic. American Indians used its bark in poultices for treating wounds, burns, sore muscles, sprains, and tumors, and they chewed it for stomach and heart trouble. The leaves also contain some of the medicine but are not as strong as the roots. You can dry the flower heads as well as the individual flowers for use in craft projects. To retain their color, dry them as quickly as possible in a dark place or dry them in silica gel. The flowers are also very attractive when pressed.

PRECAUTIONS

Hydrangea may cause dizziness and indigestion when ingested in large amounts. Lower the dose if this occurs. The wood is reported to cause skin reactions in woodworkers, and the flowers have been known to make children sick when they ate the buds.

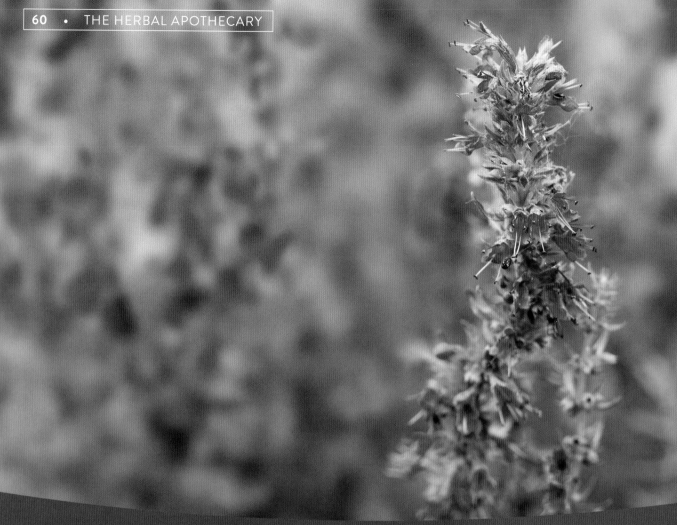

HYSSOP

BOTANICAL NAME: *HYSSOPUS OFFICINALIS*

Hyssop has been a favorite medicinal herb since it was used in ancient Greece. With its strong camphor-like odor, the herb was strewn on floors to freshen homes in the Middle Ages. Hyssop baths were once used in England to treat rheumatism. Hyssop, which has a chemistry similar to horehound, has been used mostly to treat bronchitis, flu, colds, and sore throats. It reduces inflammation, so it makes a good throat gargle. In laboratory tests, it destroys herpesvirus. A poultice of the fresh leaves promotes healing of wounds. The herb's essential oil is a prime flavoring of liqueurs, including Benedictine and Chartreuse. Add leaves to salads, chicken soup, fruit dishes, lamb, and poultry stuffing. Hyssop essential oil is expensive and found in quality perfumes. Use the herb or essential oil in a cleansing facial steam. Hyssop is said to repel flea beetles and other pests.

PRECAUTIONS

Use hyssop in small doses and not at all if you are pregnant or have high blood pressure. It can also induce epileptic seizures.

JUNIPER

BOTANICAL NAME: *JUNIPERUS COMMUNIS*

The berries give gin its distinct flavor. American Indians used the leaves and berries externally to cure infections, relieve arthritis, and treat wounds. Adding a handful of crushed juniper leaves to a warm bath soothes aching muscles. A compress of juniper berries is sometimes recommended for gout, rheumatoid arthritis, and nerve, muscle, joint, and tendon pain. The berries were once chewed by doctors to ward off infection when treating patients. Chewing them also improves bad breath.

Juniper's essential oils relieve coughs and lung congestion. Its tars and resins treat psoriasis and other skin conditions. In both treatments, juniper has a warming, circulation-stimulating action. Juniper also relieves gas in the digestive system, increases stomach acid, and is a diuretic. The essential oil in its berries has antiseptic properties and is sometimes used for chronic urinary tract infections.

In the kitchen, you can use juniper berries to flavor patés and sauerkraut. Crushed berries spice game dishes, stews, sauces, and marinades. Toss juniper branches on the grill to impart a distinctive smoky taste to meats.

PRECAUTIONS

Don't use juniper if you're pregnant or have a kidney infection or chronic kidney problems. Overdose symptoms may include diarrhea, intestinal pain, kidney pain, blood in urine, rapid heartbeat, and elevated blood pressure. Some hay fever sufferers develop allergic reactions to juniper. Don't use juniper if you develop any reactions.

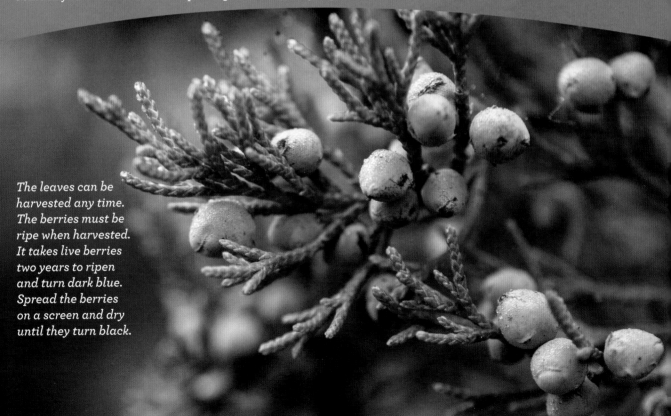

The leaves can be harvested any time. The berries must be ripe when harvested. It takes live berries two years to ripen and turn dark blue. Spread the berries on a screen and dry until they turn black.

LAVENDER

BOTANICAL NAME: *LAVANDULA ANGUSTIFOLIA*

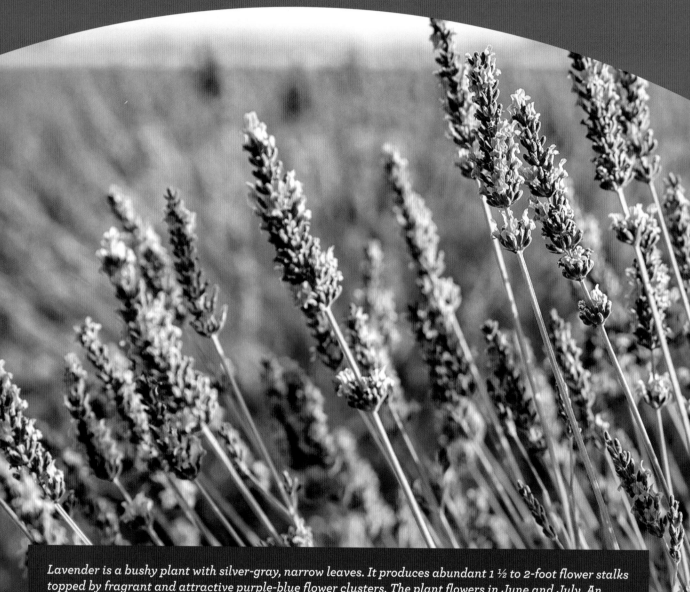

Lavender is a bushy plant with silver-gray, narrow leaves. It produces abundant 1 ½ to 2-foot flower stalks topped by fragrant and attractive purple-blue flower clusters. The plant flowers in June and July. An outstanding addition to any garden design, the herb also makes a nice edging or potted plant. There are a number of species and cultivars of lavender. Differences focus primarily on flower color (some have white, others, pink flowers), size, and growth habits.

Perhaps the smell of lavender reminds you of soap. That's because lavender is a prime ingredient of many soaps. Its name, in fact, derives from the Latin "to wash." The Romans and Greeks used lavender in the bath. Lavender is also found commercially in shaving creams, colognes, and perfumes. It is used in many cosmetics and aromatherapy products because it is so versatile, and its fragrance blends so well with other herbs. Studies show that the scent is very relaxing. Lavender's scent is also a remedy for headache and nervous tension.

Lavender cosmetics are good for all complexion types. It is an excellent skin healer: It promotes the healing of burns, abrasions, infected sores, and other types of inflammations, including varicose veins. It is also a popular hair rinse. The herb is a carminative and antispasmodic. It is most often used for sore muscles in the form of a massage oil. As recently as World War I, lavender was used in the field as a disinfectant for wounds; herbalists still recommend it for that purpose. Lavender destroys several viruses, including many that cause colds and flu. It also relieves lung and sinus congestion. Lavender flowers may be added to vinegars, jellies, sachets, and potpourri. Place a sprig of lavender in a drawer to freshen linens. And dried flowers make wonderful herbal arrangements, although they are fragile.

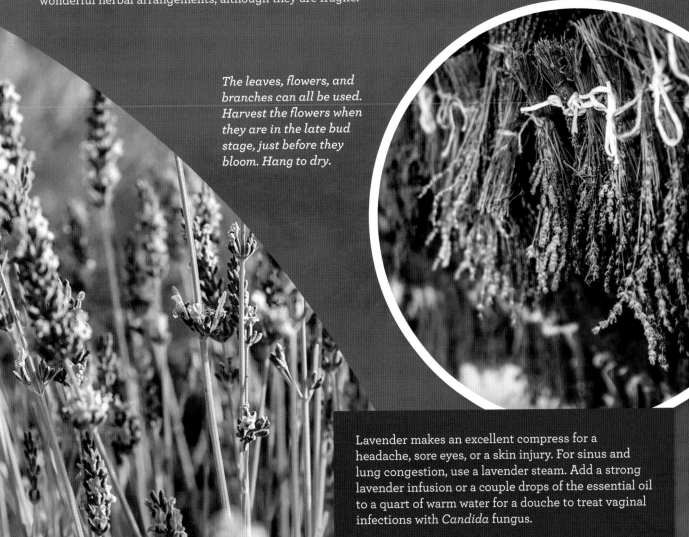

The leaves, flowers, and branches can all be used. Harvest the flowers when they are in the late bud stage, just before they bloom. Hang to dry.

Lavender makes an excellent compress for a headache, sore eyes, or a skin injury. For sinus and lung congestion, use a lavender steam. Add a strong lavender infusion or a couple drops of the essential oil to a quart of warm water for a douche to treat vaginal infections with *Candida* fungus.

LEMON BALM

BOTANICAL NAME: *MELISSA OFFICINALIS*

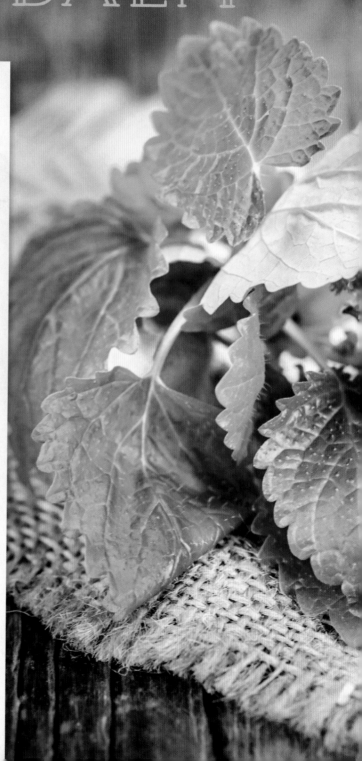

Lemon balm is an attractive plant with shield-shaped leaves that smell strongly of lemon. Like most mints, the herb produces square stems and flowers from July through September. Lemon balm is native to Europe and North Africa but has become naturalized elsewhere, including many parts of the United States. It is cultivated throughout the world.

Researchers have found that a mixture of lemon balm and valerian is as effective as some tranquilizers, without the side effects. The scent alone has long been used to reduce nervous tension. Compounds in it may even prove useful to people with hyperthyroidism, although the herb itself shouldn't replace thyroid medication. Its essential oil reduces risk of infections by inhibiting growth of bacteria and viruses. Recent studies show it is effective against the herpesvirus, flu, and colds. It can also soothe a nervous stomach and relieve mild headaches.

In the kitchen, this herb, with its lemony-mint flavor, complements salads, fruits, marinated vegetables, poultry and stuffing, punch, fish marinades, and an assortment of vegetables, including corn, broccoli, asparagus, and beans. Lemon balm is employed commercially to flavor liqueurs such as Benedictine and Chartreuse. Lemon balm infusions cleanse the skin and help clear up acne. You may add leaves to your bath, and even polish furniture with them.

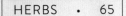
You can enjoy lemon balm tea freely. It is delicious hot or iced, by itself or mixed with other herbs. It is often blended with chamomile and mint as a digestive aid, for relaxation, or to give to children as a calmative.

AN EPIC HERB

This venerable herb has been used for at least 2,000 years. Homer mentions balm in his *Odyssey*. Greek and Roman physicians prescribed it to treat the bites of scorpions and dogs. But lemon balm's real fans were the Arabs, who believed it was good for heart disorders and dispelling melancholy. Colonists brought lemon balm to America. Thomas Jefferson grew it at Monticello, and many Old Williamsburg recipes call for its use. Lemon balm was an important medicine well into the 19th century.

Lemon balm is best harvested in midsummer. It may be dried for later use.

LICORICE

BOTANICAL NAME: *GLYCYRRHIZA GLABRA*

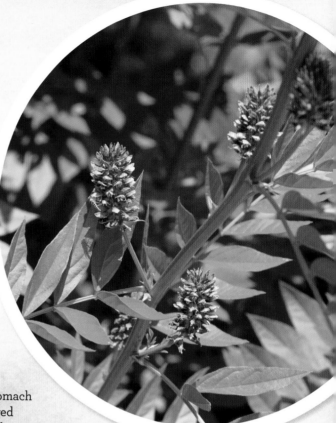

Licorice has been a popular flavoring for millennia. Archaeologists have determined that the Assyrians and Egyptians used it. Licorice's main constituent, glycyrrhizin, is 50 times sweeter than sugar. Although the herb was once a popular candy flavoring, most of the licorice candy made in the United States is actually flavored with anise. Licorice is used commercially in pastries, ice cream, puddings, soy sauce, soy-based meat substitutes, and tobacco.

As a medicine, licorice was also used by the Greeks and Romans and is still one of the most popular Chinese herbs. In the United States, licorice is in cough syrups and drops. The herb is also used to sweeten mouthwash and toothpaste. A laxative, this soothing herb has also been prescribed for stomach and bowel inflammation and peptic ulcers. Licorice reduces stomach acid and encourages the stomach to protect itself from acid. Carbenoxolene, a compound derived from licorice, was, until recently, the drug of choice to treat ulcers. Another form of licorice, deglycyrrhizinated licorice, shows promise as a future drug. Studies show it can be as effective as Tagemet and Zantac. Licorice has estrogenic effects and is useful for treating menopausal symptoms and normalizing an irregular menstrual cycle. Licorice is also an antiviral and decongestant and is used to treat dermatitis, colds, and infections. It enhances the immune system, and it may have anti-tumor properties. Several clinical studies indicate it may be useful to treat herpes, a viral condition which currently has no cure.

Like the adrenal hormone cortisone, it decreases inflammation, so it is used to reduce the symptoms of rheumatoid arthritis and other inflammatory disorders but without cortisone's side effects. And while cortisone therapy depletes the adrenal glands, licorice encourages them to function better and relieves adrenal exhaustion. Studies show licorice neutralizes liver toxins and increases the liver's ability to store glycogen, which provides muscles with energy.

PRECAUTIONS

Licorice may raise blood pressure in people who have hypertension. It may cause headaches, shortness of breath, bloating, and fluid retention in high doses or with long-term use of low daily doses. Avoid licorice if you're pregnant. Do not use as a daily laxative as it can cause excessive potassium loss.

LOVAGE

BOTANICAL NAME: *LEVISTICUM OFFICINALIS*

Herbalists have recommended lovage to increase urine flow, reduce gas and bowel pain, and treat sore throat, kidney stones, and irregular menstruation. Lovage also is used to treat stomachaches, headaches, obesity, and boils. The hot tea induces sweating. The taste of lovage's leaves, stems, and seeds resembles that of celery but is much sharper. Use leaves in salads, soups, stews, and sauces. Dried and powdered, they make a tasty addition to herbal salt substitutes. Stems may be cooked, puréed, candied, or eaten raw like celery. Add seeds to pickling brines, cheeses, salad dressings, potatoes, tomatoes, chicken, poultry stuffings, and rice. It also flavors some alcoholic beverages.

PRECAUTIONS

Do not use lovage if you are pregnant or have any kidney problems.

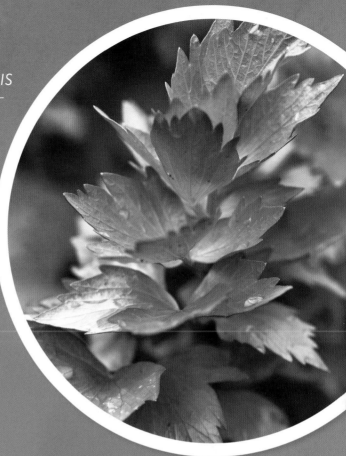

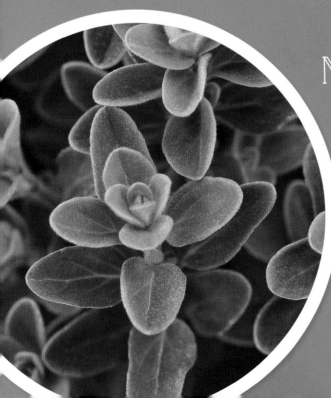

MARJORAM

BOTANICAL NAME: *ORIGANUM MAJORANA* OR *MAJORANA HORTENSIS*

Herbalists have prescribed marjoram to treat asthma, increase sweating, lower fevers, encourage menstruation, and, especially, relieve indigestion. European singers preserved their voices with marjoram tea sweetened with honey. The herb has antioxidant and antifungal properties. Recent studies show marjoram inhibits several viruses, including herpesvirus. Marjoram gargles and steam treatments relieve sinus congestion and hay fever. The diluted essential oil can be rubbed into sore gums, in place of clove oil. Its antioxidant properties are so potent they have been shown to be excellent food preservatives.

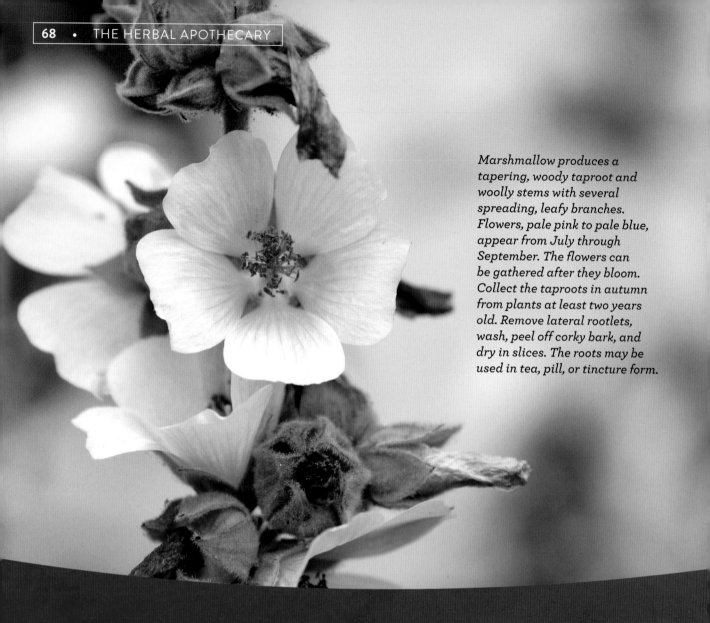

Marshmallow produces a tapering, woody taproot and woolly stems with several spreading, leafy branches. Flowers, pale pink to pale blue, appear from July through September. The flowers can be gathered after they bloom. Collect the taproots in autumn from plants at least two years old. Remove lateral rootlets, wash, peel off corky bark, and dry in slices. The roots may be used in tea, pill, or tincture form.

MARSHMALLOW

BOTANICAL NAME: *ALTHEA OFFICINALIS*

Yes, those popular campfire confections originated with these lovely plants. The Greeks used marshmallow to treat wounds, toothaches, coughing, and insect stings. The Romans valued marshmallow roots and leaves for their laxative properties. And during the Renaissance, marshmallow was used extensively to treat sore throats, stomach problems, and even venereal diseases. Marshmallow is a wonderful demulcent that soothes digestive tract inflammations and irritations; it helps heals stomach ulcers. It is also used in formulas to treat urinary and prostate infections and inflammations. It enhances immunity by stimulating white blood cells. Applied as a poultice, it helps to heal cuts and bruises. The roots are sometimes used in salves and poultices. In the kitchen, add uncooked young tops and tender leaves to spring salads, or fry roots with butter and onions.

MEADOWSWEET

BOTANICAL NAME: *FILIPENDULA ULMARIA*

The next time you take an aspirin, you can thank meadowsweet. It was from this former strewing herb that 19th-century German chemists developed the popular over-the-counter remedy. Meadowsweet's flower buds contain the pain-reliever salicin, from which researchers derived salicylic acid, aspirin's main component. Meadowsweet's ability to reduce pain is not as marked as aspirin's concentrated compounds, but the plant does not produce aspirin's main side effect: upset stomach. The herb is even used to ease the discomfort of stomach ulcers. It prevents excess acid in the stomach and is one of the best herbal treatments for heartburn.

Meadowsweet has been prescribed to treat headache, arthritis, menstrual cramps, stomach cramps and gas, low-grade fever, and inflammation. It also contains a chemical that fights diarrhea-causing bacteria. Meadowsweet promotes excretion of uric acid, so it is used to treat gout (a condition of excess uric acid) and some types of kidney stones. As an antiseptic diuretic, it is used for urinary tract infections. New research shows that meadowsweet may help prevent blood clots that can trigger heart attacks. Other studies indicate that the salicin in meadowsweet reduces blood sugar levels and may have use in managing diabetes.

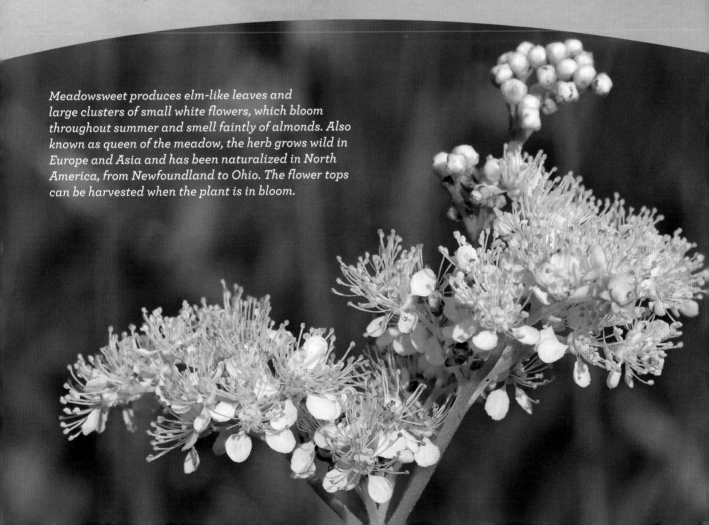

Meadowsweet produces elm-like leaves and large clusters of small white flowers, which bloom throughout summer and smell faintly of almonds. Also known as queen of the meadow, the herb grows wild in Europe and Asia and has been naturalized in North America, from Newfoundland to Ohio. The flower tops can be harvested when the plant is in bloom.

MILK THISTLE

BOTANICAL NAME: *SILYBUM MARIANUM*

Legend has it that milk thistle sprang from the milk of the Virgin Mary, and for centuries, herbalists have recommended it for increasing milk in nursing mothers. But the herb's primary use in modern times is in detoxifying and nourishing the liver. The flavonoids in milk thistle repair damaged liver cells, stimulate production of new cells, and protect existing cells. In Europe, victims of Amanita mushroom poisoning who received preparations made from a compound in milk thistle survived. This is remarkable because Amanita mushrooms are normally considered deadly—most people who eat them die of liver failure. Herbalists prescribe milk thistle to treat jaundice, hepatitis, cirrhosis, and other liver conditions caused by alcohol abuse. Benefits are noted in about two weeks.

Milk thistle contains essential oils, tyramine, histamine, and a flavonoid called silymarine. Milk thistle has antioxidant properties and counteracts some of the detrimental effects of environmental toxins. A bitter tonic, the leaves stimulate bile production—it has been prescribed to improve appetite and assist digestion. Once cultivated widely as a nutritious culinary herb, young milk thistle leaves may be eaten as a salad or potherb. To eat the leaves, cut off their sharp edges with scissors and steam. Serve as you would spinach.

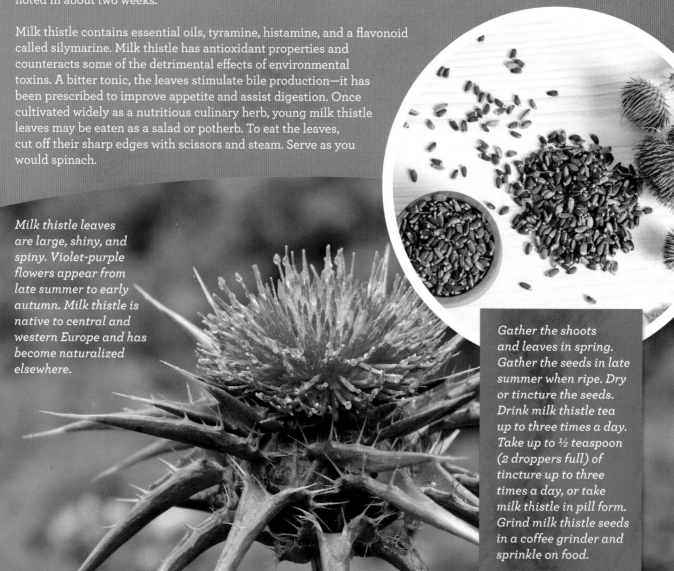

Milk thistle leaves are large, shiny, and spiny. Violet-purple flowers appear from late summer to early autumn. Milk thistle is native to central and western Europe and has become naturalized elsewhere.

Gather the shoots and leaves in spring. Gather the seeds in late summer when ripe. Dry or tincture the seeds. Drink milk thistle tea up to three times a day. Take up to ½ teaspoon (2 droppers full) of tincture up to three times a day, or take milk thistle in pill form. Grind milk thistle seeds in a coffee grinder and sprinkle on food.

MOTHERWORT

BOTANICAL NAME: *LEONURUS CARDIACA*

As its name implies, motherwort is useful for treating conditions associated with childbirth. The herb contains a chemical called leonurine, which encourages uterine contractions. Motherwort is used as a uterine tonic before and after childbirth. It has also been used for centuries to regulate the menstrual cycle, to promote the flow of mother's milk, and to treat menopausal complaints. Motherwort is a mild relaxing agent often recommended by herbalists to reduce anxiety and depression and treat nervousness, insomnia, heart palpitations, and rapid heart rate. Russian studies show that motherwort is good for hypertension because it relaxes blood vessels and calms nerves. Motherwort injections have been shown to prevent formation of blood clots, which improves blood flow and reduces risk of heart attack, stroke, and other diseases. Motherwort is also useful for headache, insomnia, vertigo, and delirium from fever. It is sometimes used to relieve asthma, bronchitis, and other lung problems, usually mixed with mullein and other lung herbs.

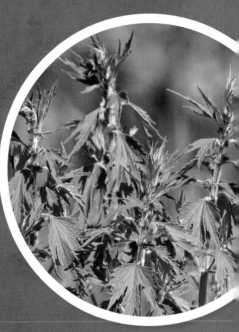

PRECAUTIONS

Don't use motherwort if you have clotting problems or take medication to thin your blood. Avoid motherwort if you are pregnant, unless a health professional recommends its use. Some people may develop a rash after handling motherwort.

MULLEIN

BOTANICAL NAME: *VERBASCUM THAPSUS*

For centuries, mullein was considered an amulet against witches and evil spirits. The plant has many uses—both medicinal and household. For example, the dried stems were dipped in suet and burned as torches. For centuries, mullein's leaves have been used to heal lung conditions. Herbalists once even recommended that patients with lung diseases smoke dried, crumbled mullein leaves. Ayurvedic physicians prescribed mullein to treat coughs. And colonists considered mullein so valuable they brought it with them to America, where Indians eventually adopted it for treating coughs, bronchitis, and asthma.

Contemporary herbalists still recommend internal use of mullein leaves to treat colds, sore throat, and coughs. The flowers and leaves reduce inflammation in the urinary and digestive tract and treat colitis, intestinal bleeding, and diarrhea. The fresh flower infused alone or with garlic in olive oil makes an ear oil for pain and inflammation associated with an earache.

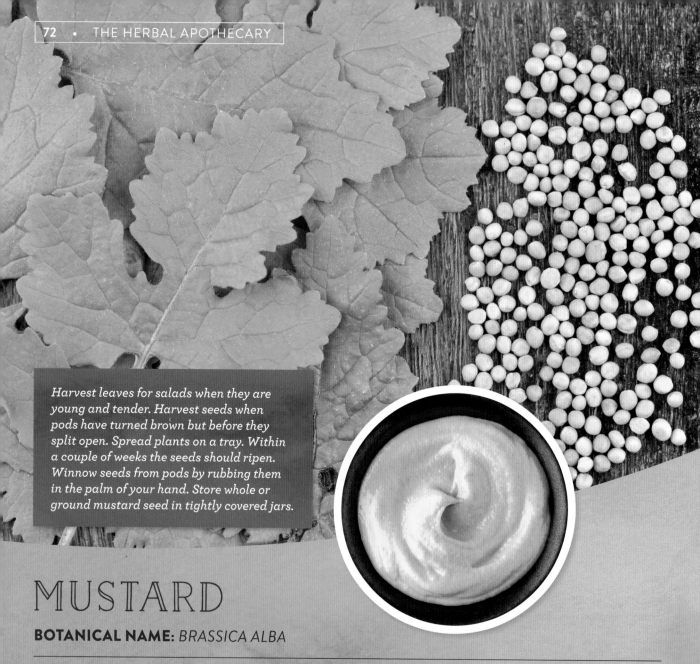

Harvest leaves for salads when they are young and tender. Harvest seeds when pods have turned brown but before they split open. Spread plants on a tray. Within a couple of weeks the seeds should ripen. Winnow seeds from pods by rubbing them in the palm of your hand. Store whole or ground mustard seed in tightly covered jars.

MUSTARD

BOTANICAL NAME: *BRASSICA ALBA*

You haven't really tasted mustard until you've made it yourself. To make mustard from seeds, boil $1/3$ cup cider vinegar, $2/3$ cup cider, 2 tablespoons honey, $1/8$ tablespoon turmeric, and up to 1 teaspoon salt. While hot, combine with ¼ cup ground mustard seeds. Blend in a food processor. After the mixture is smooth, add 1 tablespoon olive oil. This recipe makes 1 ¼ cups of mustard.

Mustard has many medicinal uses. Some of us are old enough to remember getting a mustard plaster when ill with a cold. Mustard seeds warm the skin and open the lungs to make breathing easier. Mustard plasters may also relieve rheumatism, toothache, sore muscles, and arthritis. Its chief constituent, mustard oil, gives it its heat and flavor. These constituents also make mustard an appetite stimulant and a powerful irritant. Mustard in small doses improves digestion. Young leaves are vitamin-rich additions to salads, or they can be boiled with onions and salt pork.

NASTURTIUM

BOTANICAL NAME: *TROPAEOLUM MAJUS*

Spanish conquerors brought nasturtiums from Peru to Spain. Soon these lovely flowering herbs spread across the continent. Nasturtium leaves have a peppery flavor, make good additions to salads, and can be added to sandwiches. Flower buds may be cured in vinegar and used like capers. They can also be stuffed with cream cheese or blended with butter. Pull off the individual petals to add color and flavor to a salad. The natural antibiotic in nasturtiums is effective even against some microorganisms that have built up a resistance to antibiotic drugs. The leaves and flowers fight infections of the lung and reproductive and urinary tracts. To relieve itching skin, try rubbing the juice of the fresh plant on the skin.

PRECAUTIONS

Large amounts of the seeds act as a strong laxative.

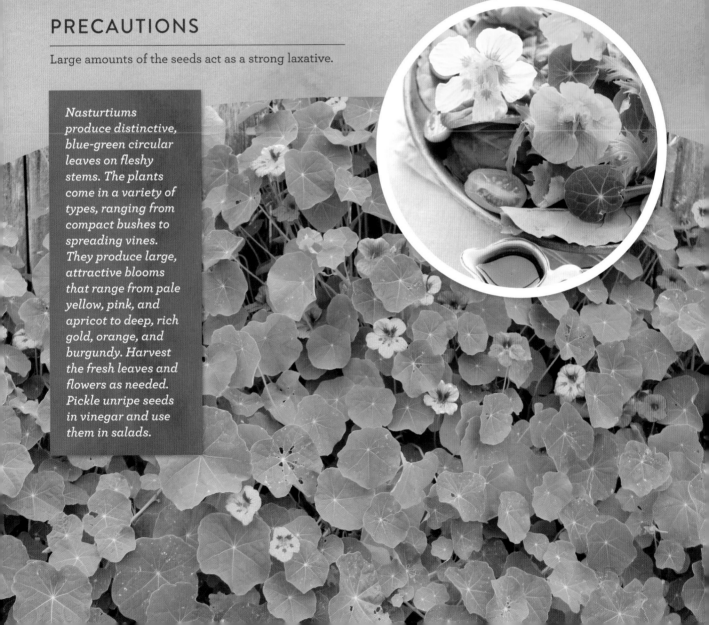

Nasturtiums produce distinctive, blue-green circular leaves on fleshy stems. The plants come in a variety of types, ranging from compact bushes to spreading vines. They produce large, attractive blooms that range from pale yellow, pink, and apricot to deep, rich gold, orange, and burgundy. Harvest the fresh leaves and flowers as needed. Pickle unripe seeds in vinegar and use them in salads.

NETTLE

BOTANICAL NAME: *URTICA DIOICA*

The Anglo-Saxons named nettle after their word for "needle." During the Bronze Age, fabric was woven from nettle. As recently as World War I, Germans wove nettle fabric when cotton supplies were low.

Nettle was once used to reduce arthritic pains and uric acid in joints and tissues (excess uric acid causes gout, a painful inflammatory condition). Nettle improves circulation and treats asthma. It is a light laxative; nettle tea has also been prescribed for intestinal weakness, diarrhea, and malnutrition. Nettle is a diuretic useful for treating bladder problems. Several studies demonstrated that the root successfully reduces prostate inflammation. Nettle treats eczema and skin rashes, increases mother's milk, slightly lowers blood sugar, and decreases profuse menstruation.

Nettle is so versatile that it has been used for centuries as a spring tonic to improve general health. The herb is rich in anti-inflammatory flavonoids and vital nutrients, including vitamins D, C, and A as well as minerals, such as iron, calcium, phosphorus, and magnesium. Thus, nettle has been used to treat malnutrition, anemia, and rickets. Hair shampoos and conditioners often include nettle because it is said to benefit the scalp and encourage hair growth.

Nettle loses its sting when cooked, dried, or ground. It is a healthy and tasty addition to scrambled eggs, pasta dishes, casseroles, and soups. Young shoots may be steamed then tossed in salads or eaten like kale or spinach. You also may juice nettle and drink it alone or combine it with other fruit or vegetable juices. Nettle leaves dye wool shades of yellow and green.

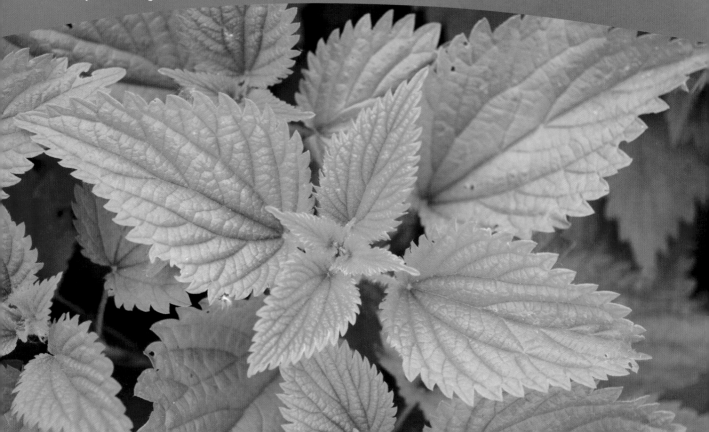

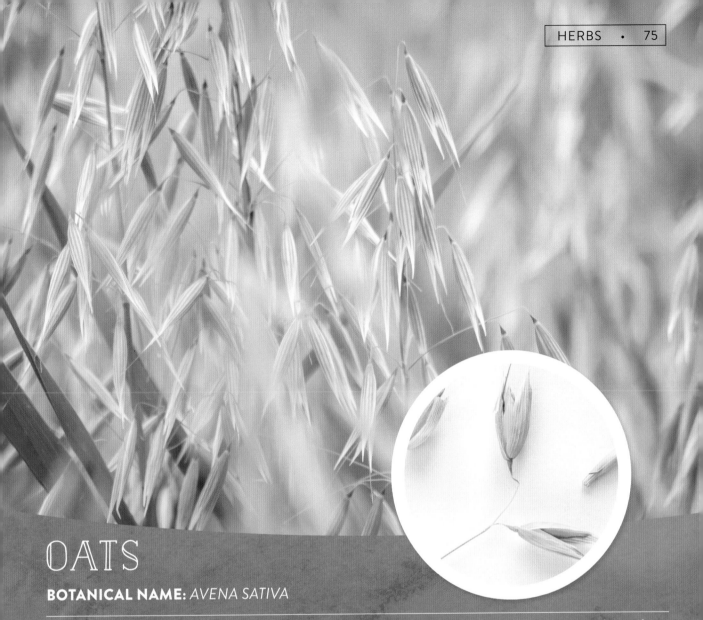

OATS

BOTANICAL NAME: *AVENA SATIVA*

The oat seed is used in two different phases of its growth: in its fresh, milky stage and as a grain once the seed is ripe and dried. Is there anyone who has not eaten oatmeal? This ubiquitous and nourishing cereal contains starches, proteins, vitamins, minerals, and dietary fiber nutritionists recommend we consume each day. Several clinical trials have found that regular consumption of oat bran reduces blood cholesterol levels in just one month. High-fiber diets may also reduce risk of colon and rectal cancer. Oats contain the alkaloid gramine, which has been credited with mild sedative properties. In its milky stage, oat tincture has been prescribed for nerve disorders and as a uterine tonic. Researchers found that fresh oats have some value in treating addiction and reducing nicotine craving. Fresh, green oats ease the anxiety that often accompanies drug withdrawal. Oat straw is sometimes made into a high-mineral tea.

Oatmeal has been used topically to heal wounds and various skin rashes. With their demulcent and soothing qualities, oats are found in soaps and bath and body products. Oatmeal baths and poultices are wonderful for soothing dry, flaky skin or alleviating itching from poison oak and chicken pox. Used in the bath, oatmeal makes a good facial scrub and helps clear up skin problems.

OREGON GRAPE

BOTANICAL NAME: *BERBERIS AQUIFOLIUM*

Oregon grape's prime constituent, the alkaloid berberine, improves blood flow to the liver and stimulates bile to aid digestion. Thus, Oregon grape root may be used to boost liver function and treat jaundice, hepatitis, poor intestinal tone and function, and gastrointestinal debility. Berberine effectively kills *Giardia* and *Candida* organisms and several other intestinal parasites, which are responsible for intestinal upsets and vaginal yeast infections. Oregon grape root is useful to treat serious cases of diarrhea and digestive tract infection. Oregon grape is also useful for treating colds, flu, and numerous other infections. In the laboratory, it's been shown to kill or suppress the growth of several disease-causing microbes. Oregon grape's berberine content makes it a good eye wash, douche, or skin cleanser for infections. The tincture is used to treat eczema, acne, herpes, and psoriasis.

High in vitamin C, the berries may be eaten raw or cooked in jam. Berries are also used to flavor jelly, wine, and soups. They have been used in folk medicine and seem to have some of the same medicinal properties as the root, but they are probably not as potent. Oregon grape root and bark dye wool yellow and tan; fruits impart a purplish blue color.

PRECAUTIONS

Oregon grape stimulates liver function, so if you have liver disease, use only under the care of a health practitioner. Avoid it if you are pregnant. Otherwise, use the herb for two to three weeks, abstain for several weeks, and resume if necessary.

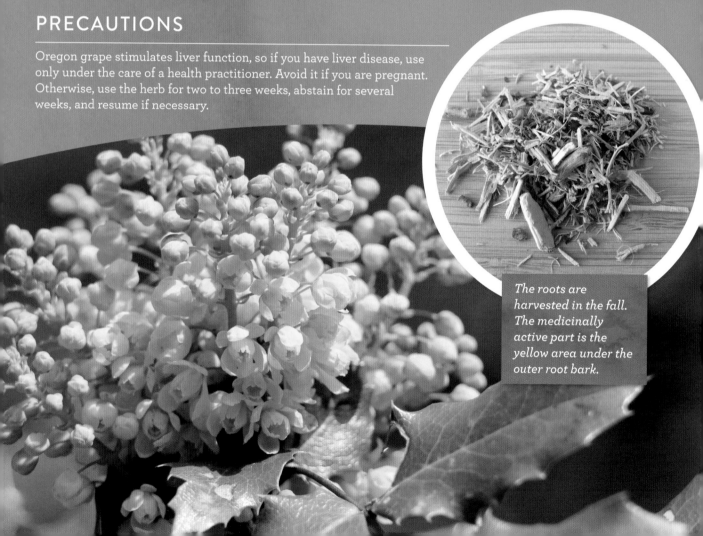

The roots are harvested in the fall. The medicinally active part is the yellow area under the outer root bark.

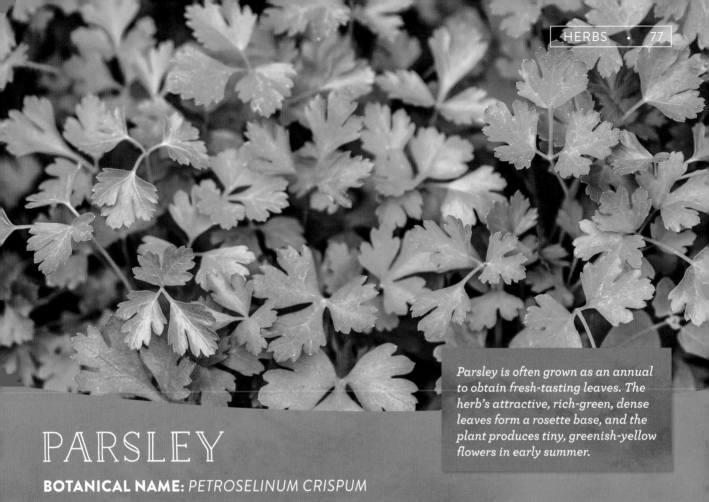

PARSLEY

Parsley is often grown as an annual to obtain fresh-tasting leaves. The herb's attractive, rich-green, dense leaves form a rosette base, and the plant produces tiny, greenish-yellow flowers in early summer.

BOTANICAL NAME: *PETROSELINUM CRISPUM*

You may think of parsley as a "throw-away" herb. It is universally used as a garnish that generally goes uneaten. But if you discard this natural breath sweetener, you'll be wasting a powerhouse of vitamins and minerals. Parsley contains vitamins A and C (more than an orange), and small amounts of several B vitamins, calcium, and iron. The leaves and root have diuretic properties and are used to treat bladder infections. Parsley's strong odor derives from its essential oils, one of which, apiol, has been extracted for medicinal uses. It is used in pharmaceutical drugs to treat some kidney ailments. Parsley seeds, or a compound in them, is used in some pharmaceutical preparations to treat urinary tract disorders. Another of parsley's compounds reduces inflammation and is a free-radical scavenger, eliminating these destructive elements. It also stimulates the appetite and increases circulation to the digestive organs. The root has more medicinal properties than the leaves.

Parsley's clean flavor blends with most foods and is often found in ethnic cuisines, including those of the Middle East, France, Belgium, Switzerland, Japan, Spain, and England. Parsley complements most meats and poultry and is a good addition to vegetable dishes, soups, and stews. It is always an ingredient in the famous bouquet garni used by cooks throughout the Western world. To make white sauce, the stems are used instead of the leaves to impart less color.

PRECAUTIONS

Avoid the root, seeds, and large amounts of the leaves if you're pregnant. Also avoid the root and seeds if you have kidney problems. Parsley is fine to eat in foods, however.

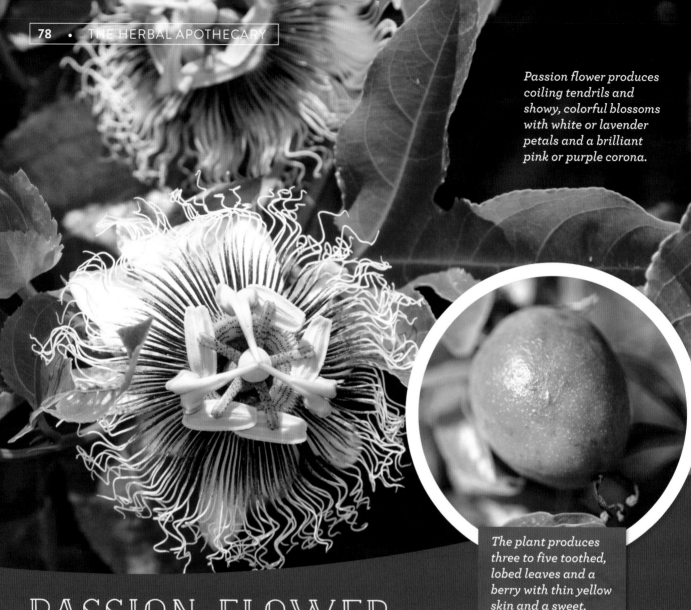

Passion flower produces coiling tendrils and showy, colorful blossoms with white or lavender petals and a brilliant pink or purple corona.

The plant produces three to five toothed, lobed leaves and a berry with thin yellow skin and a sweet, succulent pulp.

PASSION FLOWER

BOTANICAL NAME: *PASSIFLORA INCARNATE*

Few herbs have as many religious connections as passion flower. When Spanish explorers discovered the vine growing in South America, they were struck by its elaborate blossoms. Passion flower's five petals and five sepals, they reasoned, represented the 10 faithful apostles. The flower's dramatic corona looked to them like Jesus's crown of thorns. And the herb's five stamens symbolized Christ's five wounds. Curling tendrils reminded them of the cords used to whip Jesus, and the leaves were seen as the hands of his persecutors.

Passion flower's chief medicinal value is as a sedative. The Aztecs used it to promote sleep and relieve pain. Today the flowers are used in numerous pharmaceutical drugs in Europe to treat nervous disorders, heart palpitations, anxiety, and high blood pressure. It has also been prescribed for tension, fatigue, insomnia, and muscle and lung spasms. Unlike most sedative drugs, it is non-addictive, although it is not a strong pain reliever.

PEPPERMINT

BOTANICAL NAME: *MENTHA PIPERITA*

You may enjoy peppermint candies, especially after a meal, but this useful plant isn't found just in confections. A carminative and gastric stimulant, promoting the flow of bile to the stomach and aiding digestion, peppermint has been prescribed to treat indigestion, flatulence, colic, and nausea. An antispasmodic, peppermint calms muscles in the digestive tract, reduces colon spasms, and is recommended as a treatment for irritable bowel syndrome and colitis. It also reduces the inflammation of stomach ulcers and colitis. The herb—even its fragrance—eases the pain of headaches. Peppermint's main compound, menthol, is very antiseptic, killing bacteria, viruses, fungi, and parasites, while balancing intestinal flora. Menthol is found in most heating balms, vapor balms, and liniments because of its heating properties.

Experiment with peppermint in the kitchen. Use it in jellies, sauces, salads, vegetable dishes, and beverages. Peppermint is used to flavor candy, gum, and even dental products and toothpicks. Peppermint makes a good addition to sachets and potpourri. Sniffing peppermint helps clear the sinuses, so it is often used in inhalers. Studies also show that inhaling peppermint stimulates brain waves, increases concentration, and helps keep you awake. Steeped in rosemary vinegar, peppermint helps to control dandruff.

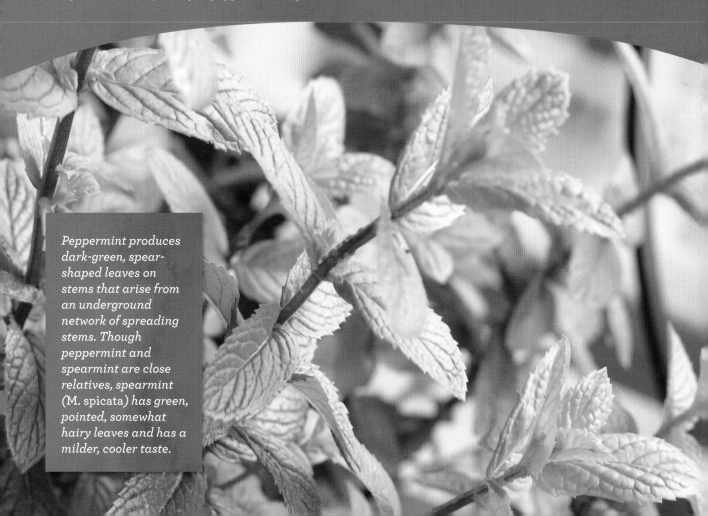

Peppermint produces dark-green, spear-shaped leaves on stems that arise from an underground network of spreading stems. Though peppermint and spearmint are close relatives, spearmint (M. spicata) has green, pointed, somewhat hairy leaves and has a milder, cooler taste.

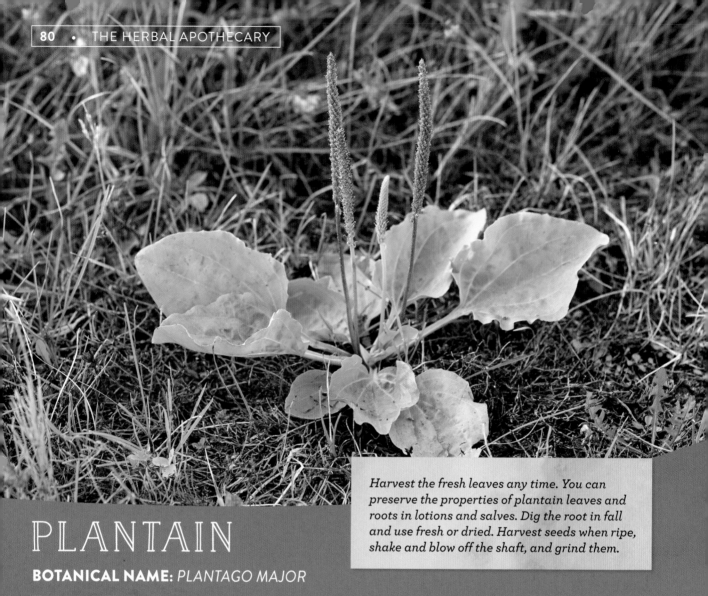

Harvest the fresh leaves any time. You can preserve the properties of plantain leaves and roots in lotions and salves. Dig the root in fall and use fresh or dried. Harvest seeds when ripe, shake and blow off the shaft, and grind them.

PLANTAIN

BOTANICAL NAME: *PLANTAGO MAJOR*

Don't consider this ubiquitous plant a nuisance. Plantain is a powerful healer and has been used for centuries to treat a variety of ailments. The ancient Saxons, in fact, regarded plantain as one of the essential herbs. If a bee stings you, apply crushed, fresh plantain leaves to the welt, which will soon disappear. And if you stumble into a patch of poison ivy, you needn't scratch and suffer. Apply a poultice of plantain leaves to relieve your discomfort. Some people, moreover, have been known to chew plantain root to stop the pain of a toothache. A diuretic, the herb is useful for treating urinary problems. Lung disorders, such as asthma and bronchitis, also respond to plantain. Research from India shows that it reduces the symptoms of colds and coughs and relieves the pain and wheezing associated with bronchial problems.

In the kitchen, steam tender young plantain leaves as you would spinach, or eat small amounts fresh in salads, although they are too fibrous for most people's tastes. The seeds are edible. Add small amounts to other grains to increase protein. The species *P. psyllium* is a popular laxative; it is used, as is *P. ovata,* in products such as Metamucil. As with other foods that provide bulk, it has been shown to reduce cholesterol levels. Applied externally, the plant stimulates and cleanses the skin and encourages wounds to heal faster. Plantain has also been used to dye wool a dull gold or camel color.

RASPBERRY

BOTANICAL NAME: *RUBUS IDAEUS*

Long revered for its healing properties, raspberry leaf is an astringent, stimulant, and tonic. Seventeenth-century English herbalist Nicholas Culpepper recommended raspberry for a number of ailments, including "fevers, ulcers, putrid sores of the mouth and secret parts . . . spitting blood . . . piles . . . stones of the kidney . . . and too much flowing of women's courses." American Indians used raspberry as a treatment for wounds. And contemporary herbalists prescribe raspberry for diarrhea, nausea, vomiting, and morning sickness. In addition, raspberry leaves are thought to tone uterine muscles and, thus, have long been used by pregnant women to prevent miscarriage and reduce labor pains. They can be used throughout pregnancy. They relieve menstrual cramps if taken as a tonic over a period of time. Raspberry leaves are also good for women with uterine problems such as fibroids, endometriosis, or excessive menstrual bleeding.

The fruit is a tonic and may be good for the blood. Fresh raspberries can have a mild laxative effect, but a tea from the leaves is a cure for diarrhea and dysentery. Fresh or frozen raspberries have many uses in the kitchen.

Native to North America and Europe, this shrubby, thorny plant, also known as hindberry and bramble, quickly spread around the world. You'll find raspberry thickets along the edges of woods and in untended fields. The raspberry plant produces a prickly stem. Its flowers are white and appear in the spring and summer of its second year.

Harvest berries in summer. Harvest leaves any time, but the best time is before the plant bears fruit; use fresh or dried.

RED CLOVER

BOTANICAL NAME: *TRIFOLIUM PRATENSE*

Red clover, a favorite of honey bees, is one of the world's oldest agricultural crops. This ubiquitous field flower has been used as a medicine for millennia, revered by Greeks, Romans, and Celts. But it's in the last 100 years that red clover has gained prominence as the source of a possible cancer treatment. Researchers have isolated several antitumor compounds such as biochanin A in red clover, which they think may help prevent cancer. The herb also contains antioxidants and a form of vitamin E. There is some evidence that it helps prevent breast tumors.

Some of red clover's constituents are thought to stimulate the immune system. Another constituent, coumarin, has blood-thinning properties. Its hormone-like effect makes red clover a potential treatment for some types of infertility and symptoms of menopause. A diuretic, sedative, and anti-inflammatory herb, red clover has been recommended for the skin conditions eczema and psoriasis. It also has some antibacterial properties.

You may pick flowers and add them to salads throughout the summer. Tiny florets are a delightful addition to iced tea. Eat red clover's nutritious leaves cooked since they are not digestible raw.

PRECAUTIONS

Avoid red clover if you're pregnant or have a history of bleeding easily. Also, because it is a blood thinner, avoid it just before surgery.

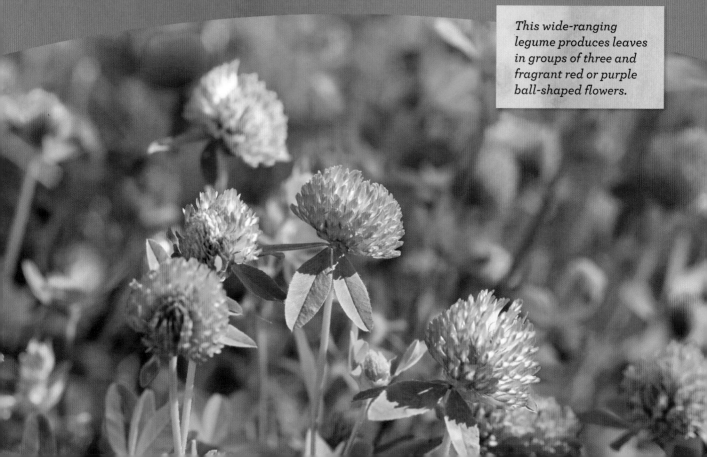

This wide-ranging legume produces leaves in groups of three and fragrant red or purple ball-shaped flowers.

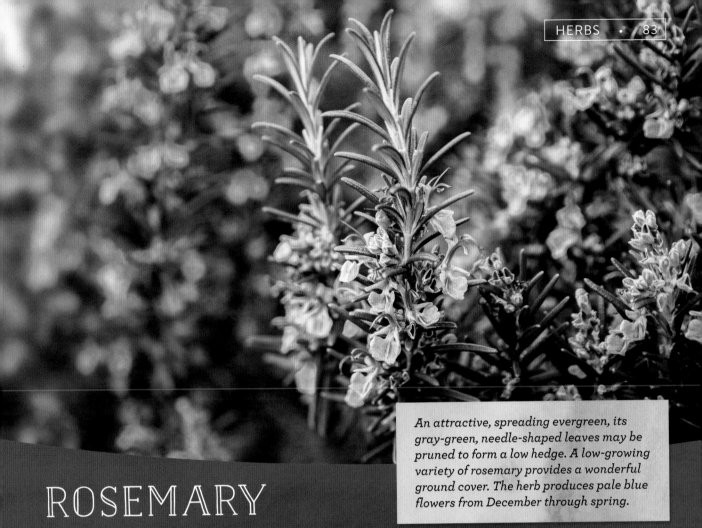

ROSEMARY

BOTANICAL NAME: *ROSMARINUS OFFICINALIS*

An attractive, spreading evergreen, its gray-green, needle-shaped leaves may be pruned to form a low hedge. A low-growing variety of rosemary provides a wonderful ground cover. The herb produces pale blue flowers from December through spring.

Before the advent of refrigeration, cooks wrapped meat in rosemary leaves to preserve it. The herb's strong piney aroma has prevented commercial use as a preservative, but efforts are underway to create a preservative without the scent. Modern studies show that rosemary has potent antioxidant properties. It is an astringent, expectorant, and diaphoretic (induces sweating). It promotes digestion and stimulates the activity of the liver and gallbladder to aid both in digestion of fats and the detoxification of the body. It also inhibits formation of kidney stones. The herb has been prescribed to treat muscle spasms. Rosemary oil helps reduce the pain of rheumatism when used as a liniment. An antiseptic, it can be applied to eczema and wounds. It strengthens blood vessels and improves circulation, so it is useful to treat varicose veins and other problems related to poor circulation. For this reason, it can also relieve some headaches. A foot bath containing rosemary is good for swollen ankles and feet that tend to be numb or cold often—both signs of poor circulation. It makes a good gargle for sore throats, gum problems, and canker sores. New studies indicate that compounds in rosemary may help to prevent cancer.

In the kitchen, rosemary's pungent taste—something like mint and ginger—complements poultry, fish, lamb, beef, veal, pork, game, cheese, and eggs, as well as many vegetables, including potatoes, tomatoes, spinach, peas, and mushrooms. The oil and herb are added to cosmetics to improve skin tone. The herb makes a fragrant, refreshing bath additive and hair rinse. It stimulates the scalp and helps control dandruff. And dried branches make good arrangements and wreaths.

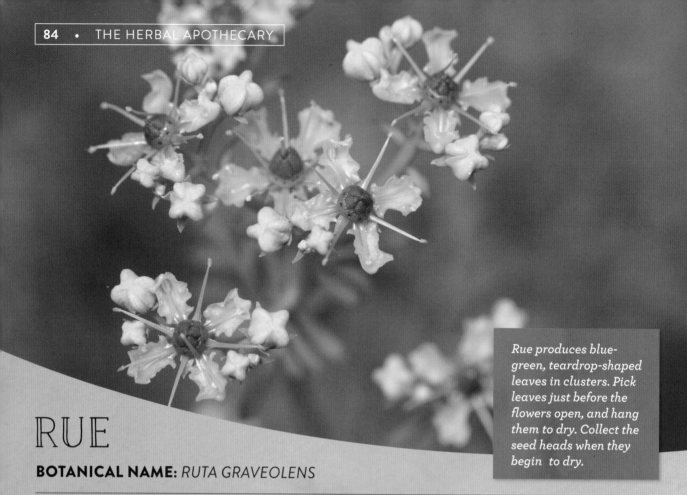

Rue produces blue-green, teardrop-shaped leaves in clusters. Pick leaves just before the flowers open, and hang them to dry. Collect the seed heads when they begin to dry.

RUE

BOTANICAL NAME: *RUTA GRAVEOLENS*

The Greeks believed that rue cured nervous indigestion, improved eyesight, was an antidote to poison, and treated insect bites. Today, rue is more popular as a medicine in several countries other than the United States. The exception is the Latino community in the United States which uses *ruta* to relieve menstrual cramps and to regulate menstruation. Throughout Latin America, people use rue tea to treat colds and rue compresses applied to the chest to treat congestion. Rue is also used topically as a liniment to relieve the pain of rheumatoid arthritis and sore muscles. In traditional Chinese medicine, rue is used to decrease the inflammation of sprains, strains, and bites. Rue contains rutin, which strengthens fragile blood vessels, so the herb helps diminish varicose veins and reduces bruising when used internally or topically. Rue eardrops decrease the pain and inflammation of an earache.

Taken internally, rue relaxes muscles and nervous indigestion and improves circulation in the digestive tract. People in the Middle East use it to kill intestinal parasites, and in India, they say it improves mental clarity, which is possible because of its action on circulation.

Although it is bitter, minute amounts are used to flavor some baked goods. The Italians use rue as a bitter digestive, eating small amounts with other bitter greens and using it in a liqueur, *grappa con ruta*.

PRECAUTIONS

Use rue internally with extreme caution. It may cause gastrointestinal pains. Large amounts cause vomiting, mental confusion, and convulsions. In rare cases, exposure to sunlight after ingesting rue causes sunburn.

SAGE

BOTANICAL NAME: *SALVIA OFFICINALIS*

The Arabs associated sage with immortality, and the Greeks considered it an herb that promotes wisdom. Appropriately enough, a constituent in sage was recently discovered to inhibit an enzyme that produces memory loss and plays a role in Alzheimer's disease. However, it's unlikely that use of the herb alone will benefit these conditions. Sage's essential oils have antiseptic properties, and the tannins are astringent. It has been used for centuries as a gargle for sore throat and inflamed gums. The herb is useful in treating mouth sores, cuts, and bruises. Sweating is decreased about two hours after ingesting sage; in fact, it is used in some deodorants and a German antiperspirant. It is also useful to prevent hot flashes, and it has some estrogenic properties. It decreases mother's milk so is useful while weaning children. It decreases saliva flow in the mouth and has successfully been used by people who have overactive salivary glands. It is a strong antioxidant and may prove useful against cell degeneration in the body. As a hair conditioner, a sage infusion reduces overactive glands in the scalp, which are sometimes responsible for causing dandruff. It also gives gloss to dark hair.

Sage is sometimes found in perfumes and cosmetics. Dried leaves on the branches make a good ornamental that complements arrangements and wreaths. Sage dyes wool shades of yellow or green-gray.

PRECAUTIONS

In large amounts, thujone, a constituent of sage, may cause a variety of symptoms, culminating in convulsions, but it is safe in the small amounts found in sage leaves.

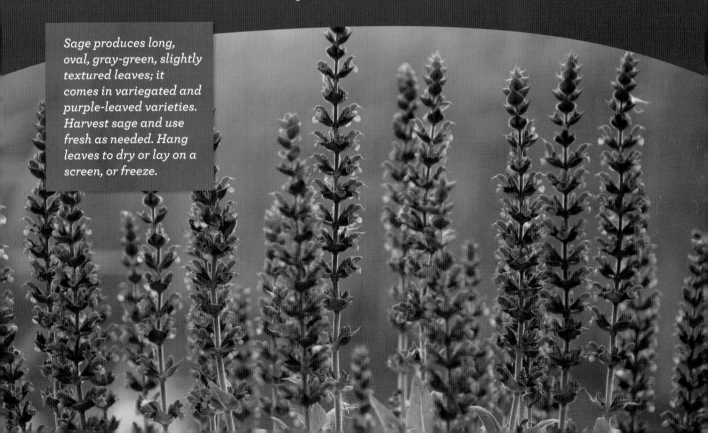

Sage produces long, oval, gray-green, slightly textured leaves; it comes in variegated and purple-leaved varieties. Harvest sage and use fresh as needed. Hang leaves to dry or lay on a screen, or freeze.

ST. JOHN'S WORT

BOTANICAL NAME: *HYPERICUM PERFORATUM*

St. John's wort has been used as a medicine for centuries. Early European and Slavic herbals mention it. It has long been used as an anti-inflammatory for bruises, varicose veins, hemorrhoids, strains, sprains, and contusions. It is used internally and topically (in tincture, oil, or salve form) for these conditions. The plant, especially its flowers, is high in flavonoid compounds that reduce inflammation.

Studies show that St. John's wort relieves anxiety and is an antidepressant. Some researchers believe that one of its constituents, hypericin, interferes with the body's production of a depression-related chemical called monoamine oxidase (MAO). In one study, it relieved depression in menopausal women in four to six weeks.

The herb has also been used to treat skin problems, urinary conditions such as bedwetting, painful nerve conditions such as carpal tunnel syndrome, and symptoms of nerve destruction. The tannin and oil in the plant have antibacterial properties. Scientists investigating the potential of one of its constituents as a treatment for AIDS discovered it also fights viral infection. It is also effective against flu. The National Cancer Institute has conducted several preliminary studies showing that constituents in St. John's wort also may have potential as a cancer-fighting drug.

PRECAUTIONS

After consuming large quantities of the herb, cattle develop severe sunburn and become disoriented; however, there are no documented reports of humans having this reaction. Recent testing among AIDS patients showed that St. John's wort is nontoxic. Avoid St. John's wort if you take an MAO inhibitor drug.

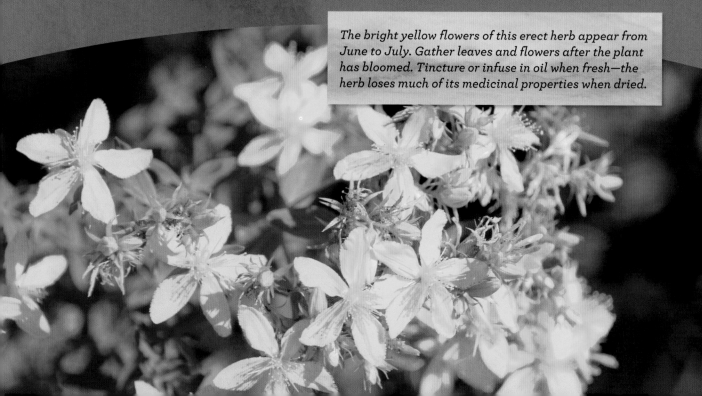

The bright yellow flowers of this erect herb appear from June to July. Gather leaves and flowers after the plant has bloomed. Tincture or infuse in oil when fresh—the herb loses much of its medicinal properties when dried.

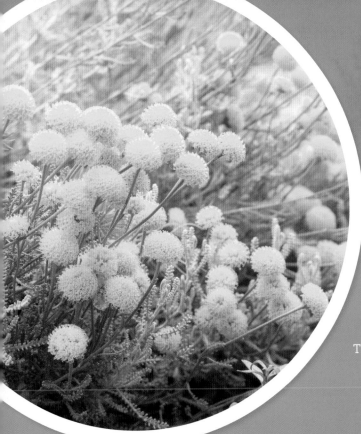

SANTOLINA

BOTANICAL NAME:
SANTOLINA CHAMAECYPARISSUS

Once used to expel parasitic worms, this astringent herb is rarely prescribed for medicinal purposes in the West, but it is an antiseptic for bacterial and fungal skin infections. It can be rubbed into sore muscles as a liniment. Small quantities of this herb taken internally act as a digestive bitter that stimulates appetite and digestion. Santolina has a musky fragrance that enhances potpourri and sachets. The strong scent of the leaves also repels wool moths.

SAVORY, SUMMER

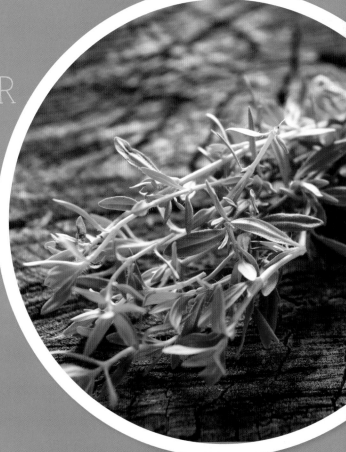

BOTANICAL NAME:
SATUREJA HORTENSIS

The Romans believed savory was sacred to satyrs. They planted it near beehives to increase honey production. They used savory to flavor vinegars and introduced the herb to England, where the Saxons adopted and named it for its spicy taste. Winter savory was said to curb sexual appetite; summer savory, to increase it. Guess which variety was most popular? Summer savory has antiseptic and astringent properties, so it has been used to treat diarrhea and mild sore throats. Like many culinary herbs, it aids digestion, stimulates appetite, and relieves a minor upset stomach and eliminates gas—probably one reason it is so popular to flavor bean dishes. It also kills several types of intestinal worms.

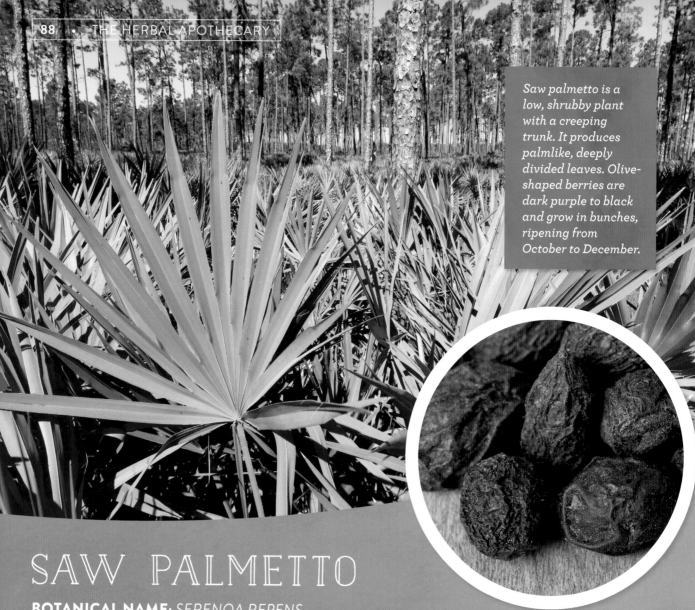

Saw palmetto is a low, shrubby plant with a creeping trunk. It produces palmlike, deeply divided leaves. Olive-shaped berries are dark purple to black and grow in bunches, ripening from October to December.

SAW PALMETTO

BOTANICAL NAME: *SERENOA REPENS*

Saw palmetto has long been considered an aphrodisiac, sexual rejuvenator, and treatment for impotence. The action of saw palmetto has been well studied, and the herb is popular for treating prostate enlargement. In one study, participants experienced significant improvement in prostate enlargement in only 45 days, with almost no side effects, and certainly none of the serious side effects seen with the drugs normally prescribed. Saw palmetto is recommended for weakening of urinary organs and resulting incontinence.

Saw palmetto also has been touted as a steroid substitute for athletes who wish to increase muscle mass, although no documentation supports this claim. Herbalists agree, however, that saw palmetto may benefit cases of tissue wasting, weakness, and debility. It was prescribed by Eclectic physicians in the early 19th century for frail people or those who were weak from chronic illness to make them stronger. This may be because saw palmetto improves digestion and absorption of nutrients. The herb is a diuretic, expectorant, and tonic, making it useful for treating colds, asthma, and bronchitis.

SHEPHERD'S PURSE

BOTANICAL NAME: *CAPSELLA BURSA-PASTORIS*

The Greeks and Romans used the seeds of shepherd's purse as a laxative. By the 16th century, the herb was prescribed to stop bleeding and eliminate blood in urine. Colonists introduced shepherd's purse to America, where it quickly became a common weed.

Shepherd's purse contains substances that hasten coagulation of blood—thus it has long been prescribed for treating excessive menstrual flow. During World War I, wounded soldiers were given shepherd's purse tea. The herb also may benefit those with ulcers, colitis, and Crohn disease. Used topically, shepherd's purse heals lacerations and other skin injuries. Some herbalists have prescribed it for treating eczema and skin rashes. The herb's peppery-tasting young leaves may be added to soups and stews or eaten like spinach.

PRECAUTIONS

Because shepherd's purse constricts blood vessels and appears to induce clotting, people with a history of hypertension, heart disease, or stroke should avoid it.

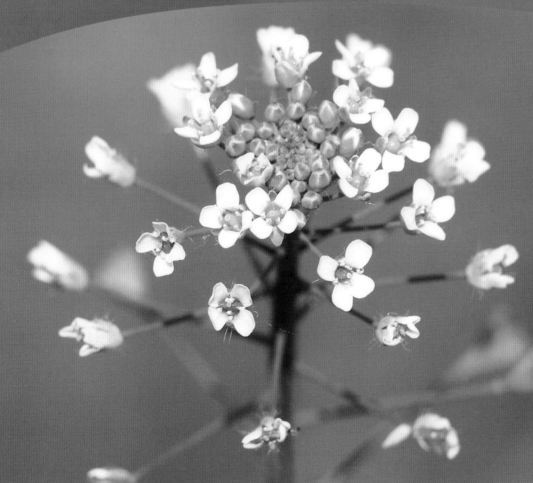

This herb's name alludes to the shape of its fruits, which resemble the purses that Europeans once hung from their belts. Smooth, slightly hairy stems arise from a basal rosette of leaves. The herb produces white flowers throughout the year, followed by triangular-shaped fruits. Harvest the leaves and flower tops as flowers open. The fresh plant is more potent than the dried plant.

SHIITAKE MUSHROOM

BOTANICAL NAME: *LENTINUS EDODES*

Shiitake mushrooms have long been a staple of Chinese cuisine. Now research has found that lentinan, a chemical in shiitake mushrooms, slows the growth of cancerous tumors in animals. Scientists hope that lentinan may one day be used to enhance the human immune system and help people fight off cancer and infections.

In China and Japan, shiitake mushrooms have been used for hundreds of years as a medicine to lower blood cholesterol as well as to fight cancer. Shiitake mushrooms also contain cortinelin, a strong antibacterial agent, which kills a wide range of disease-causing germs. A sulfide compound extracted from shiitake mushrooms has also been found to have antibiotic properties. Shiitakes have been used to treat depressed immune-system disorders, including AIDS. Shiitake mushrooms are a nutritious food source, packed with protein and full of vitamins B1, B2, B12, niacin, and pantothenic acid.

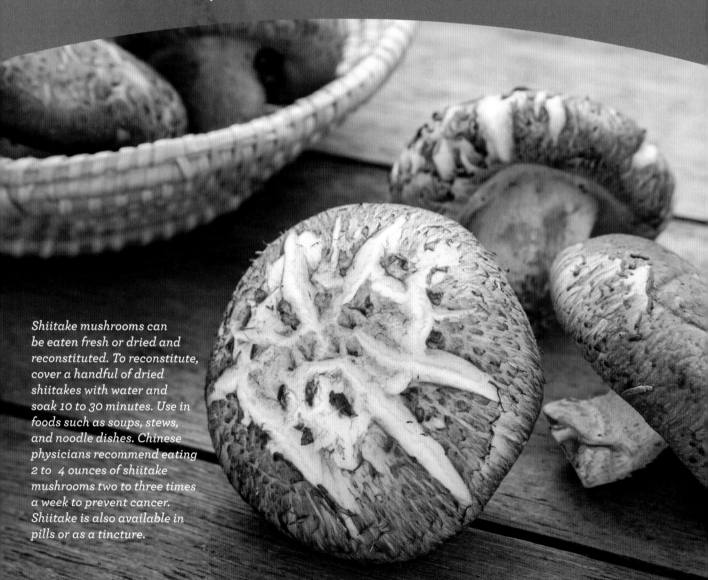

Shiitake mushrooms can be eaten fresh or dried and reconstituted. To reconstitute, cover a handful of dried shiitakes with water and soak 10 to 30 minutes. Use in foods such as soups, stews, and noodle dishes. Chinese physicians recommend eating 2 to 4 ounces of shiitake mushrooms two to three times a week to prevent cancer. Shiitake is also available in pills or as a tincture.

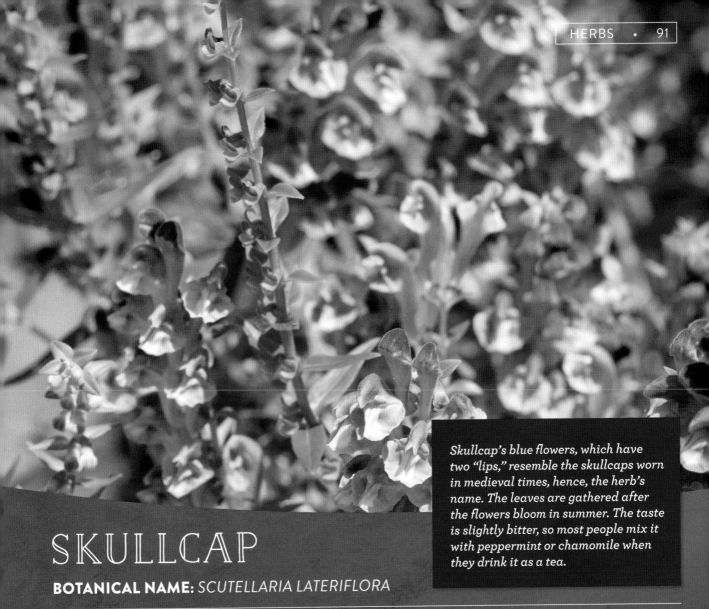

Skullcap's blue flowers, which have two "lips," resemble the skullcaps worn in medieval times, hence, the herb's name. The leaves are gathered after the flowers bloom in summer. The taste is slightly bitter, so most people mix it with peppermint or chamomile when they drink it as a tea.

SKULLCAP

BOTANICAL NAME: *SCUTELLARIA LATERIFLORA*

Skullcap received its common name, mad dog weed, in the 18th century, when the herb was widely prescribed as a cure for rabies, although no scientific evidence supports its use for that disease. The herb is a sedative often recommended for treating insomnia, nervousness, nervous twitches, and anxiety. Russian researchers have found that skullcap helps stabilize stress-related heart disease. Herbalists have also employed skullcap to treat symptoms of premenstrual syndrome (PMS). Skullcap has been found to have anti-inflammatory properties. The herb inhibits release of acetylcholine and histamine, two substances released by cells that cause inflammation and symptoms of allergic reactions. Japanese studies indicate that skullcap increases levels of HDL (high-density lipoprotein, or "good" cholesterol). And Chinese researchers report that the Chinese species, *S. baicalensis*, is useful in treating hepatitis, improving liver function, reducing swelling, and increasing appetite. It is also a strong immune system herb.

PRECAUTIONS

Used in moderation, skullcap is safe. Large amounts of tincture may cause confusion, giddiness, or convulsions.

SLIPPERY ELM

BOTANICAL NAME: *ULMUS RUBRA*

American colonists learned from Indians how to employ the herb as a food and medicine. In the days before refrigerators, Americans wrapped foods in slippery elm to retard spoilage: The powdered bark contains cells that expand into a spongy mass to form a protective covering. They also used moistened slippery elm powder to form bandages, make casts for broken bones, coat pills, and make a nourishing gruel for invalids. In the 19th century, you would have been hard-pressed to find a home in America that did not contain slippery elm lozenges.

Slippery elm is used to treat sore throats, coughs, colds, and gastrointestinal disorders—in a word, anything that needs to be soothed. Mucilage, the most abundant constituent of slippery elm bark, has a moistening, soothing action. The tannins are astringent. This combination makes slippery elm ideal for soothing inflammations, reducing swelling, and healing damaged tissues.

The powder is a healing food. Stir slippery elm powder into oatmeal or applesauce for an oatmeal-like gruel that soothes an inflamed stomach or ulcer. It is often recommended as a restorative herb for people who suffer from prolonged flu, stomach upset, chronic indigestion, and malnutrition stemming from these conditions.

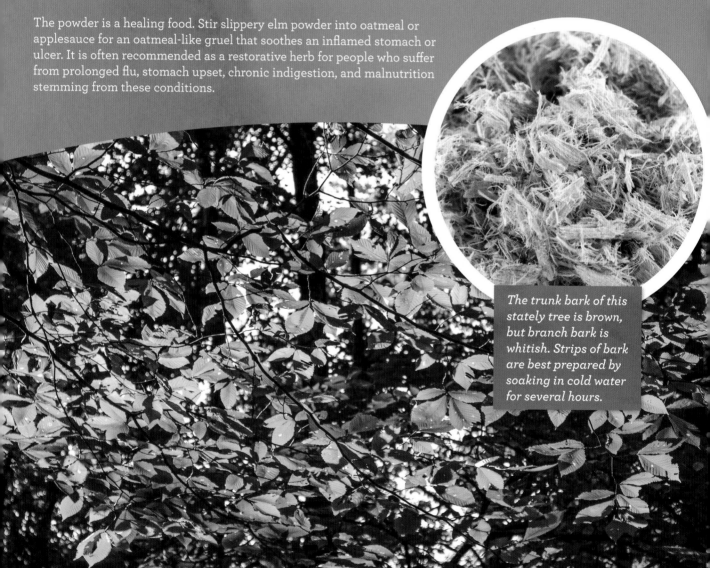

The trunk bark of this stately tree is brown, but branch bark is whitish. Strips of bark are best prepared by soaking in cold water for several hours.

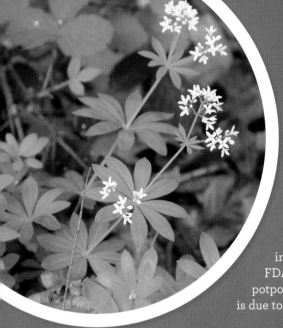

SWEET WOODRUFF

BOTANICAL NAME: *GALIUM ODORATUM*

Herbalists consider sweet woodruff a diuretic, diaphoretic, antispasmodic, and light sedative. It is especially useful to treat nervous indigestion. The herb has been used historically to treat kidney stones, nervousness, and wounds. It is also an anticoagulant, thereby reducing the risk of blood clots. Sweet woodruff has been used to flavor Scandinavian cordials, and it imparts a sort of vanilla-like bouquet to white wine. It is the flavoring in Europe's traditional May wine and other alcoholic beverages. (The FDA approves its use for alcoholic beverages.) The herb is used in potpourri and perfumes; its scent, described as like that of new-mown hay, is due to coumarin, which is also found in hay and clover.

PRECAUTIONS

Very large doses of sweet woodruff may cause vomiting and dizziness. Test animals suffered liver damage, among other effects, when fed coumarin, a constituent of sweet woodruff, but you would have to eat massive amounts daily to reach an equivalent amount.

TARRAGON, FRENCH

BOTANICAL NAME:
ARTEMISIA DRACUNCULUS

Tarragon stimulates appetite, relieves gas and colic, and makes a good local anesthetic for toothaches. Tarragon has antifungal and antioxidant properties and has been used to preserve foods. It's also found in perfumes, soaps, cosmetics, condiments, and liqueurs. One of the French *fines herbes,* tarragon has a strong flavor that may overpower foods, so use it sparingly in salads and sauces, including remoulade, tartar, and bearnaise sauces. Tarragon enhances fish, pork, beef, lamb, game, poultry, patés, rice, barley, vinegars, mayonnaise, and butter. It also goes well with a number of vegetables, including potatoes, tomatoes, carrots, onions, beets, asparagus, mushrooms, cauliflower, and broccoli.

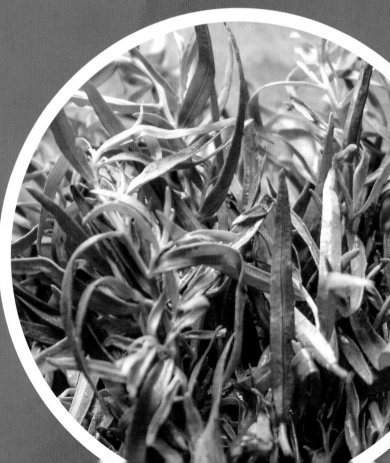

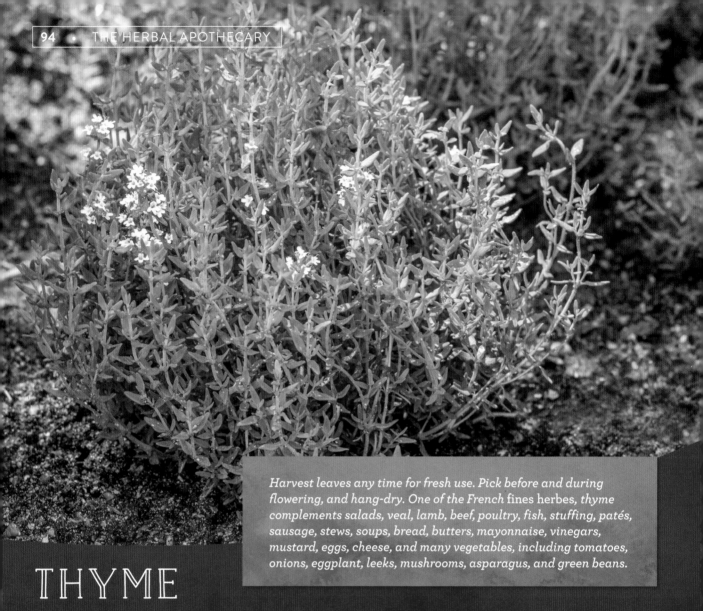

Harvest leaves any time for fresh use. Pick before and during flowering, and hang-dry. One of the French fines herbes, thyme complements salads, veal, lamb, beef, poultry, fish, stuffing, patés, sausage, stews, soups, bread, butters, mayonnaise, vinegars, mustard, eggs, cheese, and many vegetables, including tomatoes, onions, eggplant, leeks, mushrooms, asparagus, and green beans.

THYME

BOTANICAL NAME: *THYMUS VULGARIS*

You may have noticed thyme's distinctive flavor in cough medicines. Thymol, a prime constituent, is found in a number of them. Thymol is also used commercially to make colognes, aftershaves, lotions, soaps, detergents, and cosmetics. Thyme also was used as an antiseptic to treat wounds as recently as World War I. In fact, it is one of the most potent antiseptics of all the herbs. Thymol is found in many mouthwashes and gargles for sore throats and mouth and gum infections. It is one of the main ingredients in Listerine, along with compounds from eucalyptus and peppermint. This commercial mouthwash was found to cause 34 percent less gum inflammation than other brands and decrease plaque formation on the teeth. Vapor balms, used to rub on the chest to relieve congestion, also contain thymol.

Thyme destroys fungal infections. Its antispasmodic qualities make it useful for treating asthma, whooping cough, stomach cramps, gas, colic, and headache. It also reduces compounds in the body that produce menstrual cramps. Thyme preparations increase circulation in the area where applied.

UVA URSI

BOTANICAL NAME: *ARCTOSTAPHYLOS UVA URSI*

Uva ursi leaves contain up to 40 percent tannic acid, enough to make them once useful in tanning leather. Tannins and the glycoside arbutin give uva ursi its astringent and antiseptic properties.

Herbalists suggest uva ursi primarily to treat bladder infections. Uva ursi is particularly indicated for illnesses caused by *Escherichia coli (E. coli)*, a bacterium that lives in the intestines and can invade the urinary tract. It works particularly well in the alkaline environment this bacteria produces. Externally, the herb has been used to treat sprains, swellings, and sore muscles.

PRECAUTIONS

Because uva ursi may stimulate the uterus, don't take it if you're pregnant. Also don't use it if you have an active kidney infection since it will be too irritating.

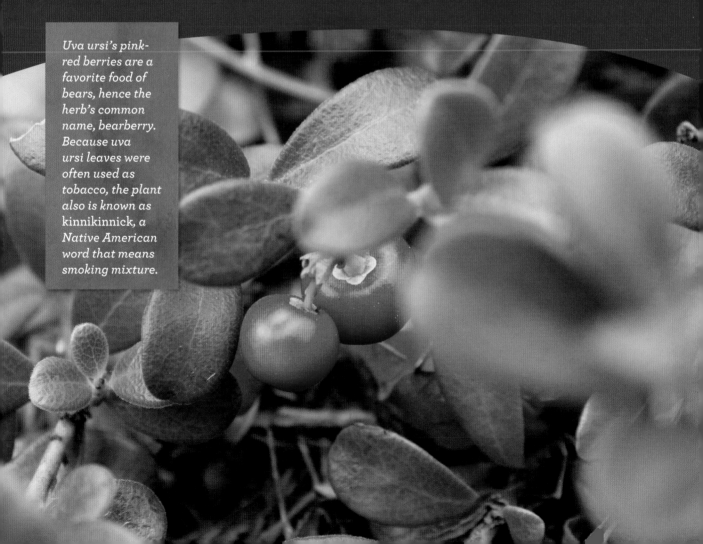

Uva ursi's pink-red berries are a favorite food of bears, hence the herb's common name, bearberry. Because uva ursi leaves were often used as tobacco, the plant also is known as kinnikinnick, *a Native American word that means smoking mixture.*

VALERIAN

BOTANICAL NAME: *VALERIANA OFFICINALIS*

Ask most people what the smell of valerian reminds them of and they're likely to say old socks. Nonetheless, cats go wild over valerian and so do rats. Lore has it, in fact, that the Pied Piper used valerian to rid Hamelin of rodents. In ancient times, valerian was widely used as a treatment for epilepsy. Today valerian finds its chief value in soothing anxiety and promoting sleep. Clinical studies have identified constituents in valerian known as valepotriates, which appear to affect the central nervous system but produce few, if any, side effects. Several studies show that valerian shortens the time needed to fall asleep and improves quality of sleep. Unlike commonly used sedatives, valerian does not cause a drugged or hung-over sensation or affect dream recall in most people. In one study, it even calmed hyperactive children.

The relaxing action of valerian also makes it useful for treatment of muscle cramps, menstrual cramps, and high blood pressure. Valerian relaxes vein and artery walls and is especially indicated for blood pressure elevations caused by stress and worry. Valerian is recommended for tension headaches as well as heart palpitations.

Valerian mildly stimulates the intestines, can help dispel gas and cramps in the digestive tract, and is weakly antimicrobial, particularly to bacteria. More than a hundred soothing valerian preparations are sold in Germany. Valerian improves stomach function and relieves gas and painful bowel spasms. The herb has been used commercially to flavor tobacco and some beverages.

PRECAUTIONS

Valerian occasionally has the opposite effect of that intended, stimulating instead of sedating. Reducing the dosage usually alleviates the problem. Valerian may cause headaches, dizziness, and heart palpitations when taken in large doses. Don't take valerian if you're pregnant.

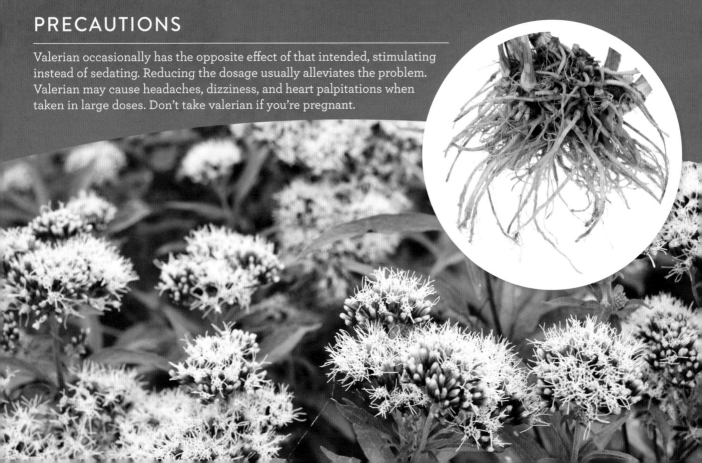

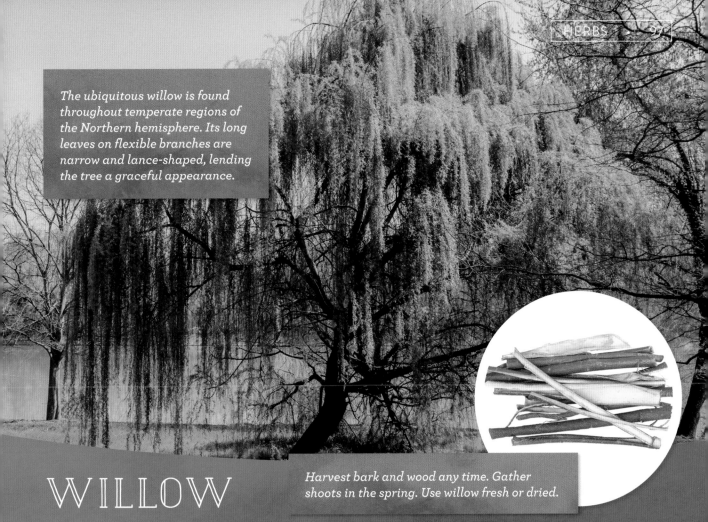

The ubiquitous willow is found throughout temperate regions of the Northern hemisphere. Its long leaves on flexible branches are narrow and lance-shaped, lending the tree a graceful appearance.

WILLOW

Harvest bark and wood any time. Gather shoots in the spring. Use willow fresh or dried.

BOTANICAL NAME: *SALIX SPP.*

Although their long billowing branches bring to mind "weeping," willows were considered a symbol of joy by the ancient Egyptians, who prized the trees that grew along the banks of the Nile. And well they should have. This attractive shade tree is also a potent healer. The various species of willow contain salicin, from which salicylic acid, the main ingredient of aspirin, is derived, and herbalists often recommend the plant to relieve pain. The Chinese have been putting it to this purpose since 500 BC. It's also a useful herb for women with painful periods. Willow contains enough salicylate to suppress chemicals known as prostaglandins, one cause of painful menstrual cramps.

Willow is also used to treat fever, headache, hay fever, neuralgia, and inflammation of joints. The inner bark is an astringent and antiseptic: Decoctions of white willow bark are valued in facial lotions and baths for their astringent properties.

PRECAUTIONS

In animal studies, aspirin has been associated with increased risk of birth defects, thus, avoid willow if you are pregnant. Also, the use of aspirin in children has been linked to Reye syndrome, a rare but potentially fatal disease. Although willow has not been associated with Reye syndrome, it's still best not to give willow to children with colds, flu, or chicken pox.

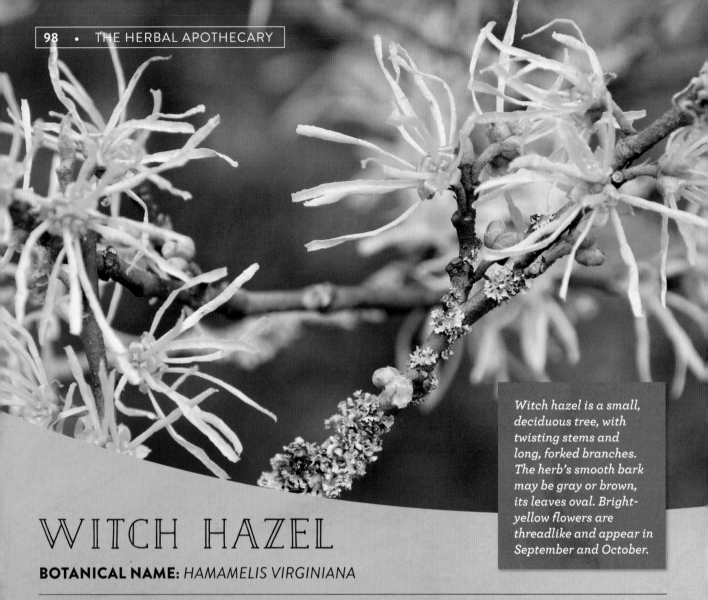

Witch hazel is a small, deciduous tree, with twisting stems and long, forked branches. The herb's smooth bark may be gray or brown, its leaves oval. Bright-yellow flowers are threadlike and appear in September and October.

WITCH HAZEL

BOTANICAL NAME: *HAMAMELIS VIRGINIANA*

Witch hazel has long been prized as an astringent cosmetic and medicinal herb. Its leaves, twigs, and bark contain tannic and gallic acids and essential oils. Witch hazel dries weeping, raw tissues. A cloth soaked in strong witch hazel tea and applied to the skin reduces the swelling and pain of hemorrhoids, bruises, wounds, and sprains and promotes speedy healing. It can also tighten and soothe aching varicose veins and reduce inflammation associated with blood clots (phlebitis) in the legs.

Witch hazel lotions are useful on rough, swollen hands. And the herb is a popular skin cleanser and body lotion; it is also effective in treating insect bites, sunburns, and poison oak and ivy rashes and is an ingredient in aftershaves. The herb is also used as a mouthwash, gargle, and douche.

PRECAUTIONS

The tannins in witch hazel may produce nausea if consumed in large quantities. Pay attention to the label of any witch hazel preparation you purchase. While you can ingest the tincture made with grain alcohol, many preparations are made from the poisonous rubbing (isopropyl) alcohol.

WORMWOOD

BOTANICAL NAME: *ARTEMISIA ABSINTHIUM*

Wormwood is steeped in mystique. It is said to have grown up in the trail left by the serpent as it slithered from the Garden of Eden. The herb is a prime ingredient of the addictive alcoholic drink called absinthe, which is illegal in most countries, including the United States. Wormwood got its name because it expels intestinal worms. The plant also is an antiseptic, antispasmodic, and carminative, and it increases bile production. It has been used to treat fever, colds, jaundice, and gallstones.

Compresses soaked in the tea are said to be good for irritations, bruises, and sprains. Wormwood oil has been used as a liniment to relieve the pain of rheumatism, neuralgia, and arthritis. The plant is also an antifungal and antibacterial, and new research indicates that compounds in one of the species of wormwood, *A. annua,* could be a cure for malaria. Wormwood is also a flea and moth repellant. Although it is brittle when dried, it makes a beautiful foundation for a wreath or swag.

PRECAUTIONS

In large doses, wormwood's active constituent, thujone, is a convulsant, poison, and narcotic. The herb is not very water-soluble, but tinctures are high in thujone, so don't use tinctures internally. Topical use is generally considered safe, but wormwood may cause dermatitis in some people. Do not use wormwood internally for more than a couple days unless you are under the supervision of a physician or qualified herbalist and not at all if you are pregnant.

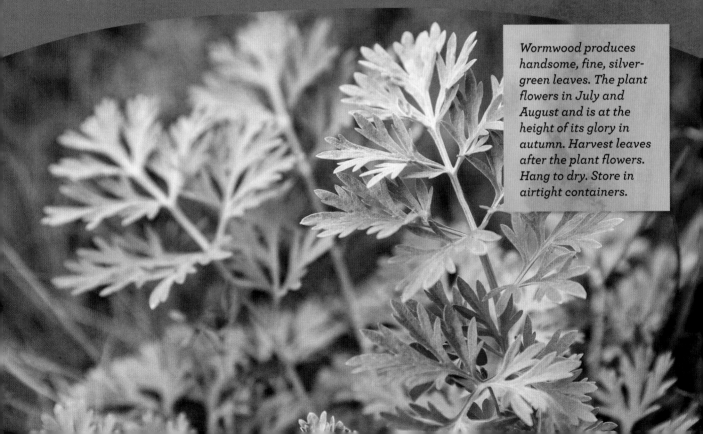

Wormwood produces handsome, fine, silver-green leaves. The plant flowers in July and August and is at the height of its glory in autumn. Harvest leaves after the plant flowers. Hang to dry. Store in airtight containers.

YARROW

BOTANICAL NAME: *ACHILLEA MILEFOLIUM*

In the epic *Iliad*, Homer reports that legendary warrior Achilles used yarrow leaves to treat the wounds of his fallen comrades. Studies show that yarrow is a fine herb indeed for accelerating healing of cuts and bruises. The Greeks used the herb to stop hemorrhages. Gerard's famous herbal cited yarrow's benefits in 1597. And after colonists brought the plant to America, Indians used it to treat bleeding, wounds, infections, headaches, indigestion, and sore throat.

Clinical studies have supported the longstanding use of yarrow to cleanse wounds and make blood clot faster. Yarrow treats bleeding stomach ulcers, heavy menstrual periods, and bleeding from the bowels. An essential oil known as azulene is responsible for yarrow's ability to reduce inflammation. Traditional Chinese medicine credits yarrow with the ability to nurture the spleen, liver, kidney, and bladder. Several studies have shown that yarrow improves uterine tone and reduces uterine spasms in animals. Apigenin and flavonoid constituents are credited with yarrow's antispasmodic properties. The herb also contains salicylic acid, aspirin's main constituent, making it useful for relieving pain. Chewing the leaves or root is an old toothache remedy. Yarrow fights bacteria and dries up congestion in sinus and other respiratory infections and allergies. The plant has long been a standby herb for promoting sweating to bring down fevers in cases of colds and influenza. It also relieves bladder infections. Because of its astringent and cleansing properties, yarrow is sometimes added to skin lotions. Flowers and stalks dry well, making attractive decorations. The flowers dye wool shades of yellow to olive.

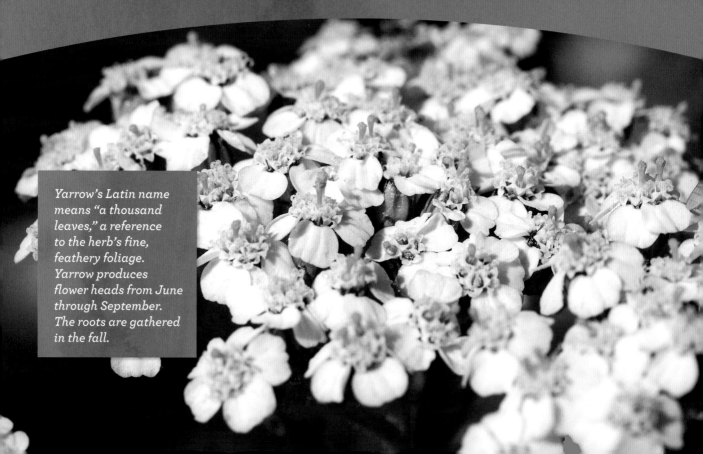

Yarrow's Latin name means "a thousand leaves," a reference to the herb's fine, feathery foliage. Yarrow produces flower heads from June through September. The roots are gathered in the fall.

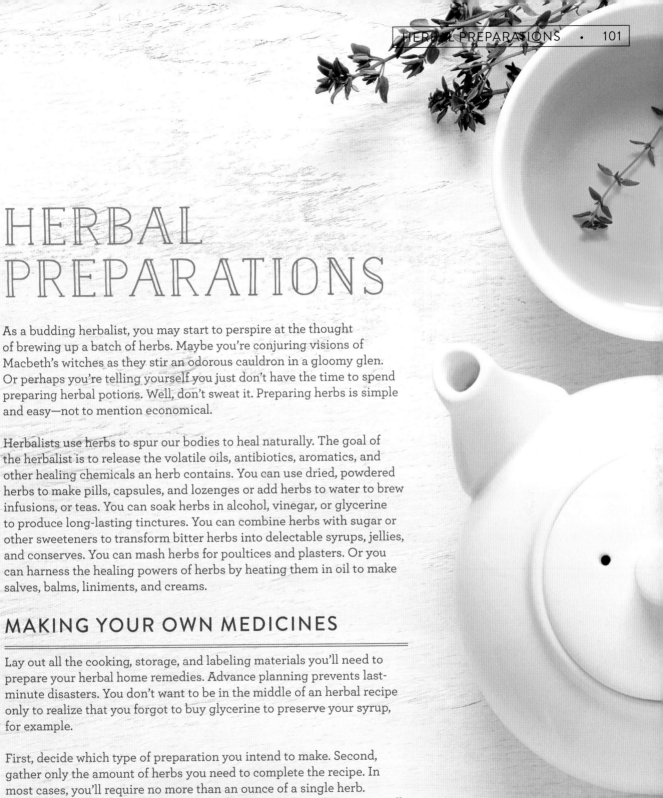

HERBAL PREPARATIONS

As a budding herbalist, you may start to perspire at the thought of brewing up a batch of herbs. Maybe you're conjuring visions of Macbeth's witches as they stir an odorous cauldron in a gloomy glen. Or perhaps you're telling yourself you just don't have the time to spend preparing herbal potions. Well, don't sweat it. Preparing herbs is simple and easy—not to mention economical.

Herbalists use herbs to spur our bodies to heal naturally. The goal of the herbalist is to release the volatile oils, antibiotics, aromatics, and other healing chemicals an herb contains. You can use dried, powdered herbs to make pills, capsules, and lozenges or add herbs to water to brew infusions, or teas. You can soak herbs in alcohol, vinegar, or glycerine to produce long-lasting tinctures. You can combine herbs with sugar or other sweeteners to transform bitter herbs into delectable syrups, jellies, and conserves. You can mash herbs for poultices and plasters. Or you can harness the healing powers of herbs by heating them in oil to make salves, balms, liniments, and creams.

MAKING YOUR OWN MEDICINES

Lay out all the cooking, storage, and labeling materials you'll need to prepare your herbal home remedies. Advance planning prevents last-minute disasters. You don't want to be in the middle of an herbal recipe only to realize that you forgot to buy glycerine to preserve your syrup, for example.

First, decide which type of preparation you intend to make. Second, gather only the amount of herbs you need to complete the recipe. In most cases, you'll require no more than an ounce of a single herb. Salves and other preparations made with oil tend to keep better in small batches. If you intend to save these medicines for longer than a few months, keep them refrigerated.

TEAS

One of the easiest and most popular ways of preparing an herbal medicine is to brew a tea. There are two types of teas: infusions and decoctions. If you have ever poured hot water over a tea bag, you have made an infusion; an infusion is simply the result of steeping herbs in hot water. A decoction is the result of boiling herbs gently in water. When you simmer cinnamon sticks and cloves in apple cider, you're making a decoction.

In general, delicate leaves and flowers are best infused; boiling may cause them to lose the volatile essential oils. To prepare an infusion, use 1 teaspoon of dried herbs per 1 cup of hot water. (If you use fresh herbs, use 1 to 2 teaspoons or more.) Pour the hot water over the herbs in a pan or teapot, cover with a lid, and allow to steep for about ten minutes. Strain and drink. Finely cut herbs in tea bags steep much faster—in about five minutes. You can make your own herbal tea bags, too. Tie up a teaspoon of herbs in a small muslin bag (sold in most natural food stores) or piece of cheesecloth, and drop it in a cup of hot water. Let the tea steep for 15 minutes. To make larger quantities of hot infusions, use 5 tablespoons of herbs per gallon of water.

Extremely volatile herbs such as peppermint and lemon balm lose a lot of essential oils with high heat. These herbs can be infused with cold water. It is easy to recognize volatile herbs because they are highly fragrant. Allow a cold tea to infuse overnight. These herbs are suitable for making the popular "sun" tea. Using 1 teaspoon of herbs per cup of water, put herbs and water in a jar, and place in the sun for a couple of hours. Strain and serve.

To decoct an herb root such as this fresh ginger root, slice it thin, then boil it gently to extract its constituents.

Roots, barks, and seeds, on the other hand, are best made into decoctions because these hard, woody materials need significant boiling time to get the constituents out of the fiber. Fresh roots generally should be sliced thin. To prepare a medicinal decoction, use one teaspoon of herbs per cup of water, cover, and gently simmer for 15 to 30 minutes. Strain the decoction. Use glass, ceramic, or earthenware pots to make your decoction—aluminum may taint herbal teas. A tea will remain fresh for several days in the refrigerator. To preserve teas, make a concentrated brew, three times as strong as an ordinary remedy. Then add one part of drinking alcohol (not rubbing alcohol) or glycerine to 3 parts of the infusion. Store in covered container. When ready to use, dilute with 3 parts water. How much of an infusion or decoction should you take at one time? In general, drink 1 cup three times a day. A rule of thumb is, if you don't notice any benefits in three days, change the treatment or see your doctor or herbalist. Rely on professional care immediately in the case of potentially life-threatening conditions, such as difficulty breathing, irregular heartbeat, allergic reactions, or severe injuries.

LEMON MINT TEA

This remedy is excellent for colds.

- ¼ cup dried peppermint leaves
- ¼ cup dried lemon balm leaves
- 3 Tbsp dried organic lemon rind, grated

Combine ingredients. Bring 1 cup of water to a boil. Remove from heat, and steep 1 to 2 Tbsp of the herb mixture in the water for 15 minutes; strain and drink. This tea is delicious either hot or iced.

COFFEE SUBSTITUTE CONCOCTION

This hot beverage is the perfect substitute for coffee if you're trying to kick the caffeine habit. If you take your coffee with cream, you can even add milk or a milk substitute, such as soy or rice milk, to this brew.

- 3 oz dandelion root
- 1 oz roasted chicory root
- 1 oz cinnamon bark
- 1 oz licorice root, shredded (optional)*
- 2 oz organic orange peel
- ½ oz carob powder
- 1 heaping tsp nutmeg

Combine the herbs. Gently simmer 1 tsp of the herb mixture in 1 cup water for 15 minutes. Remove from heat and steep 15 minutes longer. Strain and drink.

*Licorice is not recommended for individuals with high blood pressure.

STOMACH RELIEF TEA

Here's a remedy that can quiet stomach discomfort, from indigestion to a spastic colon.

- 1 Tbsp dried chamomile flowers
- 1 tsp fennel seeds
- 2 Tbsp dried mint leaves

Combine ingredients. Steep 1 tsp of the mixture in 1 cup of hot water for 15 minutes; strain and drink.

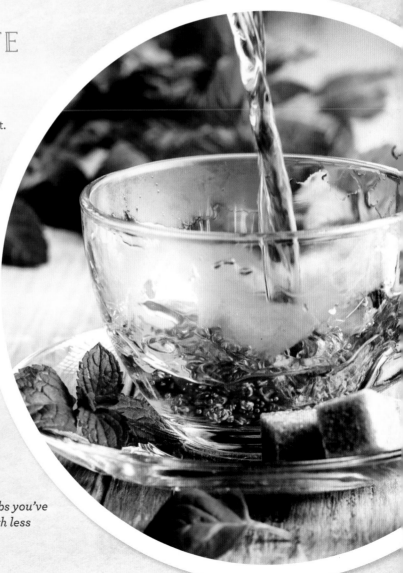

Relax with a cup of herbal tea made from herbs you've grown yourself. Adding mint to teas made with less palatable herbs improves their flavor.

TINCTURES

Commercial tinctures are made by carefully weighing the ingredients and adjusting them according to the individual herb. However, with common kitchen utensils and very little effort, you can easily prepare suitable tinctures for your own use. First, clean and pick over dried or fresh herbs, removing any insects or damaged plant material. Remove leaves and flowers from stems. Cut or chop the plant parts you want to process into small pieces, or chop them in a blender or food processor. Cover with just enough drinking alcohol to completely submerge the herbs. The spirit most commonly used is 80 to 100 proof vodka. Some herbs, such as ginger and cayenne, require the higher alcohol content to fully extract their constituents.

Puree the plant material and transfer it to a glass jar. After the plant material settles, make certain the alcohol covers the plants, and add more alcohol if it does not. This is especially important if you use fresh herbs. Plant materials exposed to air can mold or rot. Store the jar at room temperature out of sunlight, and shake the jar every day. After two weeks, strain the liquid with a kitchen strainer, cheesecloth, thin piece of muslin, or paper coffee filter. If particles eventually settle after the tincture has been stored, shake the mixture to redistribute them. Tinctures will keep for many years without refrigeration.

DANDELION ROOT TINCTURE

Place dried, chopped dandelion roots in a food processor with enough 80 to 100 proof vodka to process. Once blended, store in a glass jar, shake daily, and strain in two weeks. Take ½ to 1 tsp three times a day before meals for chronic constipation, poor digestion, or urinary tract problems, or as a spring tonic.

Because the usual dose of a tincture is 30 drops, you receive enough herb to benefit from its medicinal properties with very little alcohol. If you're allergic to alcohol—or simply don't wish to use it—try making vinegar- or glycerine-based tinctures. Vinegar and glycerine dissolve plant constituents almost as effectively as spirits. Glycerine is available at most pharmacies.

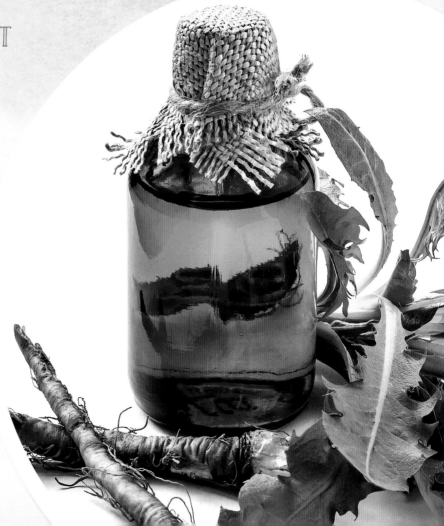

VINEGAR TINCTURES

Vinegar, which contains the solvent acetic acid, is an alternative to alcohol tinctures. You can use herbal vinegars medicinally or dilute them with more vinegar to make great-tasting salad dressings and marinades. Use any vinegar, such as apple cider, rice vinegar, red wine vinegar, or balsamic vinegar.

Vinegar is also a potent antifungal agent and makes a good athlete's foot soak when combined with antimicrobial herbs.

ATHLETE'S FOOT VINEGAR

- 2 garlic bulbs
- ½ cup fresh or dried calendula petals
- ¼ cup fresh comfrey root
- Hulls of 3 fresh black walnuts, chopped, or ½ oz black walnut tincture
- Vinegar, about 2 cups
- 2 tsp tea tree oil

Place garlic in a blender along with the calendula petals, comfrey root, and black walnut hulls or tincture. Pour enough vinegar over the herbs to blend. Pour the mixture into a jar, and add tea tree oil. Keep in a dark place for two weeks. Strain. Shake well before using.

To treat athlete's foot, dab solution on affected area several times a day. You may wish to wear dark socks when undergoing this treatment as the black walnut can stain white socks.

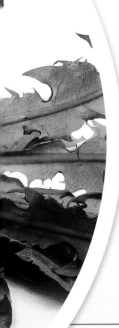

VINEGAR OF THE FOUR THIEVES

Here's a recipe handed down from the Middle Ages. Herbal lore has it that four men caught ransacking empty homes infested with bubonic plague were tried before a court in Marseilles. Asked by the judge how the men had avoided contracting the plague, the accused men said they had washed themselves with a special herbal vinegar. The thieves were granted freedom in return for the recipe.

You can add this vinegar to a bath, or take 1 teaspoon internally—no more than 1 tablespoon an hour—to protect yourself during flu season.

- 2 quarts apple cider vinegar
- 2 Tbsp lavender
- 2 Tbsp rosemary
- 2 Tbsp sage
- 2 Tbsp wormwood
- 2 Tbsp rue
- 2 Tbsp mint
- 2 Tbsp garlic buds, unpeeled

Cover the herbs with vinegar. Keep at room temperature for two weeks. Strain and bottle. You can also make a vinegar syrup by adding 4 ounces of glycerine. Sweeten to taste.

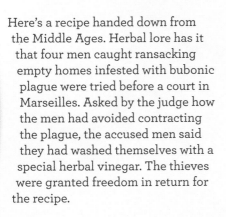

GLYCERINE TINCTURES

The advantage of using a glycerine-based tincture is that it does not contain alcohol. The disadvantage is that glycerine doesn't dissolve an herb's constituents as well as alcohol does. To make a glycerine tincture, mix 4 ounces water and 6 ounces glycerine. Pour the mixture over 1 ounce of dried or fresh chopped herbs in a clean jar. As with alcohol tinctures, make sure the herbs are submerged under the glycerine and water mixture. Shake daily. Let stand at room temperature for two weeks, then strain and bottle.

PILLS AND CAPSULES

We have come to rely on pharmaceutical pills to cure many of our ailments. There is nothing inherently wrong with taking pills. But if you're uncomfortable with the notion of ingesting synthetic chemicals, you can turn to herbal capsules, tablets, or lozenges. Capsules and tablets provide a convenient method of ingesting herbs that have strong, harsh flavors. They're also an alternative for people who do not enjoy drinking herbal teas or using alcohol-based tinctures. You can buy capsules and tablets at a natural food store or even make your own.

CAPSULES

You can find empty gelatin capsules at health food stores, online herbal houses, and some pharmacies. Fill the capsules with powdered herbs. Remember, it's best to store your herbs whole, then powder them immediately before encapsulating them. You can powder them with a mortar and pestle or in a coffee grinder or food processor. If the method you use does not produce a fine powder, strain the herbs through a sieve or strainer first.

Fill half the capsule with the powdered herb and pack tightly. A chopstick is a good tool for packing the powder into the capsule. Close with the other capsule half. Many natural food stores also sell capsule makers that speed up the process.

Decorative as well as useful, mortars and pestles come in a variety of shapes and sizes.

PILLS

To make herb pills, simply blend powdered herbs with a bit of honey to bind the mixture. Then just pinch off bits of the resulting sticky substance and roll into balls. (If the balls seem too moist, roll them in a mixture of slippery elm and licorice powder to soak up excess moisture.) Dry the herbal pills in a dehydrator, an oven set to preheat, or outdoors on a warm day covered with a cloth. Store the dried pills in an airtight container.

RELAXATION PILLS

These pills contain herbs commonly recommended to reduce tension and calm anxiety. The pills may also help relieve tension headaches.

Combine equal parts of powdered skullcap, valerian, rosemary, chamomile, and peppermint. Blend with enough honey to bind. Roll off pill-sized pieces, dry, and store in a tightly sealed container.

LOZENGES

To make herbal lozenges, combine powdered herbs with sugar and a mucilaginous binding agent such as marshmallow root, licorice root, or slippery elm bark.

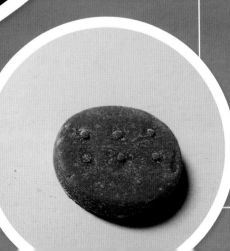

THROAT LOZENGES

- 3 Tbsp licorice powder
- 3 Tbsp slippery elm powder
- 1 Tbsp myrrh powder
- 1 tsp cayenne powder
- Honey as needed
- 20 drops orange essential oil
- 2 drops thyme essential oil
- Sugar
- Cornstarch

Mix herbal powders. Stir in honey until a gooey mass forms. Add essential oils. Mix very well. Spread the paste on a marble slab or other nonstick surface coated with sugar or cornstarch. With a rolling pin, roll the mixture flat to about the thickness of a pancake. Sprinkle with sugar and cornstarch. With a knife, cut into small, separate squares. Or pinch off pieces and roll into ¼-inch balls. Flatten the balls into round lozenges. Allow lozenges to air-dry in a well-ventilated area for 12 hours. Suck on lozenges to help soothe sore throats or calm coughs.

SYRUPS

In syrup form, even the most bitter herbs taste good. Syrups are ideal for soothing sore throats and respiratory ailments. You can make herbal syrups by combining sugar, honey, or glycerine with infusions, decoctions, tinctures, herbal juices, or medicinal liquors. (Refined sugar makes a clearer syrup with a better flavor.) Preserve syrups by refrigerating or adding glycerine.

Make syrups in small quantities. To make a simple syrup, dissolve the sweetener of your choice in a hot herb infusion. You can add herbal tinctures to increase the syrup's medicinal value. Add 1 to 2 ounces of tincture to the following formula if you wish.

HERBAL SYRUP

- ¼ cup sugar or honey
- 1½ cups strong herb infusion
- ½ cup glycerine

Combine sweetener and infusion in a pan and bring mixture to a boil. Add glycerine. Pour mixture into clean bottles and let cool. Keep refrigerated. Makes about 2 cups of syrup.

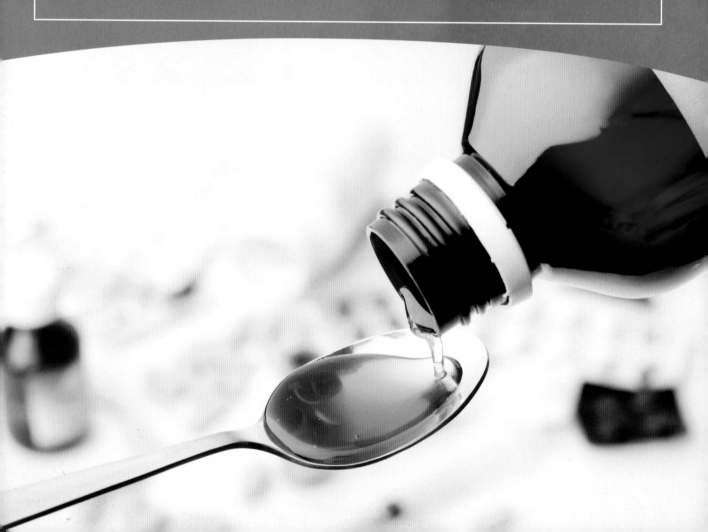

TOPICAL PREPARATIONS

It is fairly simple to create your own herbal skin preparations. Commercial oils, salves, creams, and lotions often contain byproducts and chemicals you may not wish to use. When you make your own topical preparations, you can tailor the recipes to suit your particular needs. Use your favorite kind of oil or your favorite scent.

HERBS TO SOFTEN AND HEAL SKIN

ALOE VERA	COMFREY	SLIPPERY ELM
CALENDULA	MARSHMALLOW	

HERBS FOR SORE MUSCLES

ARNICA	GINGER	ST. JOHN'S WORT
CALENDULA	JUNIPER	WINTERGREEN
CHAMOMILE	LAVENDER	
EUCALYPTUS	ROSEMARY	

HERBAL OILS

Oils provide a versatile medium for extracting herbal constituents. Olive, almond, canola, and sesame oils are good choices, but any vegetable oil will do. Select an oil with a light fragrance that won't overpower the herbs. Avoid mineral oil. You can consume herbal oils in recipes or salads, or massage sore body parts with medicinal oils. Add herbs to the oil of your choice, allow to sit for a week, strain, and bottle. Refrigerate oils you plan to use in cooking.

MASSAGE OIL FOR SORE MUSCLES

- 5 or 6 cayenne peppers
- 1 cup vegetable oil
- ¼ tsp clove essential oil
- ¼ tsp eucalyptus essential oil
- ¼ tsp mint essential oil

Chop cayenne peppers and place in a jar. Cover with vegetable oil. Make sure the peppers are completely covered. Store oil in a warm, dark place. Strain after one week. Add the essential oils.

Massage on sore muscles. Be careful not to get this oil in your eyes or open wounds—it will sting like the dickens. Wash your hands after using this oil.

HERBS FOR SALVES

ARNICA	ELDER FLOWER	MARSHMALLOW	SLIPPERY ELM
COMFREY	GOLDENSEAL	PLANTAIN	YARROW

Oil bases: Lard, vegetable or nut oils such as almond, coconut, peanut, and olive oil
Additives: Cocoa butter, lanolin
Hardeners: Beeswax
Natural preservatives: Benzoin, poplar bud, glycerine, vitamin E

SALVES

Salves, also called ointments, are fat-based preparations used to soothe abrasions, heal wounds and lacerations, protect babies' skin from diaper rash, and soften dry, rough skin and chapped lips. Salves are made by heating an herb with fat or vegetable oil until the fat absorbs the plant's healing properties. Beeswax is then added to the strained mixture to give it a thicker consistency.

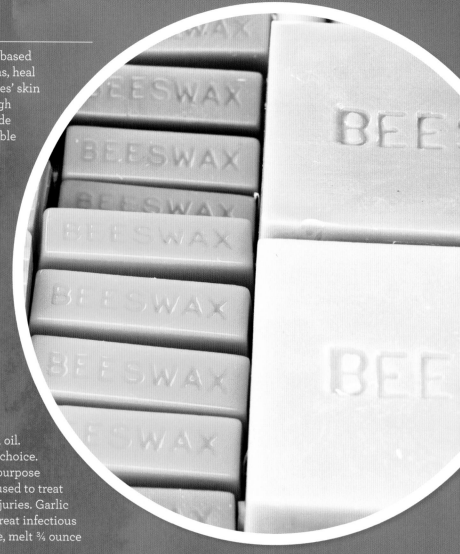

Kept in a cool place, salves last at least a year. You can preserve a salve even longer by adding a few drops of tincture of benzoin, poplar bud tincture, or glycerine. (Benzoin and glycerine are available in pharmacies; poplar bud tincture is available in some health food stores. All of these are available via online vendors) Make salves in small batches to keep them fresh. Store in tightly lidded jars.

The key ingredient of salves is herbal oil. Make your oil out of the herb of your choice. Calendula oil makes a wonderful all-purpose healing salve. St. John's wort can be used to treat swelling and bruising in traumatic injuries. Garlic oil can be used to prepare a salve to treat infectious conditions. To turn the oil into a salve, melt ¾ ounce beeswax in 1 cup herbal oil.

You can purchase beeswax from health food stores, beekeeping supply stores, and a variety of websites. Grated beeswax melts faster; use a grater or food processor to grate it. Refrigerate the wax before grating to make the job easier. (Wash utensils with very hot water to remove all the beeswax.)

Warm the herbal oil, then add the beeswax. When the beeswax melts, pour the salve into containers before the blend starts to harden. If you wish, add 500 IU of vitamin E per ounce to increase the salve's healing properties and help preserve the salve, or add a teaspoon of benzoin or poplar tincture for every cup of herbal oil to help preserve it. Other possible additives are 1 to 2 tablespoons of cocoa butter to make the consistency more creamy or ½ to 1 teaspoon hydrous lanolin per cup of herbal oil to give the salve more tack. Lanolin is especially good in a salve for diaper rash.

Note: Problems with your salve? Simply reheat it. If your salve is too runny, add a bit more beeswax. If the salve is too hard, use more oil. To test your salve before pouring it into individual containers, pour about a tablespoon of salve in a container and put it in the freezer. This "tester" will be ready in a few minutes.

ALL-PURPOSE HEALING SALVE

- ½ cup comfrey root oil
- ½ cup calendula oil
- ¾ oz beeswax
- 1 Tbsp vitamin E oil
- 20 drops vitamin A emulsion

Combine the oils and gently warm them. Melt the beeswax into the oils. Add vitamins E and A. Pour into salve containers and let stand about 20 minutes to harden.

ANTIFUNGAL SALVE

- ½ cup garlic oil
- ½ cup calendula oil
- ¾ oz beeswax
- 20 drops tea tree essential oil
- 1 tsp black walnut tincture

Combine the garlic and calendula oils and gently warm them. Melt the beeswax into the oils. Add the essential oil and tincture. Stir well. Pour into salve containers while still warm.

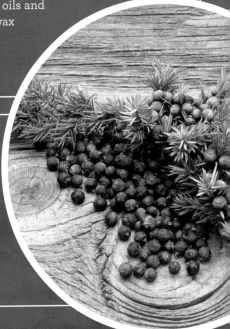

JUNIPER BERRY OINTMENT

- This ointment is good for wounds, itching, and scratches.
- 1 cup juniper berries
- 2 cups oil (olive, peanut, wheat germ, or lanolin)
- 2-3 Tbsp beeswax

Simmer berries in oil. Melt beeswax into the oil and berry mixture. Strain and pour into jars.

LINIMENTS

A liniment is a topical preparation that contains alcohol or oil and stimulating, warming herbs such as cayenne. Since liniment is for external use only, sometimes isopropyl, or rubbing, alcohol is used instead of grain alcohol. Do not take products made with rubbing alcohol internally.

Liniments warm the skin and turn it red temporarily. It is best to test your tolerance to liniments by rubbing a small amount on your wrist to make sure it does not burn. To enhance the heat, cover the area with a cloth after application.

LINIMENT FOR ARTHRITIS, LUNG CONGESTION, AND SORE MUSCLES

- ½ oz cayenne pods, chopped
- ½ oz cloves, powdered
- 1 oz eucalyptus leaves, chopped
- 1 cup isopropyl alcohol
- 60 drops wintergreen essential oil
- 20 drops peppermint essential oil
- 20 drops clove essential oil

Soak first three ingredients in alcohol for two weeks, then strain. Add essential oils. Stir well. Massage liniment into area affected by arthritis, onto back and chest for congestion, or on sore muscles.

LOTIONS

A lotion contains oil and another liquid. Add essential oils for therapeutic purposes or to give the lotion your favorite scent.

HEALING LOTION

- ½ oz calendula tincture
- 1 oz comfrey tincture
- 1 oz wheat germ oil
- 3 oz aloe vera gel or fresh pulp
- ¼ tsp vitamin C crystals
- ½ tsp essential oil, if desired

Combine ingredients in a bottle and shake vigorously. Refrigerate if made with fresh aloe pulp.

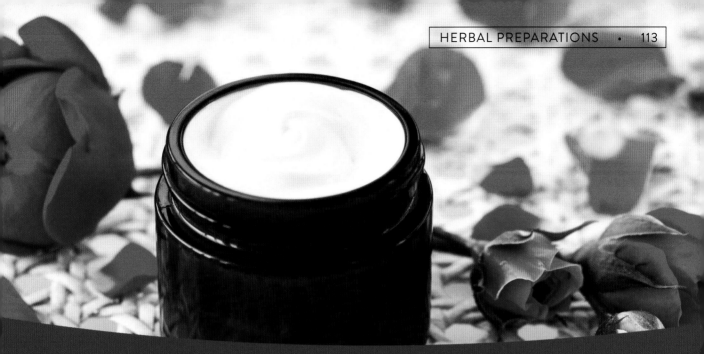

CREAMS

Creams contain water or other water-soluble liquids. They are less greasy than salves and liniments. Making a cream is similar to making mayonnaise or gravy: Slowly add liquid to the wax and oil solution until the ingredients combine smoothly. To help preserve creams, add a few drops of benzoin tincture or vitamin E, or store in the refrigerator.

CALENDULA-LAVENDER CREAM

- 2 oz comfrey oil
- 2 oz calendula oil
- ½ tsp hydrous lanolin*
- ½ oz beeswax
- 2 oz distilled water or rose water
- $^1/_{16}$ oz borax powder
- ¼ tsp lavender oil

Combine and heat comfrey and calendula oils. Melt lanolin and beeswax in oil mixture. In another pot, gently warm water and dissolve borax in it. Remove both mixtures from heat. Place oil-wax mixture in blender or food processor. Add the borax and water mixture very slowly, constantly blending, until all the water has been added. Constantly push hardened top edge of mixture back into blender or processor. Add lavender oil; blend until thickened. Pour into jars. Store any extra cream in the refrigerator. You can replace the water in this recipe with fresh plant juices, technically called succus, if they are available. Succus is usually preserved with 20 percent alcohol. But be aware that cream made from fresh plant juices tends to last only 6 to 12 months.

*Hydrous lanolin is available in pharmacies.

COMPRESSES AND POULTICES

You can use compresses to treat headaches, rashes, itching, and swollen glands, among other conditions. To make a compress, soak a cloth in a strong herbal tea, wring it out, and place it on the skin. Soak a cloth with strong peppermint tea to treat rashes that itch and burn. Soak a cloth with arnica or St. John's wort tincture and hold against a sprained ankle. A lavender compress relieves the itchy eyes caused by allergies.

To make a poultice or plaster, mash herbs with enough water to form a paste. Place the herb mash directly on the affected body part and cover with a clean white cloth or gauze.

HERBS FOR COMPRESSES

ARNICA	PEPPERMINT
GARLIC	SAGE
GINGER	ST. JOHN'S WORT
LAVENDER	WITCH HAZEL
MARJORAM	

HERBS FOR POULTICES

COMFREY	OATMEAL
MARSHMALLOW	PLANTAIN
MUSTARD	SLIPPERY ELM BARK

MUSTARD POULTICE

A mustard poultice is a time-honored therapy: Your great-grandmother may have used mustard poultices and plasters to treat congestion, coughs, bronchitis, or pneumonia. A mustard poultice, or plaster, immediately improves discomfort in the chest and actually helps to treat infectious conditions—a much-needed therapy in the days before antibiotics. It works mainly by increasing circulation, perspiration, and heat in the affected area.

The person receiving the treatment should sit or lie comfortably. To prepare a mustard poultice, mix ½ cup mustard powder with 1 cup flour. Stir hot water into the mustard and flour mixture until it forms a paste. Spread the mixture on a piece of cotton that you have soaked in hot water. Cover with a second piece of dry cotton material. Lay the moist side across the person's chest or back. Leave the moist side on for 15 to 30 minutes; promptly remove if the person experiences any discomfort. The procedure is likely to promote perspiration and reddening of the chest.

COMFREY POULTICE

Use a poultice made of fresh comfrey root or leaves to help heal cuts, abrasions, and other injuries to the skin. Place several chunks of comfrey in a blender with enough distilled water to process. Blend into a wet mass. Place the mashed comfrey directly against the skin. Leave on about a half hour. Use the comfrey poultice several times a day for an initial injury. Poultices last several days in the refrigerator. Although comfrey helps knit many minor wounds, serious injuries should be examined by a physician.

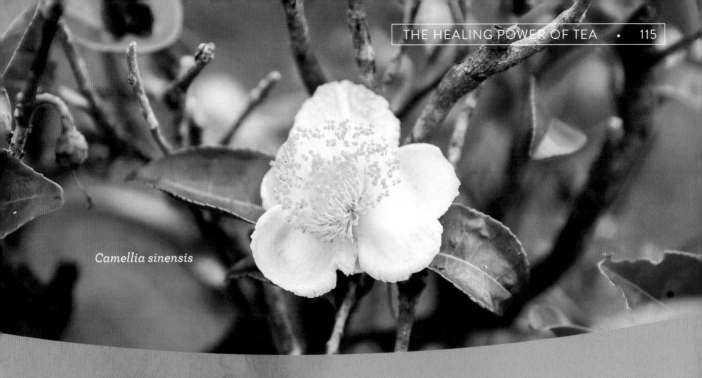

Camellia sinensis

THE HEALING POWER OF TEA

There are an estimated 3,000 varieties of tea produced worldwide. With so many different types of tea, you might think there are many different plants that produce them. But that's not the case: All tea leaves trace their roots to one plant. It's the processing the leaves undergo after they are harvested that determines whether they will become black, oolong (wu-long), green, or white tea.

All true tea comes from the leaves of an evergreen shrub, *Camellia sinensis*, a relative of the ornamental camellia plant (*Camellia japonica*) that is grown for its beautiful flowers. There are two main species: One variety, called *Thea sinensis*, is native to China, while the other, *Thea assamica*, hails from India. Other tea plant species are hybrids, made by crossbreeding *Thea sinensis* and *Thea assamica*.

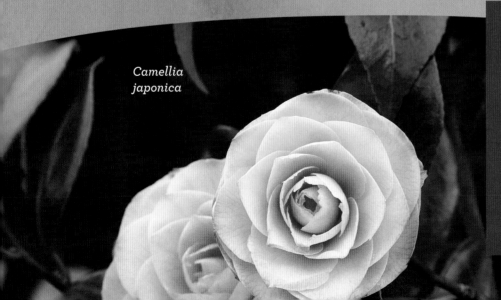

Camellia japonica

Herbal tea is not really tea because it doesn't come from the Camellia sinensis *plant. Herbal teas are tisanes, or infusions, of herb leaves, roots, seeds, or flowers in hot water. Some true teas, like Earl Grey, are black teas blended with an herb or essential oil. But unless a product contains leaves from the* Camellia sinensis *plant, it is not truly tea.*

BLACK TEA

Black tea takes the most time to make and is the most processed form of tea. First the withered leaves are rolled and bruised (the more traditional method) or cut, torn, and curled (abbreviated as the CTC method) to rupture the cells in the leaves and release some of the essential oils. As these oils come in contact with air, the leaves begin to oxidize (oils and chemicals in the leaf react with the oxygen in the air—the same thing happens when metal rusts or a cut apple turns brown). This process is also known as fermentation. Oxidizing causes the leaves to turn brown and gives a richer flavor and a darker color to the brew.

Black tea leaves are allowed to oxidize for about three to four hours. The leaves are then dried, or fired, by passing them on trays through a hot air chamber. This firing stops the oxidation process and preserves the leaves. The leaves are now dark, or black—which is why this type of tea is called black tea—and are sorted, graded, and readied for packaging.

In China, black tea is called red tea because the tea brews up a reddish color, even though the leaves are black.

OOLONG TEA

Tea leaves destined to become oolong oxidize for a shorter period of time than those for black—only about one to two hours—though growers vary the oxidation time to produce unique flavors. Oolong leaves are typically rolled and sold loose as full leaves rather than cut for tea bags. Oolong is considered the "champagne of tea" and can vary from bright amber to pale yellow in color and from light and floral or fruity to smoky in flavor.

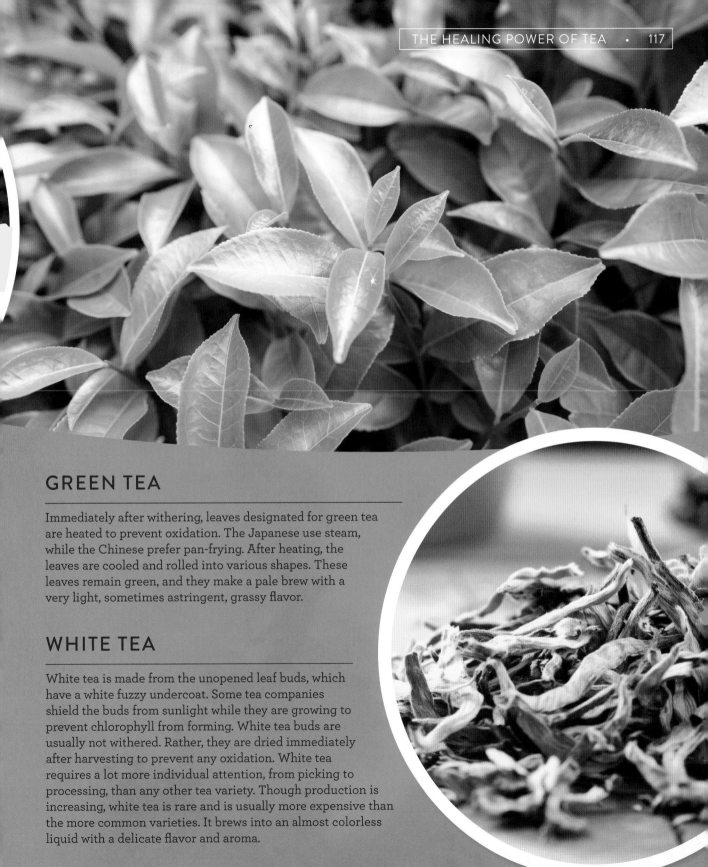

GREEN TEA

Immediately after withering, leaves designated for green tea
are heated to prevent oxidation. The Japanese use steam,
while the Chinese prefer pan-frying. After heating, the
leaves are cooled and rolled into various shapes. These
leaves remain green, and they make a pale brew with a
very light, sometimes astringent, grassy flavor.

WHITE TEA

White tea is made from the unopened leaf buds, which
have a white fuzzy undercoat. Some tea companies
shield the buds from sunlight while they are growing to
prevent chlorophyll from forming. White tea buds are
usually not withered. Rather, they are dried immediately
after harvesting to prevent any oxidation. White tea
requires a lot more individual attention, from picking to
processing, than any other tea variety. Though production is
increasing, white tea is rare and is usually more expensive than
the more common varieties. It brews into an almost colorless
liquid with a delicate flavor and aroma.

HEALING TEA

Could good health be brewing in your cup of tea? You betcha! Tea may help prevent diseases such as cardiovascular disease, cancer, diabetes, and osteoporosis. Before tea became a beloved and much sought-after beverage worldwide, it was used medicinally. The Chinese credited it as a remedy for everything from headaches to melancholy. In recent years we've come full circle, and tea is once again being touted for its healing properties. Today we know what the ancient world did not: Tea has three active ingredients that contribute to its healing power—flavonoids, fluoride, and caffeine. But the flavonoids are responsible for most of tea's health benefits.

GO GREEN—WITH FLAVONOIDS

Research has shown an indisputable link between eating plant foods and good health. Vegetables and fruits contain an array of vitamins, minerals, and phytochemicals, plant compounds that have health-protective and disease-preventive properties. Tea, which comes from the *Camellia sinensis* plant, also has an abundance of phytochemicals.

There are thousands of phytochemicals in plants. Tea leaves contain a subgroup called polyphenols, or tea polyphenols, that include flavonoids. Polyphenols—including flavonoids—are powerful antioxidants, which are critical to your health because they act as a kind of defense system for your body. Antioxidants help neutralize destructive forms of oxygen or nitrogen known as free radicals, which are unstable molecules that steal electrons from the molecules of healthy cells. Antioxidants protect cells by binding to free radicals and neutralizing them before they can damage DNA or other cell components. In addition to their antioxidant activity, flavonoids can also help regulate how cells function.

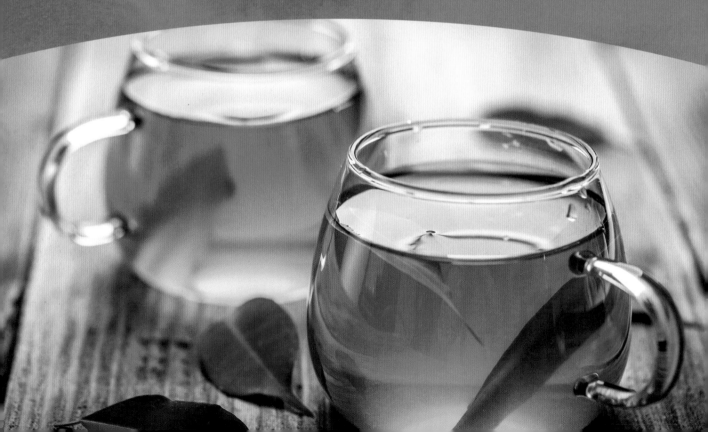

> *Better to be deprived of food for three days than tea for one.*
>
> —CHINESE PROVERB

Tea is particularly high in flavonoids, higher than many vegetables or fruits. Tea provides about 83 percent of the total intake of flavonoids in the American adult diet, followed by citrus fruit juices (4 percent), and wine (2 percent), according to a 2007 study in the *American Journal of Nutrition*.

Among the foods and beverages tested, black tea provides the largest number of flavonols—a type of flavonoid—in the U.S. diet (32 percent), according to scientists in the Nutrient Data Laboratory at the USDA Agricultural Research Service.

FLAVONOID LEVELS IN TEA—THE UPS AND DOWNS

There are thousands of flavonoids, but one type called catechins has been in the limelight in recent decades. Of special interest is epigallocatechin gallate (EGCG), a compound that is thought to be an especially powerful antioxidant. Researchers believe EGCG may be a key to the development of new drugs or complementary therapies to treat disease. Other tea catechins called epicatechin (EC), epigallocatechin (EGC), and epicatechin gallate (ECG) are also being investigated. Green and white tea have an abundance of EGCG—more than black or oolong, both of which contain many other types of antioxidants that scientists have studied for their healing benefits. In fact, a cup of green tea has more catechins than an apple.

Different kinds of tea have different kinds of flavonoids. That's important because different flavonoids appear to play different roles in protecting the body from disease. While green tea has the most EGCG, black and oolong teas have more of the complex flavonoids called thearubigins and teaflavins. These are formed during the fermentation process and have been found to offer protection against heart attacks and cardiovascular disease.

Black, green, and oolong teas are a good source of the flavonols kaempferol, quercetin, and myricetin, which help relax blood vessels, improve blood flow, and reduce inflammation in cells, among other benefits.

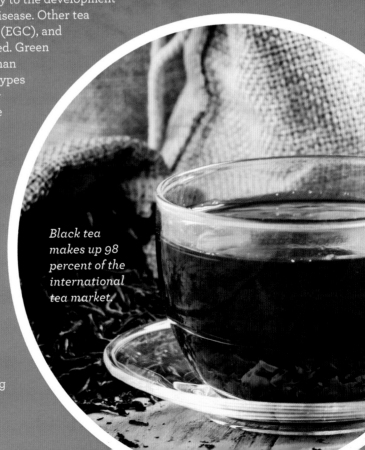

Black tea makes up 98 percent of the international tea market.

FLUORIDE

The tea plant absorbs fluoride from the soil and from fertilizers, and the mineral accumulates in the leaves over time. The amount of fluoride in brewed tea varies depending on the type of leaf, the brewing time, and the amount of fluoride in the water. In general, higher quality tea, which is made from younger leaves, contains less fluoride. That means white tea, which is made from the very youngest, unopened leaf buds, is unlikely to have much fluoride at all. Of the more common teas, oolong tea has the least fluoride (0.1–0.2 mg per 8 ounces) while black tea has the most (0.2–0.5 mg per 8 ounces). Green tea is in between the two with 0.3–0.4 mg per 8 ounces. Brick tea, a lower grade of tea made from older leaves and stems, has the most fluoride of all (0.5–1.7 mg per 8 ounces), but it is rarely consumed in the United States. The fluoride content provided above does not include the water in which the tea is brewed. In adequate doses, fluoride strengthens both teeth and bones, protecting against cavities and bone density loss. The U.S. Institute of Medicine recommends that adults get 3 to 4 mg of fluoride per day, and that children get 0.7 to 2 mg per day, depending on their age and body weight.

A recent Japanese study found that rinsing the mouth with green tea prevented the production of acid as well as the growth of bacteria that cause cavities. And a small study in Italy found that drinking black tea helped prevent cavities and plaque.

CAFFEINE

Caffeine is a stimulant that increases heart rate, makes you alert, and revs up metabolism. All *Camellia sinensis* teas naturally contain caffeine, but the amount varies depending on the grade and type of tea, whether it is brewed from loose leaves or a tea bag, and how long it is brewed. Black tea has the most caffeine (42 to 72 mg per 8 ounces) while green, white, and oolong teas have less (9 to 50 mg per 8 ounces). Compare those amounts with the caffeine content of coffee, which has 110 to 140 mg per 8 ounces. Decaffeinated teas only have 1 to 4 mg per 8 ounces.

A HEALING CUP—
TEA AND DISEASE

Research has begun to prove what the ancients divined: Tea does have properties that can help prevent or lower the risk of certain diseases. It's the constituents in tea that we discussed at the beginning of the chapter, particularly the flavonoids and other polyphenols, that give tea its healing power. All types of tea—black, green, oolong, and white—as well as tea extracts, have been studied, and each has its own particular disease-fighting and disease-preventing constituents.

Evidence supporting the health benefits of tea consumption continues to mount, but the following is what research shows thus far to be tea's contributions to good health.

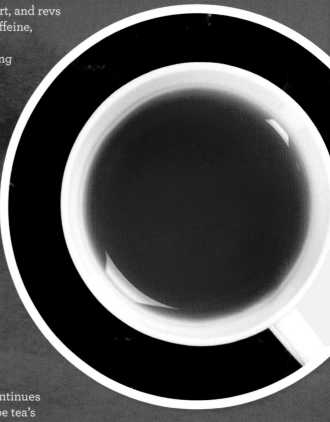

HEART DISEASE

Heart disease is the leading cause of death in the United States, but tea drinking may be able to shrink that number. Some research shows that black and green tea both help fight the development of cardiovascular diseases including heart attack and stroke. A number of studies have shown that tea consumption can slow down the progression of atherosclerosis, or hardening of the arteries. Tea has also been shown to lower LDL, or "bad," cholesterol and relax blood vessels, which can lower blood pressure. These are all important steps in preventing heart disease.

A 2002 University of North Carolina statistical review of many different tea studies found that people who drink three or more cups of black tea each day have a moderately reduced risk (about 11 percent) of heart disease and stroke compared to those who do not drink tea. The results of a Saudi national study, published in 2003, show a significantly lower incidence of heart disease among those who drank more than six cups of black tea per day compared to those who did not, even after adjusting for other risk factors such as smoking and age.

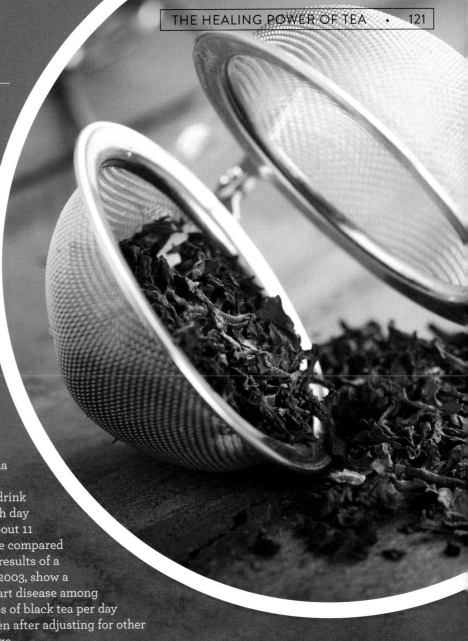

Green tea seems to offer cardiovascular protection, too. An 11-year study that followed the tea consumption of more than 40,000 people in Japan found that people who drank more than five cups of green tea a day were 26 percent less likely to die of cardiovascular disease during the study period and 16 percent less likely to die from any cause at all.

Another large study of overall diet in Japan found that people who drank green tea in addition to eating a traditional Japanese diet of fruits, vegetables, soy, and seaweed had a significantly lower incidence of cardiovascular disease than those whose diets were higher in red meat and dairy and lower in tea. This was evident despite the healthier group's tendency to consume more sodium and to have high blood pressure.

CANCER

All kinds of tea have been studied for their effects against various cancers, both in laboratory and human studies, with mixed results. Scientists caution that it's too soon to tell for sure if tea will help battle cancer.

The best results have been seen in the laboratory. EGCG, the powerful antioxidant most abundant in green tea, inhibits cancer in a number of ways in lab experiments. It binds to free radicals and neutralizes them before they can damage healthy cells. It also seems to slow, and even reduce, the size of tumors in some animal models. There's also evidence that EGCG reduces the growth of new blood cells that would feed tumors, at least in lab experiments. And it seems that EGCG can inhibit the production of COX-2, an enzyme produced by tumors that causes inflammation and can lead to further tumor growth.

Laboratory studies are a first step, but the findings aren't always replicated in human studies. Studies of people who drink green, black, or oolong tea don't always show a clear-cut benefit. Some studies show a protective effect against certain cancers, while others do not. The differences in these studies may be explained by the variations in overall diet, environment, and genetics among the study groups. And since no two pots of tea are exactly the same, the participants aren't taking in a standardized number of flavonoids.

DIABETES

Observational studies conducted in large populations have shown that people who consume green tea have a lower risk of developing type 2 diabetes, the most common form of diabetes among adults. A couple of smaller studies suggest that black and oolong teas may be preventive as well.

IMMUNE SYSTEM

Green tea may help prevent rheumatoid arthritis or other immune system disorders. Researchers have been prompted to look at green tea's potential because the incidence of these health problems is significantly lower in China and Japan, the two leading consumers of green tea.

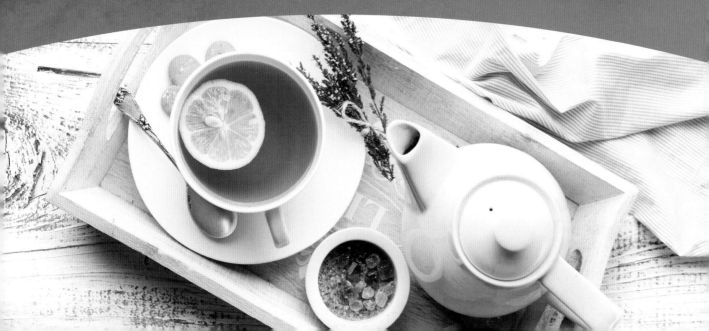

Tea may also boost the body's power to fight bacterial infections. A small study at Brigham and Women's Hospital in 2003 found that patients who drank 20 ounces of black tea per day for two weeks had stronger resistance to infections than did a similar group of coffee drinkers. In fact, the immune system's output of an infection-fighting substance called interferon gamma was doubled or tripled. Researchers noted that the amino acid responsible for the effect, L-theanine, is also present in green and oolong teas.

MIND YOUR MEMORY

In ancient China, green tea was thought to provide mental clarity, and now evidence of that is turning up in laboratory studies. Experiments on mice and rat brain cells show that green tea antioxidants seem to prevent the formation of an Alzheimer's-related protein, beta-amyloid, which accumulates in the brain as plaque and leads to memory loss. This finding has been duplicated in a number of other cell-culture experiments. In one of these types of studies the antioxidants in black tea also were protective, although not as much as those in green tea.

In humans, green tea has been associated with a lower risk of dementia and memory loss. A Japanese study published in 2006 in the *American Journal of Clinical Nutrition* surveyed more than 1,000 people older than age 70. Those who drank two or more cups a day of green tea were half as likely to develop dementia and memory loss as those who drank fewer than two cups per week. This effect was much weaker for black and oolong teas.

SLIMMING DOWN WITH TEA

Ads touting green tea's ability to help you lose weight may be more than hype. A growing body of research suggests a possible benefit, not just for green tea but for oolong as well. A study reported in the journal *Obesity* in 2007 found that 31 healthy, lean young participants who drank a mixture of green tea catechins, calcium, and caffeine for three days burned 4.6 percent more calories than when they drank plain water. Although this wasn't a huge increase in metabolism, the researchers said it could be enough to help someone succeed at controlling their weight, especially in combination with a healthy diet and exercise. The effects in older, more overweight people have not been demonstrated.

The ancient Chinese believed oolong tea helped control body weight, and at least one modern study suggests this, too. In 2001, researchers at the USDA Agricultural Research Service gave 12 male volunteers four separate oolong tea formulas (full-strength tea, colored water with the equivalent amount of caffeine to full-strength tea, half-strength tea, and plain colored water) for three days in a row. They measured the men's energy expenditure before and after the experiment and found that the participants burned, on average, 67 more calories per day when they drank tea instead of water. Even more significant to the researchers was that fat oxidation was significantly higher (12 percent) after the full-strength-tea consumption than after the plain-water consumption. The beverage containing water plus caffeine also increased energy expenditure and fat oxidation compared to water alone. It is not clear, then, whether the effects of the tea were due solely to its caffeine content. The researchers tentatively concluded that a component other than caffeine played a role.

Despite these positive studies, others show little or no effect of tea on weight loss. Green tea is a healthy drink, and evidence suggests it might help you burn a few calories, but exercise and a healthful diet are still the best way to slim down.

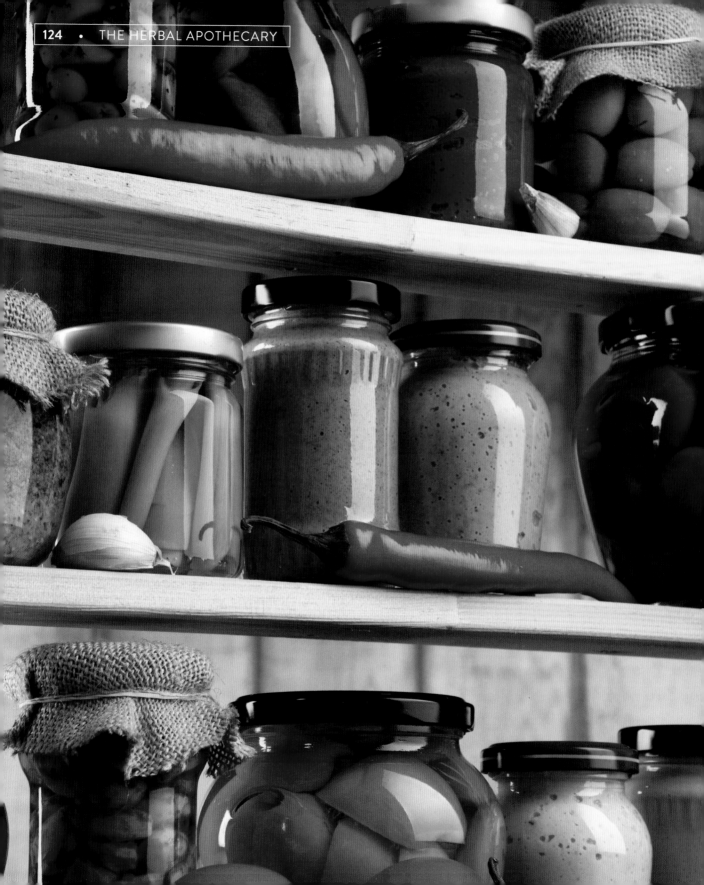

THE COMMON CUPBOARD

Don't forget your own kitchen—it's already filled with superfoods that will keep you healthy and sometimes reverse health issues you already have. Food is medicine, as they say, so let's take a look at some of the healthy kitchen standouts you're sure to have on hand already.

APRICOTS

Apricots are chock-full of beta-carotene and other carotenoids, the beautiful pigments that color fruits and vegetables. There are more than 400 different kinds and most, if not all, are antioxidants. Some of apricots' carotenoids such as lycopene, gamma carotene, and cryptoxanthin pack a much more powerful antioxidant punch than does beta-carotene, making them even more useful as cancer-fighters.

Apricots contain some vitamin C, which keeps skin and tissues supple and healthy. Vitamin C also has antioxidant properties and supports the immune system, helping the body make substances to fight off illnesses. Apricots are rich in fiber for their size, especially soluble fiber. This heart-healthy fiber lowers blood cholesterol levels and helps people with diabetes maintain stable blood sugar levels. You can count on apricots' insoluble fiber to keep the colon free of toxins and your bowels moving regularly.

Dried apricots, because they are concentrated, are a good source of iron. Three and a half ounces provide about 47 percent of the recommended dietary allowance for men and 31 percent for women.

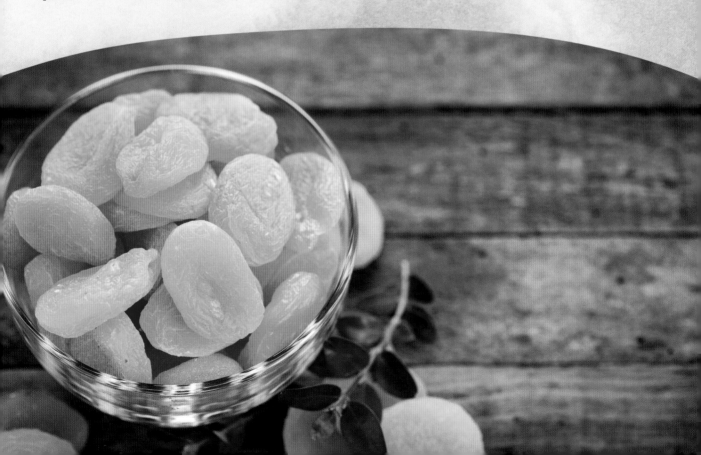

BEETS AND BEET GREENS

Beets have long been valued for their rich flavor, sweet taste, and vital nutrients. Beets are particularly rich in the B vitamin folate, which is essential for preventing a certain type of anemia and birth defects that affect the spinal column. Folate may prevent cancer, too, by protecting the DNA in cells from damage and mutation. Mutated cells are often the beginning of cancerous cells. Beets contain a wealth of soluble and insoluble fiber—great for keeping the intestines toned.

Beet greens are packed with healing nutrients, including disease fighters such as vitamin A and potassium. Calcium, too, is available from this nutritional powerhouse. The variety of vitamins and minerals make these leafy greens an all-around heart-healthy vegetable. If you are trying to quit smoking, beet greens may become your new friend. Just like soil, human blood has a pH value, and a slightly alkaline condition apparently triggers nicotine to stay in the blood longer, reducing the craving for more cigarettes. At the University of Nebraska Medical Center, researchers found that beet greens push blood pH slightly toward the alkaline side. Smokers who are trying to quit might try eating plenty of alkaline foods to reduce their need for nicotine. Other high-alkaline foods include dandelion greens, spinach, and raisins.

Beet greens are abundant in folate. This B vitamin protects lung cells from damage that can trigger cancer, so smokers get a double dose of prevention from these greens.

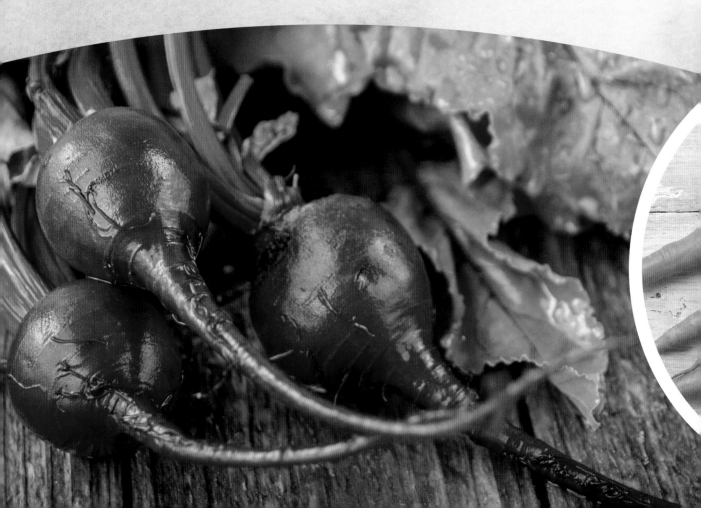

CABBAGE

Cabbage juice has been used to prevent and heal ulcers for more than 40 years. Current research at the Stanford University School of Medicine revealed that when ulcer patients drank 1 quart of raw cabbage juice each day, ulcers in the stomach and small intestine healed in about five days. People who ate cabbage instead of drinking the juice also had faster healing times than those who did not eat cabbage.

Cabbage accomplishes this by killing bacteria, including the ulcer-causing *H. pylori*. Secondly, it contains a phytochemical called gefarnate that coaxes stomach cells into making extra mucus, which protects the stomach wall from digestive acid.

As a cruciferous family member, cabbages of all types help fight the war on cancer. Two types of darker-colored cabbage—savoy and bok choy—also provide beta-carotene.

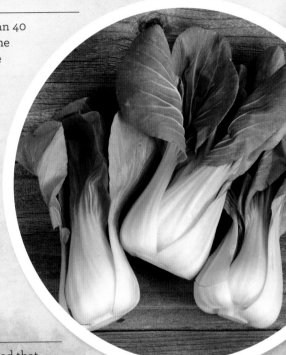

CARROTS

Modern science has determined that carrots do much more than help eyesight. They offer a natural defense against heart disease, strokes, cancer, cataracts, and even constipation. And it only takes one carrot a day to dramatically reduce health risks. Studies show that a humble carrot a day reduced the risk of heart attack in women by 22 percent, and a carrot a day five days per week reduced women's stroke risk by 68 percent. Women who did have a stroke were less likely to die or be disabled. Scientists believe that phytochemicals (plant chemicals) in carrots protect oxygen-deprived brain cells.

Lung cancer risk plunged by 60 percent in a different study when a carrot was eaten twice a week. The incidence of other cancers, such as stomach, mouth, and those of the female reproductive tract, are also decreased by eating carrots.

One raw carrot or ½ cup cooked carrots supplies two to three times the recommended daily intake of vitamin A in the form of protective beta-carotene. Carrots contain other carotenoids that are even more potent cancer warriors than beta-carotene: alpha-carotene, gamma-carotene, lycopene, and lutein.

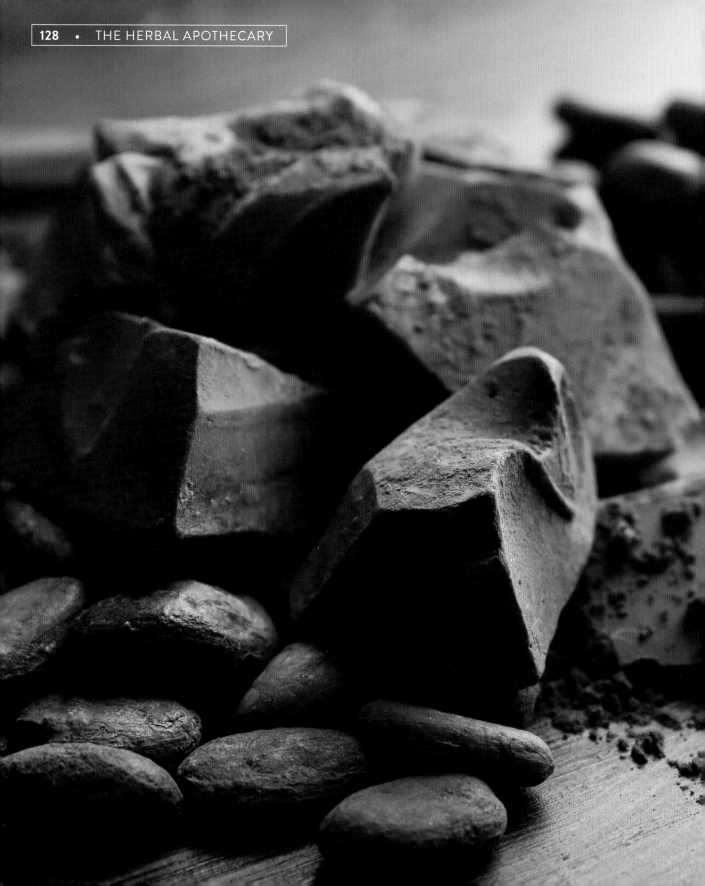

CHOCOLATE

Chocolate comes from the seeds of the fruit of the cacao tree. The seeds are fermented, dried, and roasted. Cacao, as the bitter dark stuff is known at this stage, is the source of chocolate's many amazing health benefits. Researchers have discovered that cacao is rich in antioxidant phytochemicals, especially a type called polyphenols. Polyphenols are found not only in chocolate products but in fruits and fruit juices, vegetables, tea, coffee, red wine, and some grains and legumes. And the available research seems to strongly point to some role for polyphenols in preventing a variety of diseases.

The largest and most important class of polyphenols are the flavonoids. More than 5,000 flavonoids have been identified so far, and they have begun to attract a lot of attention for their potential health benefits. Among the flavonoid-rich foods that have shown promise lately are strawberries and blueberries, garlic, red wine, and tea. But these plant foods can't hold a candle to cacao-rich cocoa products when it comes to flavonoid content and antioxidant power. Cocoa, for example, has almost twice the antioxidants found in red wine and close to three times the antioxidants in green tea, when compared in equal amounts.

One of the flavonoids in cacao (known as cocoa flavonoids, or cocoa polyphenols) gaining a particular reputation for healing is epicatechin. One Harvard Medical School scientist is so impressed by epicatechin's effects that he has said it should be considered essential for human health and, therefore, raised to the status of a vitamin. He's also stated that the health benefits of epicatechin are so striking that it may rival penicillin and anesthesia in terms of importance to public health.

Flavonoids, however, also give natural chocolate a very bitter taste. So in an effort to please their sweet-toothed consumers, chocolate manufacturers have traditionally tried to tame that natural bitterness by removing flavonoids and/or masking their taste. Nearly every step of the typical processes that turn cacao beans into chocolate and cocoa—including fermenting, roasting, and Dutching—removes some of the flavonoids. Likewise, adding ingredients such as sugar and milk to chocolate or cocoa—again, to mask or replace bitterness—leaves less room for cocoa solids and therefore results in a lower-flavonoid product. Therefore, when looking for products that have the most health benefits, opt for cocoa and chocolates with the most cocoa solids and the least sugar and milk. Better yet, look for cacao powder, found in health food stores and some grocery stores.

Blood pressure. Multiple studies have shown that eating dark chocolate helps individuals lower mild high blood pressure. For example, a 2007 review of ten different studies of chocolate's effects on blood pressure indicated that flavonoid-rich cocoa and chocolate can indeed have a place in a blood-pressure lowering diet as long as the total calorie count of the diet stays the same. On average, chocolate products lowered systolic pressure by 4 to 5 points and diastolic by 2 to 3—enough to lower heart disease risk by 10 percent and stroke risk by 20 percent. The scientists did note, however, that because the studies were short term, it's unclear if the same effects would occur with consumption of small amounts of chocolate over the long term.

Blood vessel function. In studies that were published in the *Journal of the American College of Cardiology* in 2005 and in *Proceedings of the National Academy of Sciences* in 2006, researchers demonstrated that the flavonoids (specifically, epicatechin) in flavonoid-rich cocoa beverages trigger the production of a natural substance called nitric oxide. Nitric oxide, in turn, causes blood vessels to dilate (relax), allowing for smoother blood flow. Flavonoid-rich cocoa may even benefit the compromised blood-vessel function of smokers, to the point of potentially reversing some of the vessel damage caused by smoking. And scientists have also discovered a similar improvement in blood vessel health in mildly obese adults who add dark chocolate cocoa to their diet.

Blood clotting. When the inner walls of arteries are narrowed by deposits of cholesterol and other debris, a blood clot can easily shut down the blood supply to the organ fed by the artery—leading to a heart attack, stroke, or other serious tissue damage. For that reason, many heart patients are prescribed a daily 81 milligram aspirin tablet, which thins their blood and helps prevent clots. In a 2002 study, scientists were astonished to find that drinking a flavonoid-rich cocoa drink could be just as effective as the aspirin at preventing clots. The research found similar reactions to both treatments in a group of 20- to 40-year-olds. Both the cocoa drink and the aspirin kept blood platelets from sticking together and forming clots. The researchers stopped short of suggesting that heart patients who have been prescribed a daily aspirin should drink cocoa instead. (And you should **NOT** stop taking any medication that has been prescribed for you without first consulting your doctor.) But for people at risk who can't take aspirin every day, it's possible that eating more flavonoid-rich foods could provide similar benefits.

Blood cholesterol. Consuming saturated fat in food can increase total blood-cholesterol levels and, especially, levels of LDL cholesterol, the so-called "bad" form of blood cholesterol. Having too much LDL cholesterol is a risk factor for cardiovascular diseases, including heart attack and stroke, because LDL molecules tend to deposit excess cholesterol on the inner lining of artery walls, narrowing the arteries and setting the stage for a clot to cut off blood flow to the heart or brain. Scientists have discovered, however, that not all LDL molecules are equally damaging. It appears that LDL molecules that have been oxidized are the true culprits in clogging arteries. And that's where cocoa flavonoids may help. First, research suggests cocoa flavonoids may lower LDL levels. For example, in one 2005 study of Italians with high blood pressure, the subjects who consumed flavonoid-rich dark chocolate experienced a 10 percent decrease in their LDL levels, in addition to a drop in blood pressure. Second, two 2001 studies showed that cocoa flavonoids can actually protect LDL molecules from oxidation.

In another bit of good news, scientists have determined that even the fat in cacao isn't so bad. Although cocoa butter is technically a saturated fat, it does not appear to increase LDL levels in the blood the way other saturated fats do. Half the saturated fat in cocoa butter is stearic acid, which studies indicate has a neutral effect on blood cholesterol. Chocolate also contains some oleic acid—the same type of monounsaturated fat found in olive oil, which can actually help lower LDL levels and boost levels of high-density lipoproteins (HDLs)—the "good" form of cholesterol that helps remove excess cholesterol from the blood.

FENNEL

This familiar culinary herb is considered a digestive aid and a carminative, or agent capable of diminishing gas in the intestines. It is recommended for numerous complaints related to excessive gas in the stomach and intestines, including indigestion, cramps, and bloating, as well as for colic in infants. Other Umbelliferae family members such as dill and caraway are also considered carminatives.

As an antispasmodic, fennel acts on the smooth muscle of the respiratory passages as well as the stomach and intestines, which is the reason that fennel preparations are used to relieve bronchial spasms. Since it relaxes bronchial passages, allowing them to open wider, it is sometimes included in asthma, bronchitis, and cough formulas.

Fennel is also known to have an estrogenic effect and has long been used to promote milk production in nursing mothers.

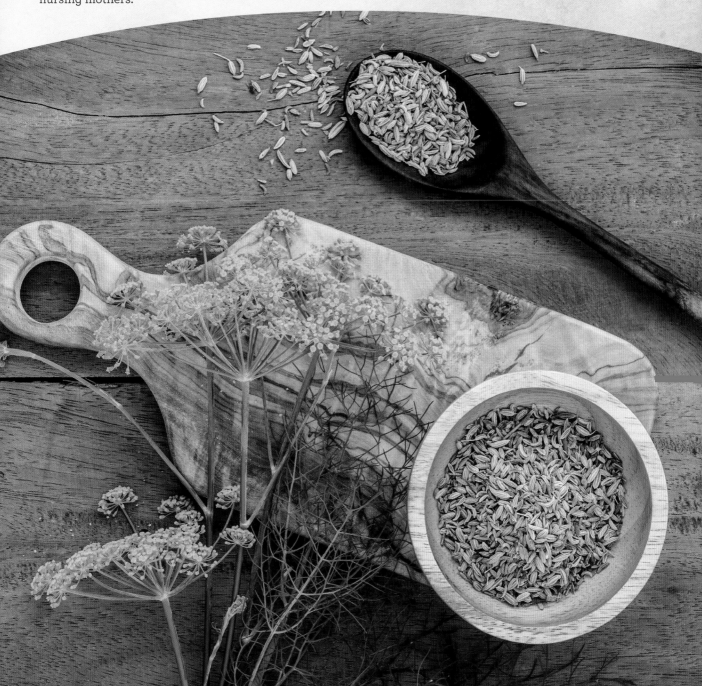

GARLIC

Help for your heart. The tiny garlic clove may play a big role in lowering cholesterol, reducing the risk of heart disease, heart attacks, and stroke. Garlic contains several powerful antioxidants—compounds that prevent oxidation, a harmful process in the body. One of them is selenium, a mineral that is a component of glutathione peroxidase, a powerful antioxidant that the body makes to defend itself. Glutathione peroxidase works with vitamin E to form a superantioxidant defense system.

Other antioxidants in garlic include vitamin C, which helps reduce the damage that LDL cholesterol can cause, and quercetin, a phytochemical. (Phytochemicals are chemical substances found in plants that may have health benefits for people.) Garlic also has trace amounts of the mineral manganese, which is an important component of an antioxidant enzyme called superoxide dismutase.

Arteries benefit greatly from the protection antioxidants provide. And garlic's ability to stop the oxidation of cholesterol may be one of the many ways it protects heart health. Garlic also appears to help prevent calcium from binding with other substances that lodge themselves in plaque. In a UCLA Medical Center study, 19 people were given either a placebo or an aged garlic extract that contained S-allylcysteine, one of garlic's sulfur-rich compounds, for one year. The placebo group had a significantly greater increase in their calcium score (22.2 percent) than the group that received the aged garlic extract (calcium score of 7.5 percent). The results of this small pilot study suggest that aged garlic extract may inhibit the rate of coronary artery calcification.

Research suggests that garlic can help make small improvements in blood pressure by increasing the blood flow to the capillaries, which are the tiniest blood vessels. The chemicals in garlic achieve this by causing the capillary walls to open wider and reducing the ability of blood platelets to stick together and cause blockages. Reductions are small—10 mmHg (millimeters of mercury, the unit of measurement for blood pressure) or less. This means if your blood pressure is 130 over 90 mmHg, garlic might help lower it to 120 over 80 mmHg. That's a slight improvement, but, along with some simple lifestyle adjustments, such as getting more exercise, garlic might help move your blood pressure out of the danger zone.

OXIDATION

Oxidation is related to oxygen, a vital element to every aspect of our lives, so why is oxidation so harmful? Think about when rust accumulates on your car or garden tools and eventually destroys the metal. That rust is an example of oxidation. Similarly, when your body breaks down glucose for energy, free radicals are produced. These free radicals start oxidizing—and damaging—cellular tissue. It's as if your bloodstream and blood vessels are "rusting out."

Antioxidants destroy free radicals, including those that are products of environmental factors, such as ultraviolet rays, air pollutants, cigarette smoke, rancid oils, and pesticides. The body keeps a steady supply of antioxidants ready to neutralize free radicals. Unfortunately, sometimes the number of free radicals can overwhelm the body's antioxidant stock, especially if we're not getting enough of the antioxidant nutrients. When free radicals harm the cells that line your arteries, your body tries to mend the damage by producing a sticky spackle-like substance. However, as mentioned earlier, this substance attracts cholesterol and debris that build up within the arteries, causing progressive plaque formation. The more plaque in your arteries, the more your health is in danger.

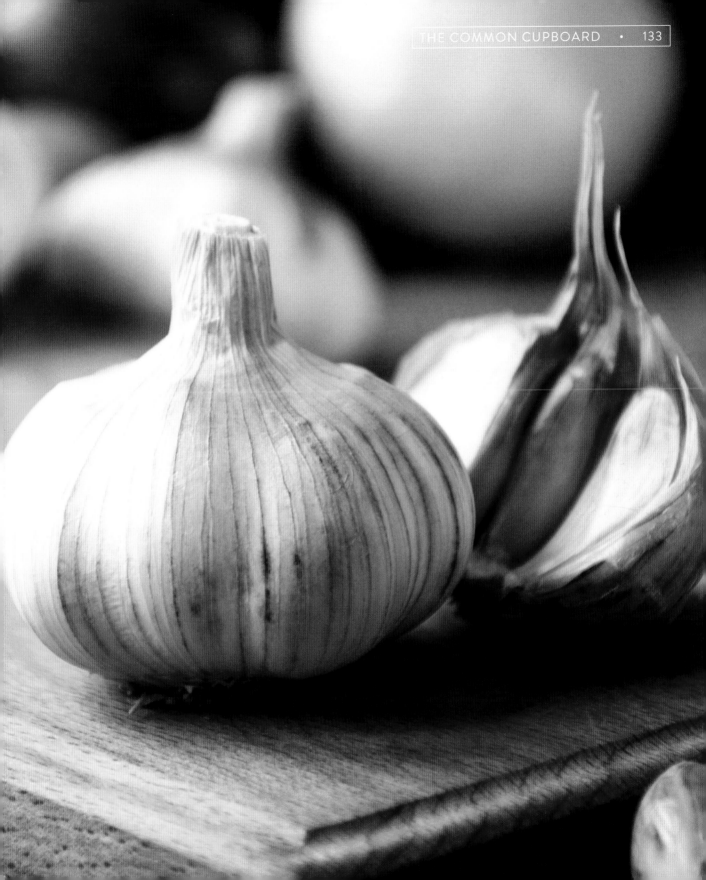

Garlic seems to deserve a spot on the battlefield in the fight against heart disease. Even if its lipid-lowering abilities are less extensive than once thought, it appears that garlic's antioxidant ability helps protect arteries from plaque formation and eventual blockage. Because garlic also appears to increase the nitric oxide in vessels and lower your blood pressure, it becomes even more valuable.

Infection fighter. Garlic's potential to combat heart disease has received a lot of attention, but it should get just as much for its antimicrobial properties. Raw garlic has proven itself since ancient times as an effective killer of bacteria and viruses. We can thank allicin.

Laboratory studies confirm that raw garlic has antibacterial and antiviral properties. Not only does it knock out many common cold and flu viruses but its effectiveness also spans a broad range of both gram-positive and gram-negative bacteria (two major classifications of bacteria), fungus, intestinal parasites, and yeast. Cooking garlic, however, destroys the allicin, so you'll need to use raw garlic to prevent or fight infections.

Eating raw garlic may help combat the pathogens that attack our bodies. Garlic has been used internally as a folk remedy for years, but now the plant is being put to the test scientifically for such uses. So far, its grades are quite good as researchers pit it against a variety of bacteria.

For eons, herbalists loaded soups and other foods with garlic and placed garlic compresses on people's chests to provide relief from colds and chest congestion. Now the Mayo Clinic has stated, "preliminary reports suggest that garlic may reduce the severity of upper respiratory tract infection." The findings have not yet passed the scrutiny of numerous, large, well-designed human studies, so current results are classified as "unclear."

External treatment. Garlic has many uses on the outside of the body, too. Applying a topical solution of raw garlic and water may stop wounds from getting infected. (Simply crush one clove of garlic and mix it with one-third of a cup of clean water. Use the solution within three hours because it will lose its potency over time.) A garlic solution used as a footbath several times a day is traditionally believed to improve athlete's foot.

A study conducted at Bastyr University, a natural health sciences school and research center near Seattle, showed that a garlic oil extract cured all warts it was applied to within two weeks. A water extract of garlic was much less effective, however. In the same study, the garlic oil extract also proved useful in dissolving corns.

Using garlic oil extract appears to work better than the old folk remedy of tying or taping a slice of garlic to a wart. If the slice of garlic is bigger than the wart or moves just a bit, it blisters the healthy surrounding skin (of course, you have the same risk when using wart-removing products that contain acid). Garlic's phytochemical compounds are strong enough to create chemical burns, so always apply externally with caution and do not use on young children. One way you can protect the surrounding healthy skin is to smear petroleum jelly on it before you apply the garlic.

Cancer crusader. Eating as few as two servings of garlic a week might be enough to help protect against colon cancer. Controlled clinical trials will help determine the true extent of garlic's cancer fighting powers. What gives garlic this wonderful gift? Several factors, including antioxidants and those same sulfur-containing agents we've discussed before, including allicin. (Antioxidants help protect cells from damage; continual cell damage can eventually lead to cancer.) Allicin appears to protect colon cells from the toxic effects of cancer-causing agents. For instance, when meat is cooked with garlic, the herb reduces the production of cancer-causing compounds that would otherwise form when meat is grilled at high temperatures.

Garlic's potential ability to decrease *H. pylori* bacteria in the stomach may help prevent gastritis (inflammation of the stomach lining) from eventually evolving into cancer. (*H. pylori* is most famous for its link to stomach ulcers, but it can also cause chronic gastritis.) Numerous studies around the world indicate that garlic's sulfur-containing compounds have the potential to help prevent stomach cancer.

DON'T FORGET ONIONS

Although less research has been done on onions than on garlic, findings show the two have many of the same anti-cancer, cholesterol-lowering properties. A Harvard Medical School study showed that "good" HDL cholesterol climbed significantly when participants ate about half of a medium-sized raw onion each day. Cooked onion did not affect HDL levels. Garlic and onions both contain the smooth-muscle relaxant adenosine. This means that onions, too, may fight high blood pressure. They play a role in preventing blood clots as well, keeping blood platelets from sticking together and quickly dissolving clots that may have already formed. Researchers in India found that when raw or cooked onions were eaten along with fatty foods, the blood's clot-dissolving ability remained intact, which doesn't usually occur after fatty foods are eaten. It's a good idea, then, always to include onions when you eat that occasional high-fat meal. Be aware, though, that onions may cause heartburn to worsen in some people.

Onions have many substances that protect you from cancer. Scallions are particularly effective at fighting stomach cancer. Onions are also good at killing bacteria and viruses, which makes them useful for fending off colds and flu. Studies suggest that the humble onion also helps insulin do its job by decreasing the liver's breakdown of insulin. This is good news for diabetics. Studies in India showed that onions—raw or cooked—help lower blood sugar levels.

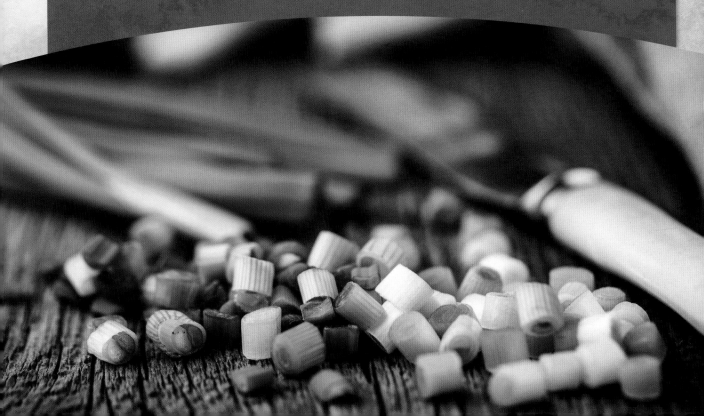

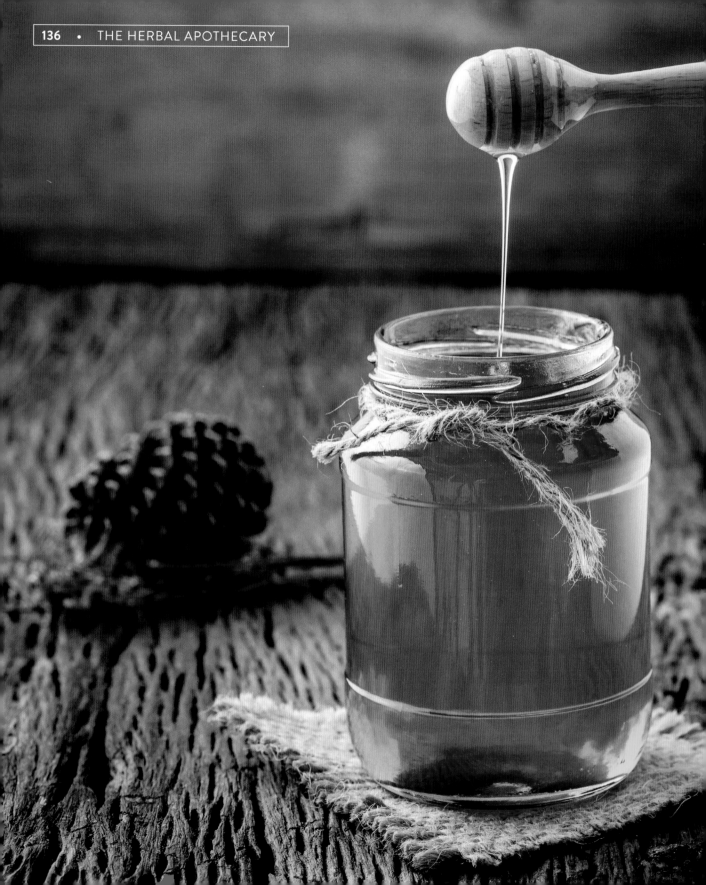

HONEY

Honey is the only food that includes all the nutrients necessary to sustain life. Honey and bee pollen contain water, as well as all 22 minerals and enzymes that the human body needs. Bonus: it's also fat- and cholesterol-free! Honey is a fantastic option for many of life's minor maladies. For example:

- Honey can help wounds heal more rapidly. Apply it directly to a scratch, scrape, or small cut, and let it go to work.

- You may be able to fend off a migraine if you feel one coming on. Just take 1 teaspoon of honey as soon as you feel the warning signs. If it's already too late, take 2 teaspoons of honey with each meal until the headache subsides.

- Obtain relief from a hangover by taking 1 teaspoon of honey every hour until you feel better. The large quantity of fructose found in honey will help speed up the metabolism of alcohol in your system.

Colds, coughs, and sore throats. Help that sore throat—and promote the flow of mucus—by drinking a cup of hot tea mixed with 1 tablespoon of honey and 2 drops of lemon juice. This even works with plain hot water instead of tea! These are good tonics to help ease laryngitis, as well. More throat relief comes when honey soothes and vinegar kills bacteria. Whip up a batch of homemade cough syrup by mixing ¼ cup each of apple cider vinegar and honey. Pour into a bottle or jar that can be sealed tightly. Take 1 tablespoon every 4 hours, shaking well before each dose. Sore throats respond well to this drink: In a glass of water, mix 1 teaspoon of honey, 3 tablespoons of lime juice, and 1 tablespoon of pineapple juice. Sip to obtain soothing relief.

Soothing a sick stomach. Digest this suggestion: a teaspoon or two of honey mixed with milk can help improve digestion. The mixture works well either warm or cold, but some people swear by warm milk. You may also prevent indigestion by taking a spoonful of honey sprinkled with a bit of cinnamon before beginning a meal. Honey taken by itself or mixed with water, milk, or tea can remedy feelings of nausea too.

Advice for a long, healthy life. What me worry? The nutrients found in honey can help you feel calmer when you're experiencing anxiety or nervousness, so mix a spoonful of honey into your oatmeal, yogurt, or cereal to start your day off right. In fact, honey has incredible nutritional value, providing several antioxidants in addition to thiamin, niacin, riboflavin, pantothenic acid, and vitamin B6.

- Don't be down in the dumps! A straight shot of honey mixed into your favorite beverage is known to alleviate symptoms of depression.

- Fight fatigue with a mix of a teaspoon of honey in tepid water. The glucose in honey is quickly absorbed into your bloodstream and your brain, providing a quick pick-me-up.

- Honey has been known to boost athletic performance. Enjoy a tablespoon before your next workout.

- Take the edge off your appetite. Thirty minutes before each meal, drink a mixture of 2 teaspoons honey in a glass of water.

- Cool it down. Mix a teaspoon of honey and a teaspoon of vinegar in a glass of tepid water to treat heat exhaustion. This mixture of honey and vinegar is such a potent combination it can also be beneficial in lowering blood pressure, reducing the effects of eczema, and treating brittle fingernails and toenails.

HORSERADISH

Have you ever bitten into a roast beef sandwich and thought your nose was on fire? The sandwich probably contained horseradish. Even a tiny taste of this potent condiment seems to go straight to your nose. Whether on a sandwich or in a herbal preparation, horseradish clears sinuses, increases facial circulation, and promotes expulsion of mucus.

Horseradish is helpful for sinus infections because it encourages your body to get rid of mucus. One way a sinus infection starts is with the accumulation of thick mucus in the sinuses: Stagnant mucus is the perfect breeding ground for bacteria to multiply and cause a painful infection. Horseradish can help thin and move out older, thicker mucus accumulations. If you are prone to developing sinus infections, try taking horseradish the minute you feel a cold coming on. Herbalists also recommend horseradish for common colds, influenza, and lung congestion. Incidentally, don't view the increase of mucus production after horseradish therapy as a sign your cold is worsening. The free-flowing mucus is a positive sign that your body is ridding itself of wastes.

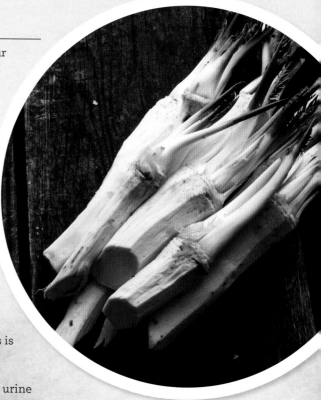

Horseradish has a mild natural antibiotic effect and it stimulates urine production. Thus, it has been used for urinary infections.

MINT

Mint is one of the most reliable home remedies for an upset stomach. Grandmas have been handing out mints for centuries to treat indigestion, flatulence, and colic. The two types of mint you're most likely to encounter are spearmint and peppermint. Although they once were considered the same plant, peppermint actually is a natural hybrid of spearmint. It's also the more potent of the herbs.

Peppermint owes part of its healing power to an aromatic oil called menthol. Spearmint's primary active constituent is a similar but weaker chemical called carvone. Oil of peppermint contains up to 78 percent menthol. Menthol encourages bile (a fluid secreted by the liver) to flow into the duodenum, where it promotes digestion. Menthol also is a potent antispasmodic; in other words, it calms the action of muscles, particularly those of the digestive system.

Menthol's medicinal value has been borne out in numerous studies with animals and with humans. German and Russian studies show that peppermint not only helps to stimulate bile secretion but also may prevent stomach ulcers. The potent oil is also capable of killing myriad microorganisms that are associated with digestive and other problems. Recent studies, moreover, suggest that menthol may be useful in treating irritable bowel syndrome, a common but hard-to-treat digestive disorder in which the bowel contracts, causing a crampy type of adult colic.

MELONS

Melons come in a wide variety of shapes, sizes, and flavors, yet have certain healing nutrients in common. Their high levels of potassium benefit the heart. Some melons have health-boosting phytochemicals and top-notch amounts of vitamins C and A. Orange-fleshed melons, such as cantaloupe, are high in beta-carotene. One cup of melon cubes supplies nearly everyone's daily requirement for vitamin A. When studying endometrial cancer, researchers at the University of Alabama reported that women who did not have this cancer had eaten at least one food high in beta-carotene, such as cantaloupe, every day. The women who had endometrial cancer had eaten less than one betacarotene food per week.

Watermelon's red pulp is teeming with a different carotenoid, lycopene. Lycopene is even more potent than beta-carotene at doing away with free radicals, those damaging molecules that can be the culprits in heart disease, cancer, and cataracts. High intakes of lycopene, though not watermelon itself as yet, are linked to a decreased incidence of prostate cancer.

OATS

You might think oatmeal is the most boring bowl of breakfast food around, but oats are a fantastic source of healing nourishment. They contain starches, proteins, vitamins, and minerals, and though they contain some fat, they are low in saturated fat, which makes them a healthy choice. A serving of hot oat bran cereal provides about 4 grams of dietary fiber (health professionals recommend we consume 20 to 35 grams of fiber each day). Some types of dietary fiber bind to cholesterol, and since this form of fiber is not absorbed by the body, neither is the cholesterol. A number of clinical trials have found that regular consumption of oat bran reduces blood cholesterol levels in just one month. High fiber diets may also reduce the risk of colon and rectal cancer.

Oats have been used topically to heal wounds and various skin rashes and diseases. The familiar sticky-but-smooth consistency of cooked oats is emulated in many oat products; as a result they have mucilaginous, demulcent, and soothing qualities. Soaps and various bath and body products made from oats are readily available. Oatmeal baths are wonderful for soothing dry, flaky skin or allaying itching in cases of poison oak and chicken pox.

Because oats are believed to have a calming effect, herbalists recommend them to help ease the frustration and anxiety that often accompany nicotine and drug withdrawal. Oats contain the alkaloid gramine, which has been credited with mild sedative properties. Scientists have conducted clinical trials to determine whether oats may help treat drug addiction or reduce nicotine craving, but the evidence is inconclusive.

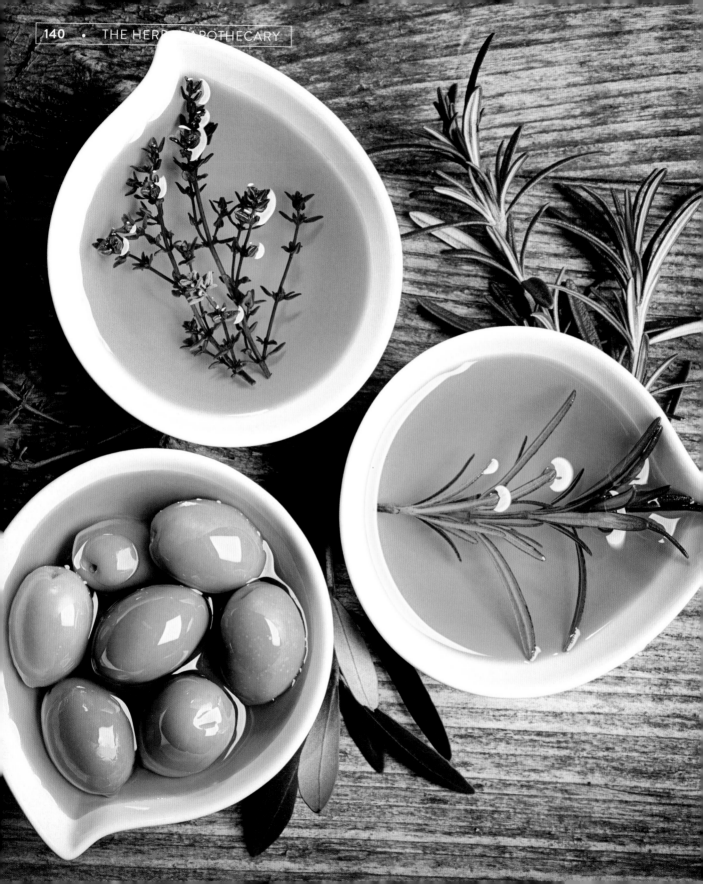

OLIVE OIL

A diet that is rich in olive oil has enhanced the health of people living in the Mediterranean region for thousands of years. Within the past century, however, olive oil's benefits have also been scientifically investigated, acknowledged, and proclaimed across the globe.

There are two important polyunsaturated fats that are essential for human health, but the body cannot make them. This means we must get them from the foods we eat. These two essential fatty acids are alpha-linolenic acid, an omega-3 fatty acid, and linoleic acid, an omega-6 fatty acid. The body gets both from olive oil. Omega-3 oils are the healthiest. They are part of a group of substances called prostaglandins that help keep blood cells from sticking together, increase blood flow, and reduce inflammation. This makes omega-3 oils useful in preventing cardiovascular disease as well as inflammatory conditions, such as arthritis.

FAT FACTS

Some fats, especially olive oil, have more healthful properties than others, so to make the right choices, it's important to know the differences among the various kinds. Let's review the four types of dietary fats, also known as fatty acids.

Monounsaturated fat. This is the healthiest type of fat. It promotes heart health and might help prevent cancer and a host of other ailments. Monounsaturated fat helps lower "bad" LDL cholesterol levels without negatively affecting the "good" HDL cholesterol. Olive oil, peanut oil, canola oil, and avocados are rich in healthy monounsaturated fat.

Polyunsaturated fat. Polyunsaturated fat is moderately healthy. It lowers LDL cholesterol, which is good, but it also reduces levels of artery-clearing HDL cholesterol. Polyunsaturated fat is usually liquid at room temperature and is the predominant type of fatty acid in soybean oil, safflower oil, corn oil, and several other vegetable oils. Olive oil contains some polyunsaturated fat.

Saturated fat. This fat is unhealthy because the body turns it into artery-clogging cholesterol, which is harmful to your heart. Saturated fat is mostly found in animal products and is solid at room temperature. It is the white fat you see along the edge or marbled throughout a piece of meat and is the fat in the skin of poultry. It is also "hidden" in whole milk and foods made from whole milk, as well as in tropical oils such as coconut oil. Dietitians recommend that people eat only small amounts of saturated fat.

Trans fat. Trans fat is the worst type of fat; you're best off avoiding it. Most trans fat is manufactured by forcing hydrogen into liquid polyunsaturated fat in a process called hydrogenation. The process can create a solid fat product—margarine is made this way. Hydrogenation gives foods that contain trans fats a longer shelf life and helps stabilize their flavors, but your body pays a big price.

Omega-6 oils are healthy, too, but they are not quite as helpful as omega-3's. Omega-6's can help form prostaglandins that are similarly beneficial to the ones produced by omega 3's, but they can also produce harmful prostaglandins. The unfavorable prostaglandins increase blood-cell stickiness and promote cardiovascular disease, and they also appear to be linked to the formation of cancer. To encourage your body to make beneficial prostaglandins from omega-6 oils, you should decrease the amount of animal fats you eat. Too many animal fats tend to push your body into using omega-6 oils to make the unfavorable prostaglandins rather than the helpful ones.

The research is inconclusive about how much omega-6 you should eat compared to the amount of omega-3. Many researchers suggest consuming one to four times more omega-6's than omega-3's. However, the typical American eats anywhere from 11 to 30 times more omega-6's than omega-3's.

The U.S. Dietary Reference Intakes for essential fatty acids recommends the consumption of omega-6 and omega-3 fats in a ratio of 10-to-1. This means consuming ten times more omega-6's than omega-3's. Lucky for us, nature provided that exact ratio of fat in each little olive. The linoleic-to-linolenic ratio is about 10-to-1.

Cholesterol combatant. Olive oil boosts heart health by keeping a lid on cholesterol levels. It lowers total cholesterol, LDL cholesterol, and triglyceride levels. Some studies show that it does not affect HDL cholesterol; others show that it slightly increases HDL levels. A 2002 article in *The American Journal of Medicine* reported that total cholesterol levels decrease an average of 13.4 percent and LDL cholesterol levels drop an average of 18 percent when people replace saturated fat with monounsaturated fat in their diets.

The polyphenolic compounds (types of phytochemicals) in olive oil appear to play a big part in protecting blood vessels. Three polyphenols, oleuropein, tyrosol, and hydroxytyrosol, are believed to be particularly helpful. Numerous studies have shown that polyphenols and monounsaturated fat help keep LDL cholesterol from being oxidized and getting stuck to the inner walls of arteries, which forms the plaque that hampers blood flow.

Polyphenolic compounds are also responsible for protecting two enzymes—glutathione reductase and glutathione peroxidase—that fight free radicals in the body. Without these enzymes, free radicals can damage healthy cells, potentially leading to cancer and other serious health problems.

Cooling inflammation. Inflammation within the body may occur in response to cigarette smoking or eating large amounts of saturated fat and trans fat. In overweight or obese people, excess fat from fat cells can float through the bloodstream and cause inflammation. Although inflammation can help the body, it can also hurt. Certain dietary fats cause more of an inflammatory response than others. Trans fat and the saturated fat in animal foods stimulate inflammation. To a smaller extent, polyunsaturated fat in foods such as safflower oil, sunflower oil, and corn oil trigger inflammation, as well. This is where olive oil helps. Olive oil's phytonutrients—in this case phenolic compounds called squalene, beta-sitosterol, and tyrosol—don't cause the inflammation that other fats do. In fact, consuming olive oil on a regular basis may help decrease the risk of conditions linked to inflammation.

SOY

When you think soy, you probably think tofu. But there's more to soy—and it's worth considering. The evidence linking soy protein and heart-disease prevention was so compelling that the Food and Drug Administration approved a health claim for use on food labels stating: "25 grams of soy protein per day, as part of a diet low in saturated fat and cholesterol, may reduce the risk of heart disease."

For many, getting this much soy in the diet is a challenge. Fortunately, soy foods are more widely available these days, and more versatile, so the choices extend far beyond the traditional tofu and soy milk. For instance, a simple substitution of soy flour for up to 30 percent of all-purpose flour is an easy way to sneak in soy. Soy protein isolate, a powdered form of soy, can be added to a smoothie, sprinkled over cereal, or mixed in a casserole dish. Even easier and especially good for the soy wary are the veggie burgers, energy bars, breakfast cereals, and snack foods made from soy commonly available today.

SPINACH

Spinach's beautiful deep green color is a tip-off that it contains plenty of betacarotene; those orange and red carotene pigments are hiding beneath the dark green chlorophyll. Spinach is also an excellent source of vitamin C, folate, and iron.

Spinach is a cornucopia of cancer fighters. For example, it has triple the amount of lutein and four times the amount of beta-carotene as broccoli. These antioxidants not only help prevent cancer, heart disease, and cataracts, but also boost the immune system. One study found that eating spinach more than twice a week was correlated with reduced risk of breast cancer. This vegetable contains a lot of folate, too. McGill University researchers found that folate improves serotonin levels in the brain, inducing a feeling of well-being. A daily dose of cooked spinach alleviated depression in study participants.

Spinach has the mineral manganese, too, which works with other minerals to strengthen bones. Although spinach is rich in calcium, the body is not able to absorb much of it. That's because spinach contains a compound called oxalic acid that binds with calcium, making it unavailable to the body. People who are prone to developing the most common type of kidney stones will want to limit their intake of spinach because the oxalic acid in this food can promote the formation of stones.

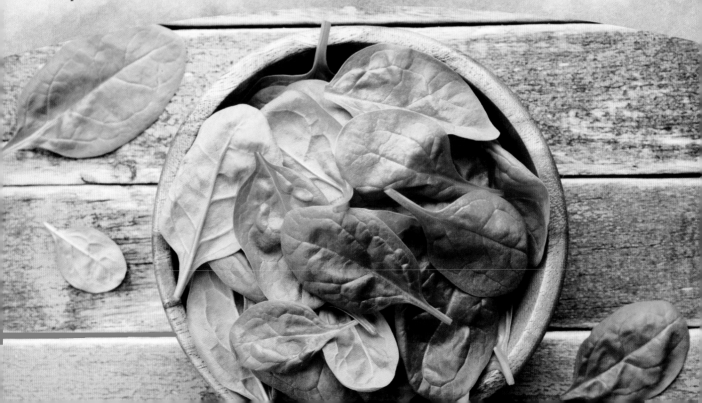

SWEET POTATOES

Sweet potatoes are among the unsung heroes of healthy eating. Nutrient-packed with only a few calories, sweet potatoes support immune function, eyesight, heart health, and cancer protection.

Teeming with beta-carotene, sweet potatoes outrank carrots by far in this healthful nutrient. This beneficial antioxidant wages a continuous battle against free radicals and the diseases they trigger, including cancer. In a study at Harvard University, people who ate ¾ cup cooked sweet potatoes, carrots, or spinach every day (all foods high in beta-carotene) had a 40 percent lower risk of experiencing a stroke. Researchers theorized that this nutrient protects blood cholesterol from undergoing damage from oxygen molecules. Damaged cholesterol begins the artery-clogging process. Other studies show that the more beta-carotene and vitamin A stroke patients have in their bloodstream, the less likely they are to die from the stroke and the more likely they are to make a full recovery.

All this beta-carotene also promotes healthy eyes and vision, since much of it gets turned into vitamin A as the body needs it. This wonder nutrient also works with certain white blood cells, tuning up your immune system to fight off colds, flu, and other illnesses.

Sweet potatoes rank right up with bananas as a source of potassium, the heart-friendly nutrient. These colorful roots are a surprisingly good source of vitamin C.

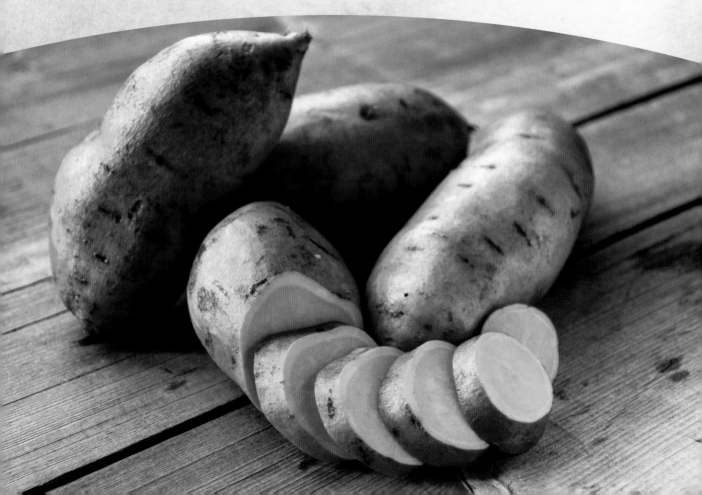

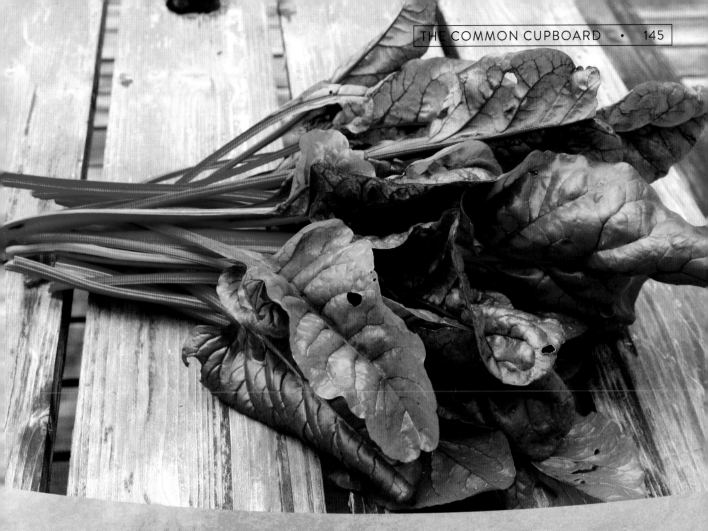

SWISS CHARD

This gently flavored vegetable is chock-full of beta-carotene and its relatives lutein and zeaxanthin, all potent disease fighters and immune boosters. The minerals potassium and magnesium, along with vitamin C, also hide in these beautifully colored, crinkled leaves.

Chard's carotenoids are strong protectors against cancer, heart disease, strokes, cataracts, and maybe even aging. Studies have not addressed whether eating chard confers these same protective benefits. Some researchers believe that antioxidants such as these prevent wear and tear on cells, thus reducing the number of times they need to reproduce within a person's lifetime and possibly slowing down the aging process. Chard also contains reasonable amounts of vitamin C, another antioxidant.

Even though chard is full of calcium and iron, like spinach, it's not very absorbable. Chard, too, is rich in oxalic acid, which binds these minerals.

Some people shy away from chard, having heard that it is high in sodium. One-half cup cooked chard does contain 158 mg of sodium, but this is just a fraction of the daily maximum recommended of 2400 mg. (However, our bodies only need 200 mg per day.) Processed foods such as crackers, chips, canned soups, and lunchmeats have many times more sodium than chard, and often without the plethora of healing nutrients.

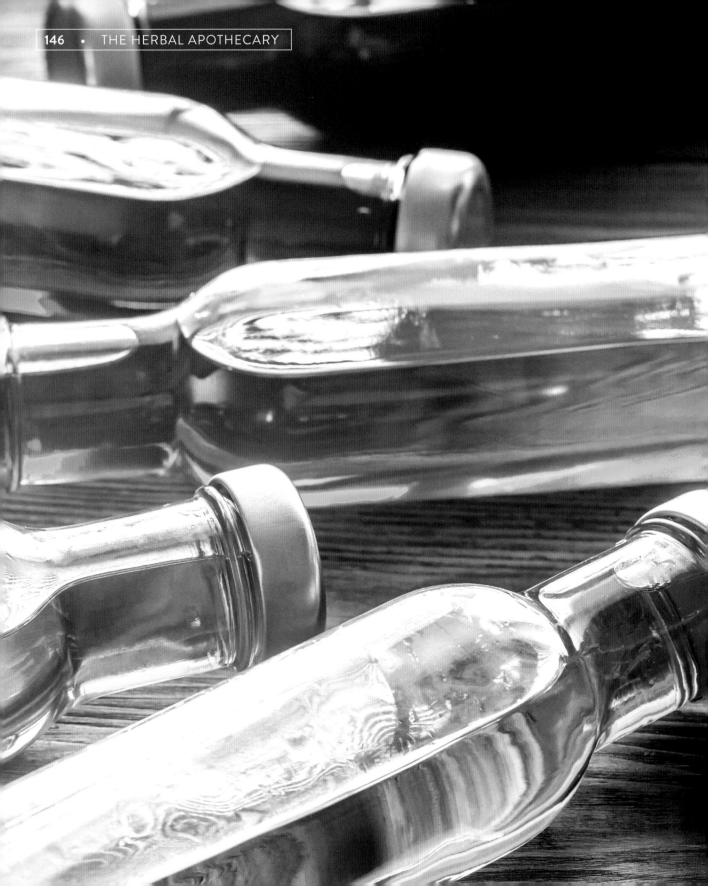

VINEGAR

Vinegar has been valued for its healing properties for about as long as garlic has, and like garlic, vinegar has found its way from the apothecary's shelf to the cook's pot. There seems hardly an ailment that vinegar has not been touted to cure at some point in history. And while science has yet to prove the effectiveness of many of these folk cures, scores of people still praise and value vinegar as a healthful and healing food. Vinegar may well contain yet-to-be-identified phytochemicals that would account for some of the healing benefits that vinegar fans swear by. Scientists continue to discover such beneficial substances in all kinds of foods.

Increasing calcium absorption. Vinegar is high in acetic acid. And acetic acid, like other acids, can increase the body's absorption of important minerals from the foods we eat. Therefore, including apple cider vinegar in meals or possibly even drinking a mild tonic of vinegar and water (up to a tablespoon in a glass of water) just before or with meals might improve your body's ability to absorb the essential minerals locked in foods. Vinegar may be especially useful to women, who generally have a hard time getting all the calcium their bodies need to keep bones strong and prevent the debilitating, bone-thinning disease osteoporosis. Although dietary calcium is most abundant in dairy products such as milk, many women (and men) suffer from a condition called lactose intolerance that makes it difficult or impossible for them to digest the sugar in milk. As a result, they may suffer uncomfortable gastrointestinal symptoms, such as cramping and diarrhea, when they consume dairy products. These women must often look elsewhere to fulfill their dietary calcium needs.

Dark, leafy greens are good sources of calcium, but some of these greens also contain compounds that inhibit calcium absorption. Fortunately for dairy-deprived women (and even those who do drink milk), a few splashes of vinegar or a tangy vinaigrette on their greens may very well allow them to absorb more valuable calcium. Don't you wish all medications were so tasty?

Controlling blood sugar levels. Vinegar has won attention for its potential to help people with type 2 diabetes get a better handle on their disease. Improved control could help them delay or prevent such complications as blindness, impotence, and a loss of feeling in the extremities that may necessitate amputation. Also, because people with diabetes are at increased risk for other serious health problems, such as heart disease, improved control of their diabetes could potentially help to ward off these associated conditions, as well.

Making a healthy diet easier to swallow. Some of our strongest natural weapons against cancer and aging are fruits and vegetables. The antioxidants and phytochemicals they contain seem to hold real promise in lowering our risk of many types of cancer. Their antioxidants also help to protect cells from the free-radical damage that is thought to underlie many of the changes we associate with aging. Protected cells don't wear out and need replacing as often as cells that aren't bathed in antioxidants. Scientists think this continual cell replacement may be at the root of aging.

We're supposed to eat several cups of fruits and vegetables a day. One way to add excitement and variety to all those vegetables is to use vinegar liberally as a seasoning.

- Rice vinegar and a little soy sauce give veggies an Asian flavor or can form the base of an Asian coleslaw.

- Red wine vinegar or white wine vinegar can turn boring vegetables into a quick-and-easy marinated-vegetable salad that's ready to grab out of the refrigerator whenever hunger strikes. Just chop your favorite veggies, put them in a bowl with a marinade of vinegar, herbs, and a dash of olive oil, and let them sit for at least an hour. (You don't need much oil to make the marinade stick to the veggies, so go light, and be sure you choose olive oil.)

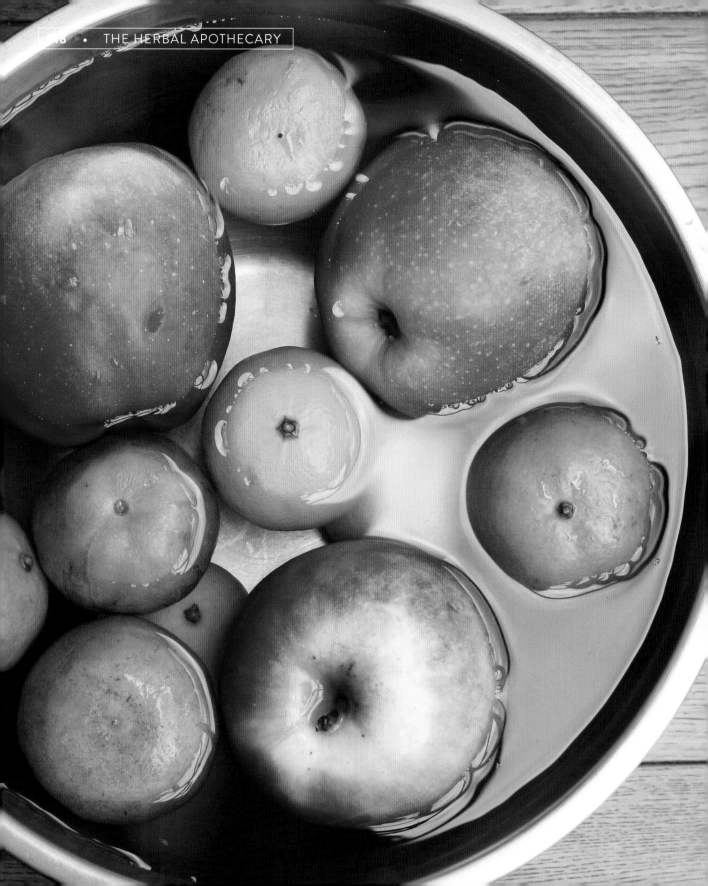

- Toss chopped vegetables in a vinegar-and-olive-oil salad dressing before loading them on skewers and putting them on the grill. The aroma and flavor will actually have your family asking for seconds.

- After steaming vegetables, drizzle a little of your favorite vinegar over them instead of adding butter or salt. They'll taste so good, you may never get to the meat on your plate.

Removing harmful substances from produce. Some people are concerned that eating large amounts of fruits and vegetables may lead to an unhealthy consumption of pesticides and other farm-chemical residues. Vinegar can lend a hand here, too. Washing produce in a mixture of water and vinegar appears to help remove certain pesticides, according to the small amount of research that has been published. Vinegar also appears to be helpful in getting rid of harmful bacteria on fruits and vegetables.

To help remove potentially harmful residues, mix a solution of 10 percent vinegar to 90 percent water (for example, mix one cup of white vinegar in nine cups of water). Then, place the produce in the vinegar solution, let it soak briefly, and then swish it around in the solution. Finally, rinse the produce thoroughly. Do not use this process on tender, fragile fruits, such as berries, that might be damaged in the process or soak up too much vinegar through their porous skins.

Remedies for minor ailments. Vinegar's potential for treating or preventing major medical problems is of interest to almost everyone. But it also has been cherished as a home remedy for some common minor ailments for centuries. Although they're not life-or-death issues, these minor health problems can be uncomfortable, and there is often little modern medicine can offer in the way of a cure. So you may want to give vinegar a shot to determine for yourself if it can help.

Stomach upset: To settle minor stomach upset, try a simple cider vinegar tonic with a meal. Drinking a mixture of a spoonful of vinegar in a glass of water is said to improve digestion and ease minor stomach upset by stimulating digestive juices.

Common cold symptoms: Apple cider vinegar is an age-old treatment for symptoms of the common cold. For a sore throat, mix one teaspoon of apple cider vinegar into a glass of water; gargle with a mouthful of the solution and then swallow it, repeating until you've finished all the solution in the glass. For a natural cough syrup, mix half a tablespoon apple cider vinegar with half a tablespoon honey and swallow. Finally, you can add a quarter-cup of apple cider vinegar to the recommended amount of water in your room vaporizer to help with congestion.

Insect bites: In the folklore of New England, rural Indiana, and parts of the Southwest, a vinegar wash is sometimes used for treating bites and stings. (However, if the person bitten has a known allergy to insect venom or begins to exhibit signs of a serious allergic reaction, such as widespread hives, swelling of the face or mouth, difficulty breathing, or loss of consciousness, skip the home remedies and seek immediate medical attention.) Pour undiluted vinegar over the area, avoiding surrounding healthy skin as much as possible.

Athlete's foot: One way to eliminate athlete's foot is to create an environment that is inhospitable to the fungus that causes the condition. The Amish traditionally use a footbath of vinegar and water to discourage the growth of athlete's foot fungus. To try this remedy, mix one cup of vinegar into two quarts of water in a basin or pan. Soak your feet in this solution every night for 15 to 30 minutes, using a fresh solution each night. Or, if you prefer, mix up a solution using one cup of vinegar and one cup of water. Apply the solution to the affected parts of your feet with a cotton ball. Let your feet dry completely before putting on socks and/or shoes.

WATER

That's right—water. Every part of your body relies on water. Without it, you wouldn't live long—four or five days at the most. Your blood, for example, is more than three quarters water. Other body fluids, such as saliva and digestive juices, are primarily water, as is urine. You couldn't get rid of body wastes without it. Almost every chemical reaction in the body takes place in a water medium; water also lubricates and protects the joints, organs, nose, and mouth. Your body needs water so that when you get hot, you can sweat. The water you sweat off then evaporates on your skin, cooling you down.

So how much do you need to drink? Generally, you should drink six to eight cups of water a day. Although you can get by on less, drinking this much water is especially kind to your kidneys and colon because it helps flush toxins out of your body. When you drink a lot of water, the toxins can't hang around long enough to cause damage to your kidneys or cancerous growths in the colon. In fact, drinking plenty of water may be the simplest of all disease prevention tips.

Why not just drink when you're thirsty? Because your body's thirst-o-meter isn't very reliable. You should drink about three cups more than your thirst tells you to. And as you get older, your body loses the ability to tell when it's thirsty, making it doubly important to drink water even when you don't crave a cool drink.

YOGURT

Yogurt (along with some of its other fermented dairy cousins, like kefir) was a long-established staple in Eastern Europe and the Middle East before it reached our shores. And there was a time when yogurt eaters in this country were considered "health nuts." Our attitudes have changed considerably. Today, yogurt is commonly consumed by men, women, and children of all ages. Walk into any supermarket today, and you'll see that the varieties and flavors of this nutritious food take up considerable space in the dairy section.

Friendly bacteria. Yogurt may not be the miracle food some have claimed, but it certainly has a lot to offer in the health department. Besides being an excellent source of bone-building calcium, it is believed that the bacterial cultures *Lactobacillus bulgaricus* and *Streptococcus thermophilus* that are used to make yogurt carry their own health benefits. For example, research has suggested that eating yogurt regularly helps boost the body's immune system function, warding off colds and possibly even helping to fend off cancer. It is also thought the friendly bacteria found in many types of yogurt can help prevent and even remedy diarrhea.

For people who suffer from lactose intolerance, yogurt is often well tolerated because live yogurt cultures produce lactase, making the lactose sugar in the yogurt easier to digest. Be sure to check the label on the yogurt carton for the National Yogurt Association's Live and Active Cultures (LAC) seal. This seal identifies products that contain a significant amount of live and active cultures. But don't look to frozen yogurt as an option; most frozen yogurt contains little of the healthful bacteria.

Selection and storage. There is a dizzying array of brands and varieties of yogurts in most supermarkets. But there are some basic traits to look for when deciding which to put in your cart. Choose a yogurt that is either low fat or fat free. It should contain no more than three grams of fat per eight-ounce carton. Some yogurts are also sugar free (these are often signaled by the term "light," but check the label to be sure, since this term might also refer to fat content) and contain an alternative sweetener instead of added sugar. Consider choosing plain, vanilla, lemon, or any one of the yogurts without a fruit mixture added. The mixture adds calories and little if anything in the way of vitamins, minerals, or fiber. Your best health bet is to add your own fresh fruit to plain fat-free yogurt.

Yogurt must always be refrigerated. Each carton should have a "sell by" date stamped on it. It should be eaten within the week following the "sell by" date to take full advantage of the live and active cultures in the yogurt. As yogurt is stored, the amount of live and active cultures begins to decline.

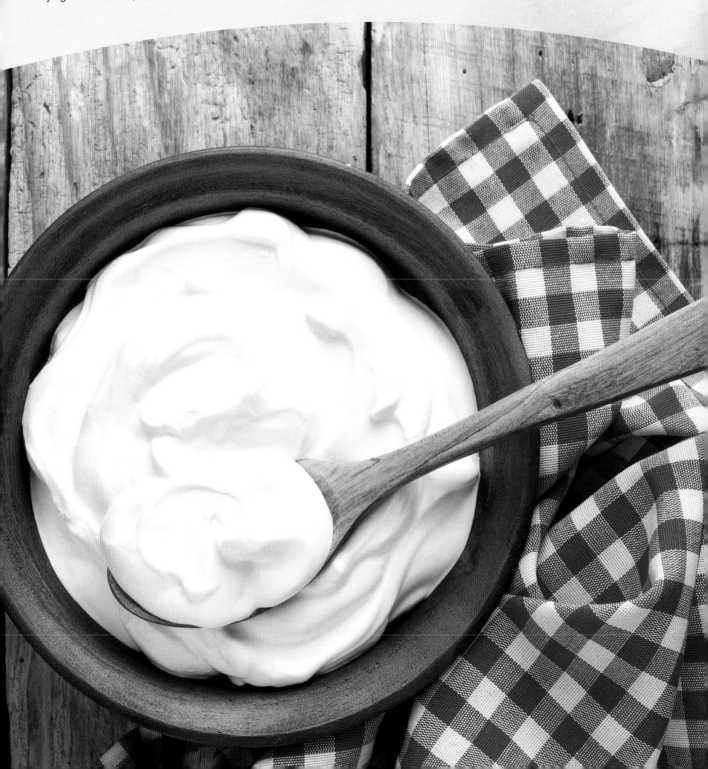

ESSENTAL OILS

Remember the heady fragrance of an herb or flower garden on a hot summer's day, or the crisp smell of an orange as you peel it? These odors are the fragrance of the plant's essential oils, the potent, volatile, and aromatic substance contained in various parts of the plant, including its flowers, leaves, roots, wood, seeds, fruit, and bark. The essential oils carry concentrations of the plant's healing properties—those same properties that traditional Western medicine utilizes in many drugs.

AROMATHERAPY

Aromatherapy simply means the application of those healing powers—it is a fragrant cure. Professional aromatherapists focus very specifically on the controlled use of essential oils to treat ailments and disease and to promote physical and emotional well-being.

Aromatherapy doesn't just work through the sense of smell alone, however. Inhalation is only one application method. Essential oils can also be diluted in a carrier oil and applied to the skin. When used topically, the oils penetrate the skin, taking direct action on body tissues and organs in the vicinity of application. They also enter the bloodstream and are carried throughout the body. Of course, when applied topically the fragrance of the essential oil is also inhaled.

There are three different modes of action in the body: pharmacological, which affects the chemistry of the body; physiological, which affects the ability of the body to function and process; and psychological, which affects emotions and attitudes. These three modes interact continuously. Aromatherapy is so powerful partly because it affects all three modes. You choose the application method based on where you most want the effects concentrated and on what is most convenient and pleasing to you.

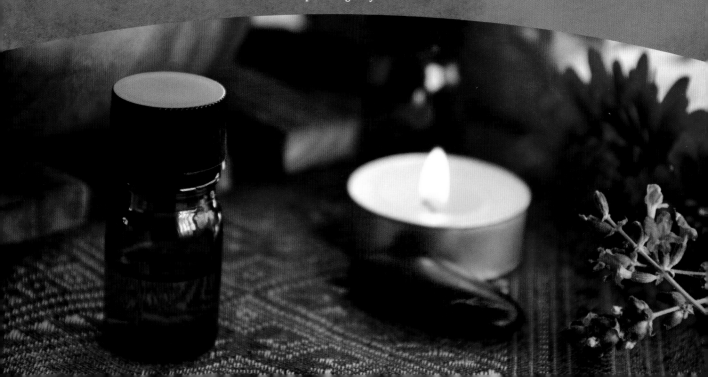

THERAPEUTIC USES OF ESSENTIAL OILS

You can treat a wide range of physical problems with aromatherapy. Almost all essential oils have antiseptic properties and are able to fight infection and destroy bacteria, fungi, yeast, parasites, and/or viruses. Many essential oils also reduce aches and pain, soothe or rout inflammations and spasms, stimulate the immune system and insulin and hormone production, affect blood circulation, dissolve mucus and open nasal passages, or aid digestion—just to mention a few of their amazing properties.

Aromatherapy can also have a considerable influence on our emotions. Sniffing clary sage, for example, can quell panic, while the fragrance released by peeling an orange can make you feel more optimistic. Since your mind strongly influences your health and is itself a powerful tool for healing, it makes aromatherapy's potential even more exciting.

CAUTION: RESPECT YOUR PLANT ALLIES

Essential oils can be purchased in health stores, some grocery stores, and of course online. Their easy availability and the fact that they are distilled directly from plants may make cautionary guidelines seem unnecessary—after all, there are no FDA warnings or lists of side effects on their labels—but you should *never* underestimate the capacity this natural pharmacy has for both beneficial and harmful results. Essential oils contain powerful chemical compounds. Misuse via direct topical application or ingestion can result in serious harm.

METHOD OF APPLICATION

The safest way to be exposed to essential oils is via diffusion. Inhalation presents a low risk level to most people. When using a diffuser, avoid prolonged exposure (over 1 hour) to high levels of diffused essential oils.

You should never ingest essential oils. There are some instances where practitioners will recommend the ingestion of small, diluted amounts to address specific conditions, but you should never do this without the guidance of a qualified professional.

When applying essential oils to the skin, always dilute them with a carrier oil (more on that at the end of this chapter). As you increase the ratio of essential oil to carrier oil, you run a greater risk of an adverse dermal reaction. Higher levels of essential oils also increase the risk of sensitization occurring. For this reason, most aromatherapists do not recommend direct (neat) application of undiluted essential oils to the skin.

While many oils are generally well-tolerated by most individuals when applied via massage in a carrier oil, others are best avoided. Essential oils known to be dermal irritants include the following:

BAY	CUMIN	TAGETES
CINNAMON BARK OR LEAF	LEMONGRASS	THYME
CITRONELLA	LEMON VERBENA	
CLOVE BUD	OREGANO	

This is a partial list. More and more essential oils are being made available commercially each year, and the effects of some are not well understood.

PHOTOSENSITIZATION

Some essential oils act as photosensitizers. Reactions may range from mild color change and irritation to extreme burning. If you have used photosensitizing essential oils topically, avoid prolonged exposure to sunlight for 24 hours. Some of the common photosensitizing essential oils include:

ANGELICA ROOT	DISTILLED OR EXPRESSED GRAPEFRUIT	ORANGE, BITTER
BERGAMOT	EXPRESSED LEMON	RUE
CUMIN	EXPRESSED LIME	

This is also a partial list, so exercise caution and good judgment when applying an essential oil.

CAUTION: HUMANS AND PETS RESPOND TO ESSENTIAL OILS DIFFERENTLY

Do not assume that what is good for you will be the equivalent (or even safe) for an animal. It is best to consult first with a veterinarian and a trained aromatherapist before administering *any* essential oil for your pet's health.

Essential oils have sometimes been used for dogs, horses, and some other farm animals. In these cases they have been used topically for spot application and hoof/paw care. Inhalation therapy has also been used.

As a general rule, do not use *any* essential oil topically on cats. Their metabolic systems do not break down many of the substances contained in essential oils. Liver or kidney damage, or worse, may result when cats are exposed to essential oils. This can even include exposure to essential oils via diffusion. You should use the same extreme caution with fish, reptiles, birds, rodents, and small mammals.

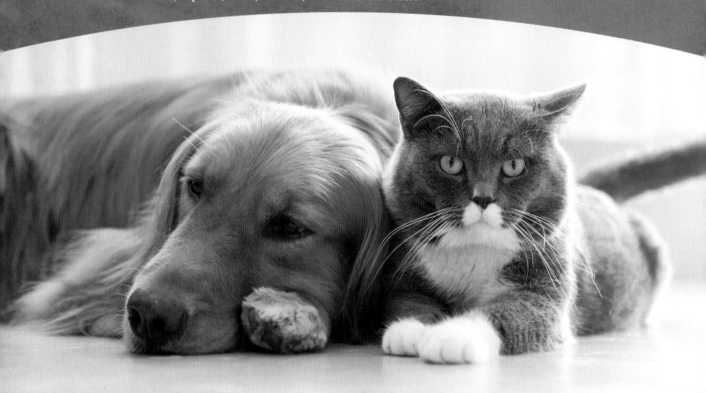

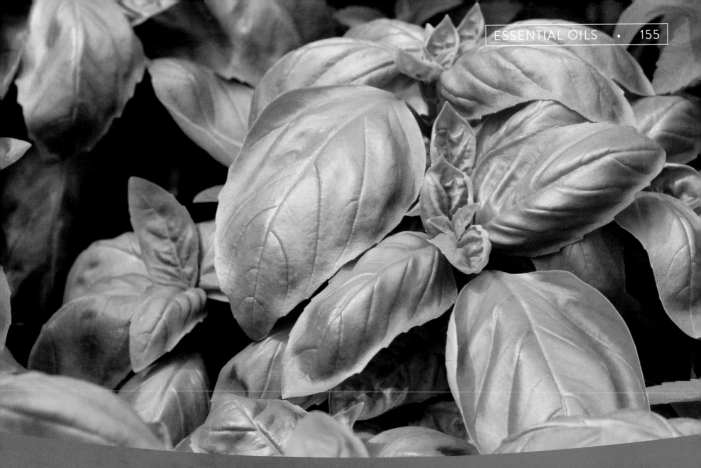

BASIL

BOTANICAL NAME: *OCIMUM BASILICUM*

Named after the Greek *basileus*, meaning "king," basil—the "king of herbs"—has been cultivated in India for at least 5,000 years. It has been used for culinary purposes in Asian and Mediterranean cultures for centuries, and today many of us know it mostly as an essential pizza and pesto ingredient. But the tasty herb was often used in ancient Chinese and Ayurvedic medicinal practices to treat coughs, fevers, indigestion, constipation, and skin rashes. The herb is also used in religious practices in the Eastern Orthodox Church and Hinduism. The spicy, herby scented oil can be diluted in olive or coconut oil and applied topically, or used in a diffuser.

THERAPEUTIC PROPERTIES

Aids digestion; has antibacterial, antiviral, and analgesic properties; muscle relaxant; repels some insects.

USED FOR

Research has shown that basil oil is effective at fighting bacteria and fungi, making it an excellent choice for a natural kitchen and bathroom cleaner. The oil also helps to kill odor-causing bacteria and mold on furniture, kitchen appliances, or in your car. You can use the oil when fighting colds or the flu by diffusing it in your home, or adding a few drops to a bath. Try adding a few drops of basil oil to coconut oil and rubbing into sore, painful muscles. The oil can also be used to make bug repellant, mouthwash, or toothpaste.

BENZOIN

BOTANICAL NAME: *STYRAX BENZOIN*

The trunk of the benzoin tree exudes a vanilla-scented gum resin when cut. Used since antiquity in medicine, it was imported by the Arabs to use as a less expensive substitute for frankincense. They made pomades that smelled like vanilla and were rubbed on the skin for fragrance and healing. Traders brought benzoin to Greece, Rome, and Egypt, where it became prized as a fixative in perfumes—still one of its uses today. Europeans highly regarded benzoin for its medicinal properties as well as its scent. Benzoin is typically sold as an absolute, but it is so thick it may be difficult for you to get it out of the bottle. If so, dilute it with a little alcohol or dissolve it in warm vegetable oil so it is easier to pour.

THERAPEUTIC PROPERTIES

Antibacterial, antifungal, antioxidant; seals wounds from infection; counteracts inflammation; decreases gas, indigestion, and lung congestion; promotes circulation.

USED FOR

Effective against redness, irritation, or itching on the skin, benzoin's most popular use is in a cream to protect chapped skin and improve skin elasticity. Since it is also a strong preservative, adding it to vegetable oil–based preparations delays their oxidation and spoilage. Benzoin essential oil can be added to chest rub balms and massage oils for lung and sinus ailments.

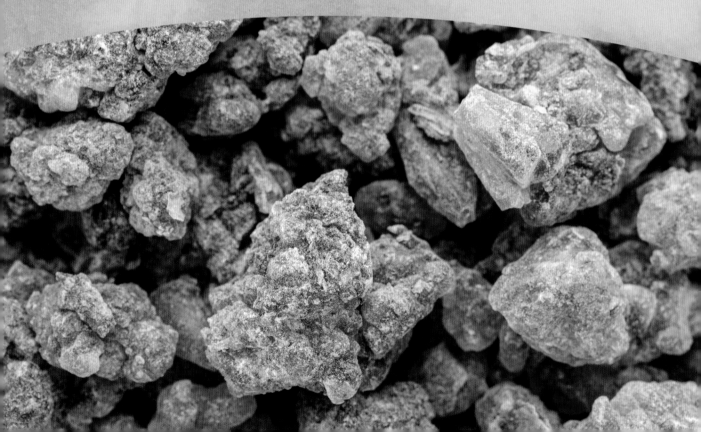

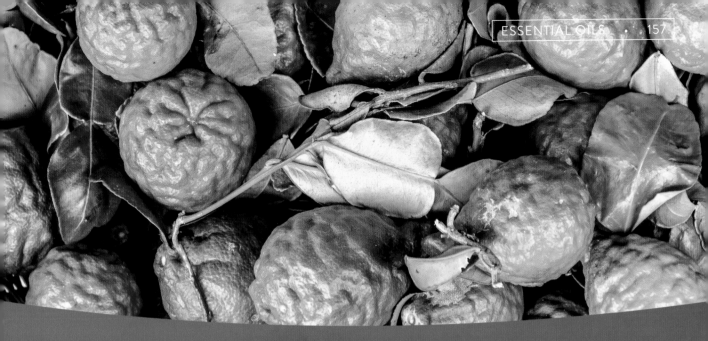

BERGAMOT

BOTANICAL NAME: *CITRUS BERGAMIA*

A small citrus tree originally from tropical Asia, it produces the round, green fruit whose oils are expressed from the rinds before ripening. While not edible or pretty, they smell truly wonderful! The green-tinted oil gained favor only after the tree was brought to Bergamot, Italy, in the fifteenth century. There it was used to treat fevers, malaria, and intestinal worms. According to legend, Christopher Columbus brought the tree to the Caribbean, where it was popularly used in voodoo practices to protect one from misfortune. Modern aromatherapists suggest placing a few drops of bergamot on a cloth and carrying it in your pocket or travel bag. Sniff the scented cloth while traveling to reduce stress, depression, anxiety, or insomnia.

THERAPEUTIC PROPERTIES

Antiseptic, anti-inflammatory, antidepressant, antiviral, antibiotic.

USED FOR

Bergamot fights several viruses, including those that cause flu, herpes, shingles, and chicken pox. Due to its versatile antibiotic properties, it also treats bacterial infections of the urinary system, mouth, and throat. It is helpful for a variety of skin conditions, including eczema. The best way to use it is diluted in a salve or massage oil that is applied externally over the afflicted area. As a natural deodorant, it not only provides a pleasant scent, but it kills bacteria that are responsible for odor.

PRECAUTIONS

Due to bergapten, bergamot can cause abnormal skin pigmentation when used externally by sensitive individuals who then go out in the sun. A bergapten-free essential oil is available; this should be noted on the bottle. While it may sound appealing to make your own Earl Grey tea, leave that up to the experts; they add only the tiniest amount of essential oil in a quantity that is safe to ingest.

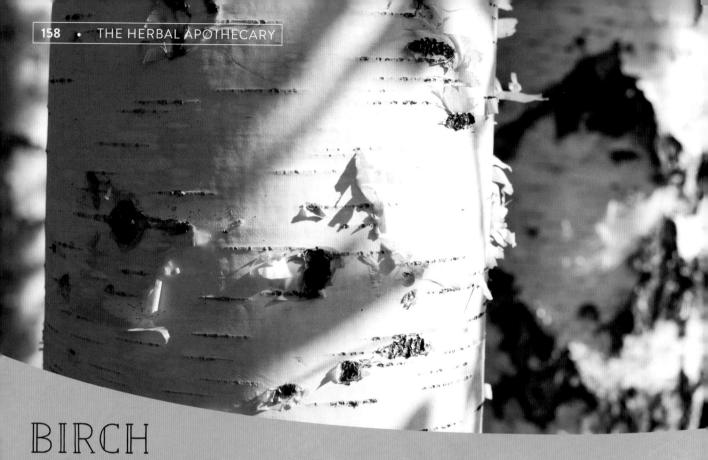

BIRCH

BOTANICAL NAME: *BETULA LENTA*

The scent and flavor of birch has been a European and North American Indian favorite for centuries. Birch drinks were favored by those suffering from consumption because the natural aspirin, methyl salicylate, in the essential oil relieves pain and makes it easier to breathe.

THERAPEUTIC PROPERTIES

Astringent, antiseptic; promotes menstruation; alleviates joint pain.

USED FOR

In a massage oil or liniment, birch can be rubbed over painful areas to ease muscular and arthritic pain and stiffness. Alternatively, a couple drops of birch essential oil, along with a drop or two of another oil such as lavender to soften birch's sharp scent, can be added to your bath for the same purpose. This type of aromatherapy bath is also useful to increase circulation and promote menstruation, especially when delayed by physical or emotional stress. A salve or lotion containing birch essential oil softens the roughness caused by psoriasis, eczema, and other skin problems.

PRECAUTIONS

Be sure not to overdo the suggested quantities of this potent essential oil, as it can be toxic in high doses. Since it smells like candy, store it safely away from children so they won't be tempted to taste it.

BLACK PEPPER

BOTANICAL NAME: *PIPER NIGRUM*

Traded more than any other spice in the world, black pepper has been prized since antiquity not only for its flavor-enhancing spiciness, but also for its medicinal usefulness. The spice has been found in ancient Egyptian tombs, was frequently used in ancient Roman cookery, and was so coveted by Europeans that it was briefly used as a form of currency. In fact, Alaric the Visigoth, famous for sacking the city of Rome in the year 410, demanded 3,000 pounds of pepper as a ransom for the city! The spice is obtained by cooking and drying the unripe fruit of the flowering vine. Once dried, oil can be extracted from the fruit by crushing it.

THERAPEUTIC PROPERTIES

Supports cell function, immune system, and circulation; antioxidant; provides a warming sensation when applied topically.

USED FOR

The warming properties of black pepper oil make it ideal for soothing sore muscles and aiding in relief from arthritis and rheumatism. A couple diluted drops rubbed into the affected area can help improve pain and ease mobility. Taken internally (again, diluted), black pepper oil protects the body from free radicals and helps to repair cell damage, and has even been shown to lower cholesterol. It may also aid digestion, and help to kill harmful bacteria in the body.

PRECAUTIONS

Black pepper oil should not be taken in large quantities, as it can cause vomiting, sleeplessness, and overheating. Also, care should be used when applying topically, as the warming sensation of the oil may be irritating for sensitive skin.

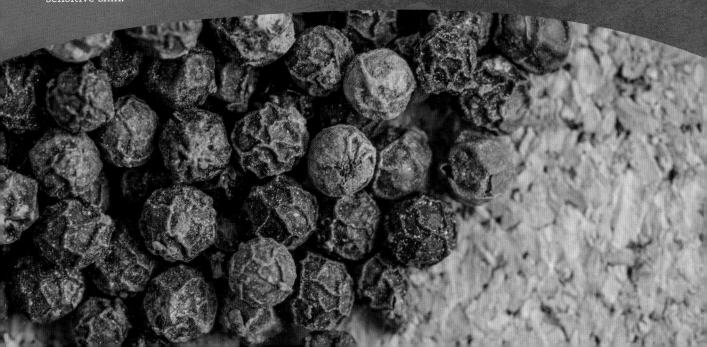

CALENDULA

BOTANICAL NAME: *CALENDULA OFFICINALIS*

Calendula—often referred to as the pot marigold—is an edible flower that has been used for centuries in European, Middle Eastern, and Mediterranean cooking. The bright yellow petals were sometimes used to add color to butter and cheese, or as a fabric dye. But calendula's usefulness goes far beyond its taste and color: the flower is mentioned in some of history's earliest medical texts, where it was recommended for aiding digestion, preventing infections, and detoxifying the liver. The flower was even used on the battlefield during the Civil War and World War I, as a remedy to prevent infection of open wounds. The sticky, syrupy oil distilled from the flowers is often extracted by steeping the petals in a hot carrier oil.

THERAPEUTIC PROPERTIES

Anti-inflammatory, antimicrobial, anti-viral; muscle relaxer; helps increase blood flow to injuries; improves skin firmness and hydration.

USED FOR

Calendula is a potent remedy for many inflammatory ailments, including dermatitis, ear infections, sore throats, ulcers, and diaper rash. Its muscle-relaxing properties can be used for abdominal cramps or constipation, and provide relief from PMS symptoms. It is also a popular additive in toothpastes, mouthwashes, and topical antiseptic ointments, due to its powerful antimicrobial properties.

PRECAUTIONS

Some people are allergic to calendula and other related plants, including ragweed, chamomile, and echinacea. Due to its muscle-relaxing properties, there is a possibility that it could interact negatively with some medications, including sedatives and diabetes or blood pressure medication. Pregnant women should also avoid calendula.

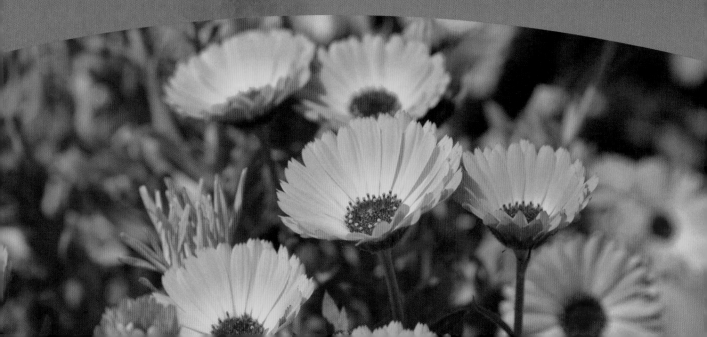

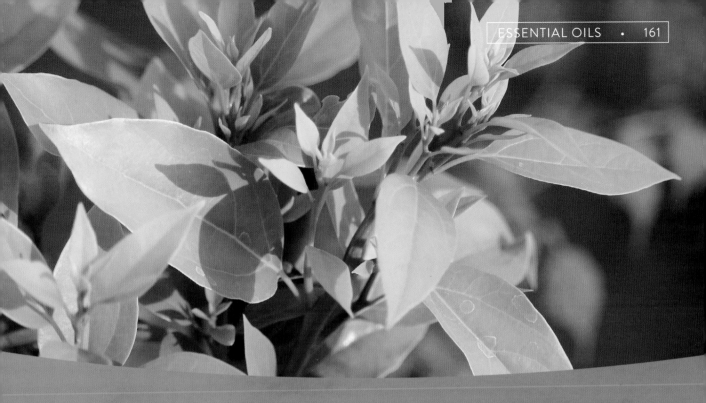

CAMPHOR

BOTANICAL NAME: *CINNAMOMUM CAMPHORA*

The camphor laurel is a large evergreen tree native to China, Japan, and other Asian countries. In fact, the third largest tree to ever grow in Japan is an 82-foot-tall camphor laurel, which is said to have first sprouted in prehistoric times! The wood and leaves of these trees are steam distilled to extract the essential oil, which has been used for centuries in everything from embalming fluid to medicines to insect repellant. Although researchers can't trace the first time the oil was ever used, they suspect that its strong scent and decongestant properties are what cemented camphor's place as a medicinal powerhouse.

THERAPEUTIC PROPERTIES

Decongestant, anesthetic, anti-inflammatory, disinfectant; insect repellant; stimulates circulatory system.

USED FOR

Camphor is popularly used as a decongestant because of its strong, sinus-clearing scent. It is also an excellent disinfectant, and can be added to ointments and lotions to aid skin conditions and kill bacteria. It provides a cooling sensation to the skin, making it ideal for mixing with bath water to escape oppressive summer heat. It works well to repel and kill unwanted insects.

PRECAUTIONS

Camphor oil is toxic when ingested. Even small amounts of the oil can be poisonous, and produce symptoms such as extreme thirst, vomiting, and dizziness. The oil should be diluted before applying topically.

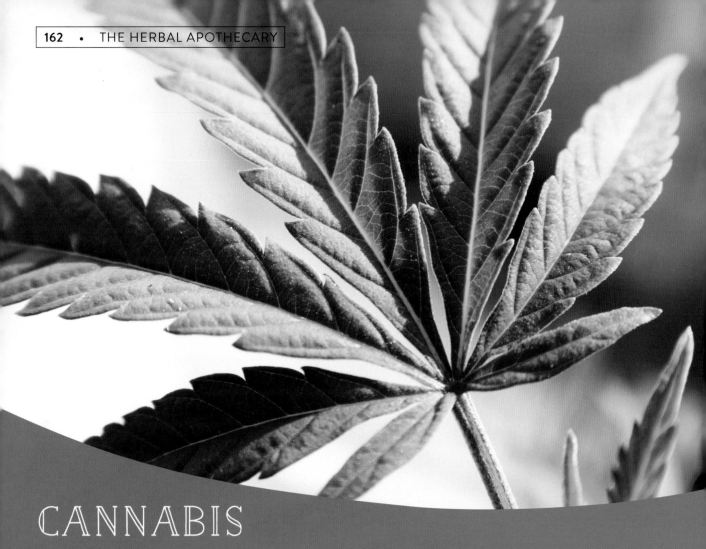

CANNABIS

BOTANICAL NAME: *CANNABIS SATIVA*

No doubt the first thing that comes to mind when we think of cannabis is the recreational drug marijuana; but the oil derived from the flowering cannabis plant is prized for its medicinal benefits. The plant has been found in the graves of ancient Europeans, and is mentioned in various texts written by ancient Egyptians, Indians, and Greeks. Cannabis was used in Chinese medicine as far back as AD 100, and the second-century Chinese surgeon Hua Tuo is the first person known to use the plant as an anesthetic. Although the benefits of the plant have been known for millennia, its association with drug use can make the non-psychoactive essential oil hard to find.

THERAPEUTIC PROPERTIES

Reduces stress and anxiety; pain reliever; improves quality of sleep.

USED FOR

There are hundreds of chemical compounds in cannabis that work together to give the oil many calming, stress-relieving properties. This makes it ideal for people who suffer with anxiety or insomnia. It may also give relief for inflammatory conditions.

CARROT SEED

BOTANICAL NAME: *DAUCUS CAROTA*

Carrot seed essential oil is derived from the seeds of the wild, rather than the domestic, carrot. This flowering plant is related to the common domesticated carrot found in grocery stores. It is also known as Queen Anne's Lace. Carrots trace their roots back to central Asia, where they were originally grown exclusively for their leaves and seeds. In fact, many of the vegetable's relatives—including parsley, cilantro, dill, and cumin—are still grown for the same reason today. Carrot seed was prized in ancient times for its ability to aid digestion and soothe stomach ailments, and today is considered one of the most underrated essential oils on the market.

THERAPEUTIC PROPERTIES

Antioxidant, antiseptic, antiviral; can aid digestion; useful in aromatherapy; anti-parasitic.

USED FOR

Carrot seed oil can be applied topically, either on its own or mixed with lotion or face cream, to rejuvenate skin or help ward off infections. When ingested, it may help fight infections of the mouth or digestive system, and can help treat colds, the flu, and bronchitis. Its soothing aroma helps relieve stress and anxiety when used in aromatherapy. The oil even helps kill intestinal parasites, but is safely consumed by humans.

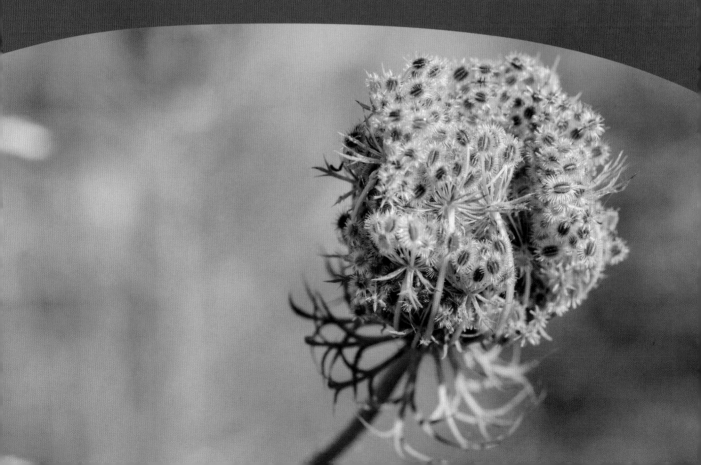

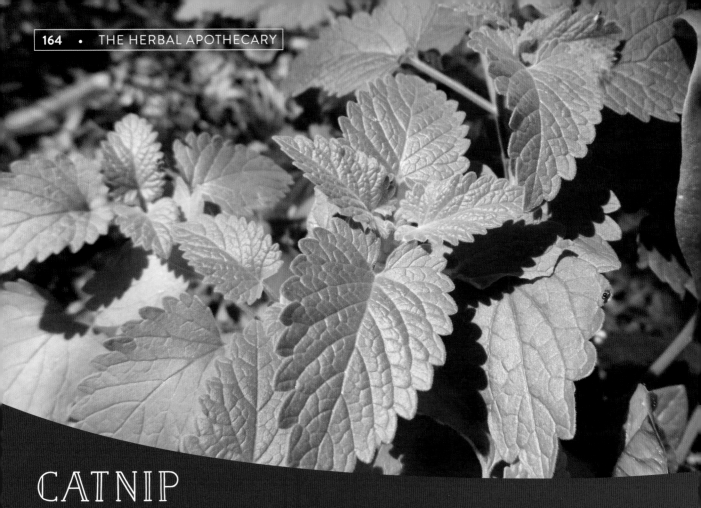

CATNIP

BOTANICAL NAME: *NEPETA CATARIA*

Native to Europe, Africa, and Asia, catnip is best known for being irresistible to our feline friends. But the herbaceous plant has many beneficial qualities that should make it irresistible to people, as well! Unlike the energizing effect it has on cats, catnip has a calming, sedative effect on humans. Ancient Romans took note of this benefit and used the plant in cooking, medicine, and catnip-infused tea. French sailors also enjoyed catnip tea before Chinese tea was readily available. Eventually, the herb was used throughout Europe to promote calm and to aid digestion. And by the 18th century, the herb made its way across the Atlantic, where Native Americans began using it for medicinal purposes.

THERAPEUTIC PROPERTIES

Anti-spasmodic, astringent, sedative; useful as an insect repellant.

USED FOR

Catnip is popular in many calming teas, and drinking it before bedtime can help promote a more restful night's sleep. The essential oil can help to relieve muscle and intestinal cramps, and helps to tone and tighten skin when applied topically. Catnip has even been shown to be more effective at repelling insects than the harmful chemical repellant DEET.

CEDARWOOD

BOTANICAL NAME: *CEDRUS DEODARA* OR *C. ATLANTICA*

The ancient Egyptians used cedar as a preservative and for embalming, in cosmetics, and as incense. Cedar is included in men's colognes and aftershaves and is used to make cigar boxes, cedar chests, and panel closets. Cedar wood and its essential oil make clothes smell great, and on a practical level, they repel wool moths. You won't find true cedar of Lebanon oil because of the shortage of trees, but Tibetan or Himalayan cedarwood (*C. deodara*, meaning "god tree"), and Atlas cedarwood (*C. atlantica*) have similar scents. The modern source of most "cedarwood" oil is juniper (*Juniperus virginiana*), known as "red cedar." Don't confuse cedarwood with thuja or cedar leaf (*Thuja occidentalis*).

THERAPEUTIC PROPERTIES

Antiseptic, astringent; brings on menstruation, clears mucus, sedates nerves, stimulates circulation.

USED FOR

Inhale the steam of cedarwood essential oil to treat respiratory infections and clear congestion. Add a few drops to a sitz bath to ease the pain and irritation of urinary infections and to cure the infection more quickly. Applied to oily skin, cedarwood essential oil is an astringent that dries and helps clear acne. Incorporate it into a facial wash, spritzer, or other cosmetic (10 drops of essential oil per ounce of preparation). Added to a salve (15 drops of essential oil per ounce of salve), it relieves dermatitis and, in some cases, eczema and psoriasis. Add two drops of essential oil to every ounce of shampoo or hair conditioner to ease dandruff.

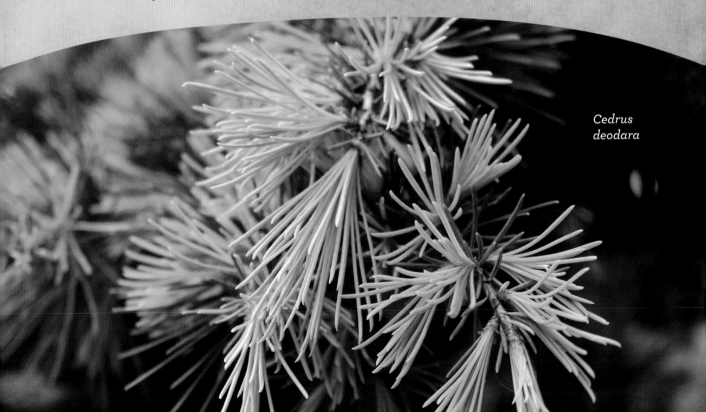

Cedrus deodara

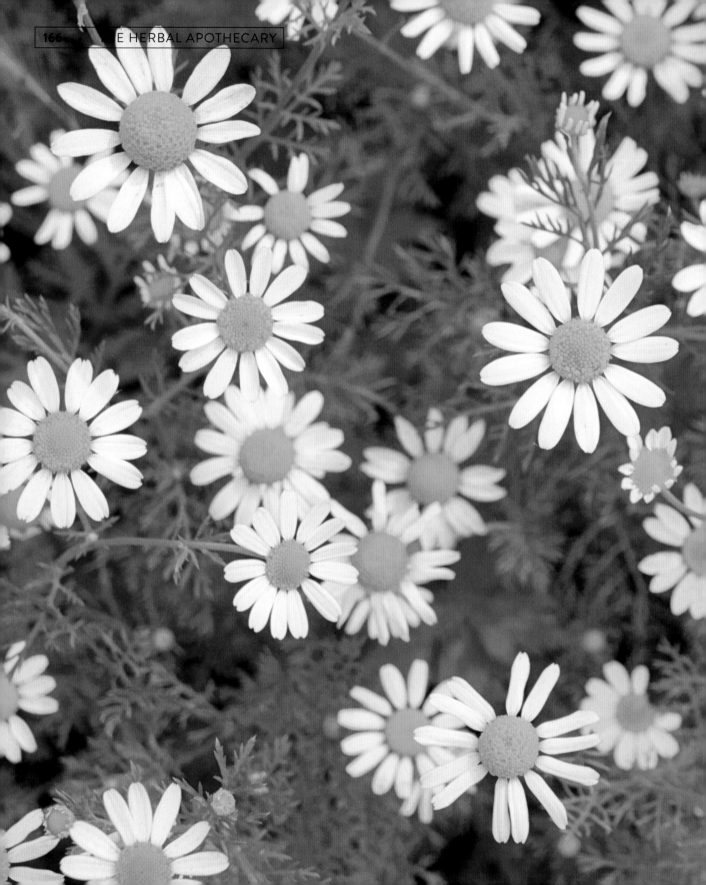

CHAMOMILE

BOTANICAL NAME: *MATRICARIA RECUTITA* (GERMAN)

Chamomile's flowers resemble tiny daisies, but one sniff will have you thinking of apples instead. The herb has long been grown for its healing properties. Its smell was thought to relieve depression and to encourage relaxation. Medieval monks planted raised garden beds of chamomile, and those who were sad or depressed lay on them as therapy. Chamomile also was once a "strewing herb," spread on bare floors so that the scent was released when people walked on it. Drinking chamomile tea made from the flowers stimulates appetite before meals; after meals it settles the stomach. Roman chamomile (*Camaemelum nobile*, formerly *Anthemis nobilis*) yields a pale yellow essential oil that is an anti-inflammatory. When German chamomile (left) is distilled, a chemical reaction produces the deep blue-green chamazulene that is even more potent an anti-inflammatory.

Inhaling chamomile tea's aroma relaxes both the mind and the body. Research studies show that chamomile relaxes emotions, muscles, and even brain waves. It eases the emotional ups and downs of PMS, menopause, and hyperactivity in children. It also helps control the pain of bruises, stiff joints, headaches, sore muscles, menstrual and digestive system cramping, as well as the pain and swelling of sprains and some allergic reactions. Chamomile is mild enough to ease a baby's colic and calm it for sleep. It is especially soothing in a massage oil, as a compress, or in a bath. Make a chamomile room spray by diluting 12 drops of the essential oil per ounce of distilled water. Chamomile is suitable for most complexion types or skin problems, from burns and eczema to varicose veins. It is especially useful for sensitive, puffy, or inflamed conditions. Add it to shampoos to lighten and brighten hair.

THERAPEUTIC PROPERTIES

Anti-inflammatory, antiseptic; promotes digestion, relieves gas and nausea, encourages menstruation, soothes nervous tension, promotes sleep.

To most people, Roman chamomile is identical to German chamomile. Roman chamomile is renowned for its soothing and sedative qualities. It is used to enhance calm and relieve tension, grief, anger, and over-sensitivity.

CINNAMON

BOTANICAL NAME: *CINNAMOMUM ZEYLANICUM*

The simple powder used in cooking starts off as the dry inner bark of a large 20-to-30-foot tree most likely growing in Sri Lanka. The Arabs, Portuguese, Dutch, and British successively controlled trade of this valuable spice. Then, as now, cinnamon flavored mouthwashes, foods, and drinks and was used as an aphrodisiac. Cinnamon's scent also stirs the appetite, invigorates and "warms" the senses, and may even produce a feeling of joy. There are several types of cinnamon oil to choose from: Oil can be distilled from the leaf or the much more potent bark, or you can obtain cassia oil, a less expensive relative of cinnamon that comes from China.

THERAPEUTIC PROPERTIES

Antiseptic, digestive, antiviral; relieves muscle spasms and rheumatic pain when used topically.

USED FOR

In general, cinnamon is used as a physical and emotional stimulant. Researchers have found that it reduces drowsiness, irritability, and the pain and number of headaches. In one study, the aroma of cinnamon in the room helped participants to concentrate and perform better. The essential oil and its fragrance help relax tight muscles, ease painful joints, and relieve menstrual cramps.

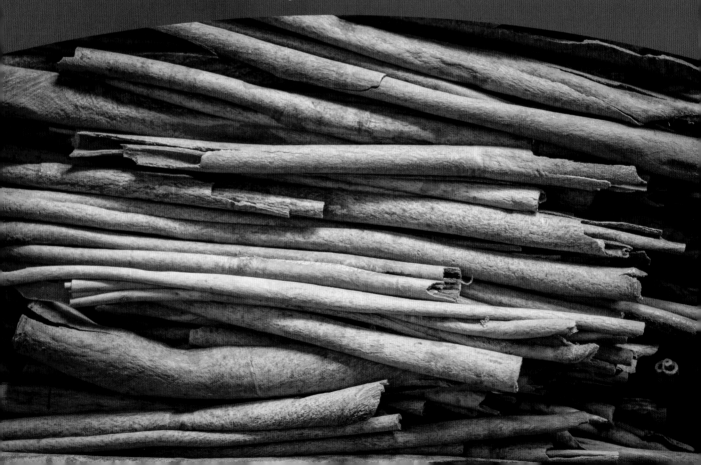

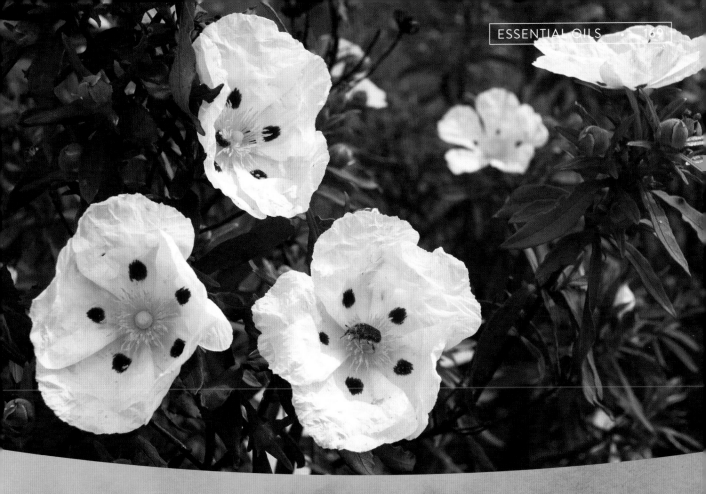

CISTUS

BOTANICAL NAME: *CISTUS LADANIFER*

Cistus, also commonly known as rockrose or labdanum, is a flowering plant found in the Mediterranean region. It has been prized for its amber-like scent since the time of the ancient Egyptians, and is even mentioned in the biblical book of Genesis. In ancient times, shepherds would collect the sweet-smelling resin of the cistus shrub by brushing it off the hair of their goats and sheep, which grazed on the plants. The resin was then used to treat colds, coughs, and arthritis, as well as for incense. By the Middle Ages, the use of the plant had spread to Europe, where it was used to treat wounds and skin ulcers.

THERAPEUTIC PROPERTIES

Antimicrobial, astringent; helps to slow bleeding; useful in aromatherapy.

USED FOR

Cistus is often used to give perfumes a warm, amber note, and is said to promote feelings of calm and peace when used in aromatherapy. It is popular in many skincare products, providing benefits for those struggling with acne, oily skin, eczema, or psoriasis. Cistus can also help to stop bleeding from fresh cuts and scrapes.

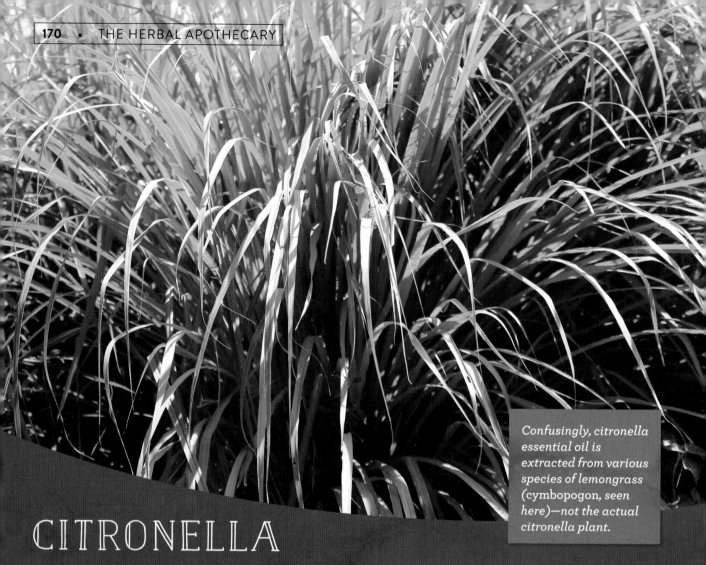

Confusingly, citronella essential oil is extracted from various species of lemongrass (cymbopogon, seen here)—not the actual citronella plant.

CITRONELLA

BOTANICAL NAME: *CYMBOPOGON NARDUS, C. WINTERIANUS,* AND OTHERS

Citronella grass is a type of lemongrass native to tropical Asia. The grass grows to about six and a half feet in length. It is a popular choice for home gardens due to its supposed ability to ward off insects—though some studies have found it ineffective for this use. The oil extracted from the plant's stems and leaves has many other uses as well. In fact, citronella oil has been used in China, Indonesia, and Sri Lanka for centuries for medicinal purposes. Many clinical studies have shown the oil to be an effective antiseptic, making it a natural bug bite remedy.

THERAPEUTIC PROPERTIES

Antiseptic, antimicrobial, antifungal; insect repellant.

USED FOR

The oil continues to be popular as a natural insect repellant, albeit with mixed results. A few drops can be added to coconut oil and then rubbed on like body lotion. It can be used as a skin remedy to help heal bug bites, eczema, or fungal infections. Its fresh scent and antiseptic properties make it an excellent kitchen and bathroom cleaner.

CLARY SAGE

BOTANICAL NAME: *SALVIA SCLAREA*

In ancient times, clary sage was praised as a panacea with the ability to render man immortal. The tea was once thought not only to clear eyesight and the brain, but also to clarify one's intuition and allow one to see more clearly into the future. Simply sniffing the oil before going to bed can produce dramatic dreams and, when you awake, a euphoric state of mind. It was an important ingredient in one of the most popular European cordials. Along with elderflowers, it still flavors high quality Muscatel wine and Italian vermouth. Distilled from the flowering tops and leaves of a three-foot-tall perennial, clary sage now is produced mostly for flavoring a large variety of foods.

THERAPEUTIC PROPERTIES

Antidepressant, anti-inflammatory, astringent, deodorant; decreases gas and indigestion, brings on menstruation, relaxes muscles and nerves, and lowers blood pressure.

USED FOR

Added to a massage oil or used in a compress, clary sage eases muscle and nervous tension and pain. Its relaxing action can reduce muscle spasms and asthma attacks and lower blood pressure. Especially good for female ailments, it helps one cope better with menstrual cramps or PMS and has established itself as a premier remedy for menopausal hot flashes. Improve your complexion by adding it to creams, especially if you have acne or thin, wrinkled, or inflamed skin.

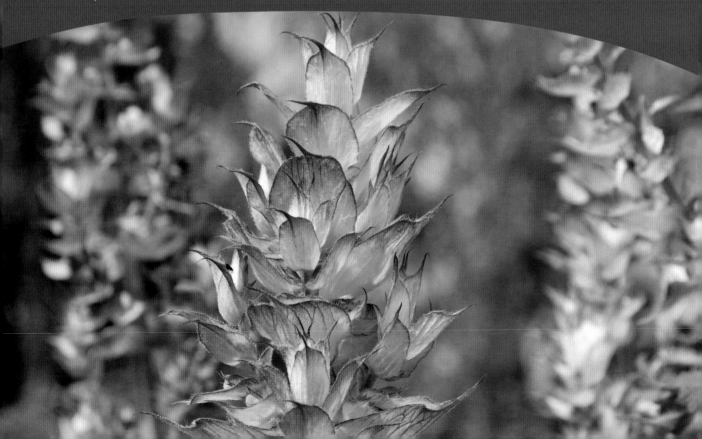

CLOVE

BOTANICAL NAME: *SYZYGIUM AROMATICUM*

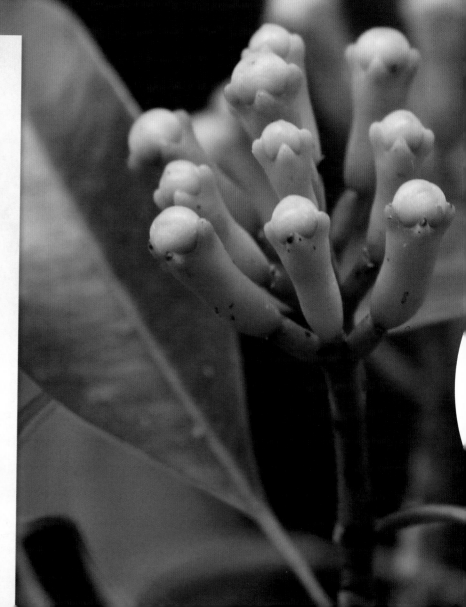

The flower buds are picked and then sorted. The buds are dried on mats in the sun for about three days.

In ancient China, courtiers at the Han court held cloves in their mouths to freshen their breath before they had an audience with the emperor. Today, cloves are still used to sweeten breath. Modern dental preparations numb tooth and gum pain and quell infection with clove essential oil or its main constituent, eugenol. Simply inhaling the fragrance was once said to improve eyesight and fend off the plague. Clove's scent developed a reputation, now backed by science, for being stimulating. The fragrance was also believed to be an aphrodisiac. Cloves were so valuable that a Frenchman risked his life to steal a clove tree from the Dutch colonies in Indonesia and plant it in French ground. Once established, the slender evergreen trees bear buds for at least a century. The familiar clove buds used to poke hams and flavor mulled wine are picked while still unripe and dried before being shipped or distilled into essential oil.

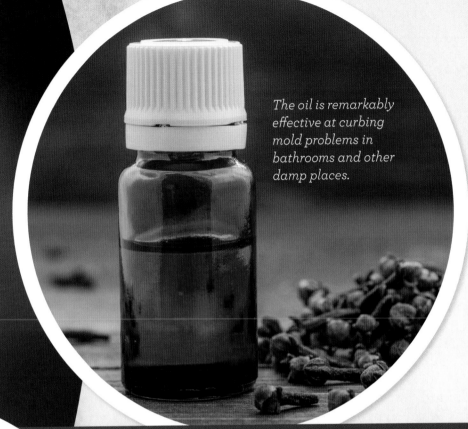

The oil is remarkably effective at curbing mold problems in bathrooms and other damp places.

As an antiseptic and pain reliever, clove essential oil relieves toothaches, flu, colds, and bronchial congestion. But don't try to use it straight on an infant's gums for teething as is often suggested, or you may end up with a screaming baby because it tastes so strong and hot. Instead mix only two drops of clove oil in at least a teaspoon of vegetable oil. It can still be hot, however, so try it in your own mouth first. Then apply it directly to the baby's gums. In a heating liniment, clove essential oil helps sore muscles and arthritis. Mix 30 drops of clove essential oil in one ounce of apple cider vinegar, shake well, and dab on athlete's foot. Researchers have found that the spicy aroma of clove reduces drowsiness, irritability, and headaches.

PRECAUTIONS

The essential oil irritates skin and mucous membranes, so be sure to dilute it before use. Clove leaf is almost pure eugenol; do not use it in aromatherapy preparations.

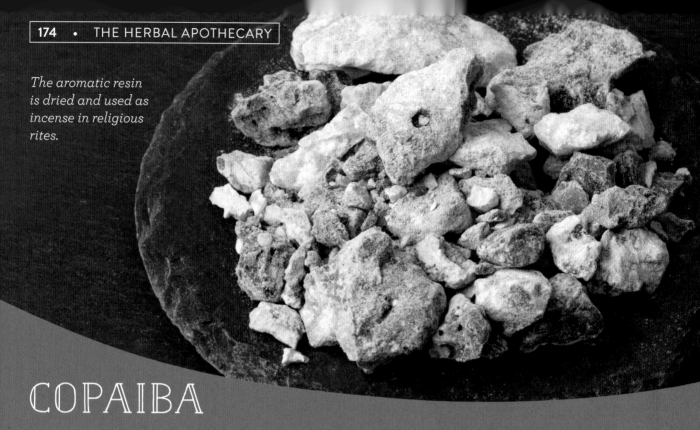

The aromatic resin is dried and used as incense in religious rites.

COPAIBA

BOTANICAL NAME: *COPAIFERA LANGSDORFFII, C. RETICULATA, AND OTHERS*

Grown in South American tropical rain forests, the tree that yields copaiba oil is often called the "diesel tree" because the oil can be used for fuel. Many people have found the oil useful for making lacquer and varnish, and it is also popularly used by artists for oil painting and pottery. But indigenous people in Brazil have used the oil medicinally since at least the 16th century, and 21st century studies have lent credence to their practices: the oil has been found to have anti-inflammatory, antiseptic, and anti-hemorrhagic properties. The popularity of this oil has been spreading around the world, and the production of copaiba oil now makes up 95 percent of Brazil's oil-resin production industry.

THERAPEUTIC PROPERTIES

Anti-inflammatory, antibacterial, astringent; may help to reduce blood pressure.

USED FOR

Copaiba oil is popularly used to tone and tighten skin, and reduce the appearance of scars and stretch marks. Its anti-inflammatory properties also make it a great choice for calming acne. It helps to to reduce pain caused by arthritis, headaches, muscle cramps, and injuries, either used as aromatherapy or applied topically. Some have described the scent of copaiba oil as being sweet like honey, and breathing in the soothing scent may help to lower blood pressure.

PRECAUTIONS

While copaiba oil is safe to ingest in minute amounts, consuming too much can cause stomach pain and symptoms similar to food poisoning. Use very sparingly.

CORIANDER

BOTANICAL NAME: *CORIANDRUM SATIVUM*

The coriander plant is native to west Asia, Europe, and the eastern Mediterranean. It has been used for centuries as an aphrodisiac, to lift spirits, assist digestion, and restore calm. The seeds were reputedly found in the tomb of the Egyptian pharaoh Rameses II.

Coriander is now cultivated across the globe. As a culinary herb, it is commonly known as cilantro. The essential oil is not distilled from the herb, but rather from the seeds (although there is also a cilantro essential oil made from the herb). The oil's smell is pungent, refreshing, sweet, and slightly woody.

THERAPEUTIC PROPERTIES

Analgesic, antispasmodic, carminative, deodorant; relieves anxiety and depression.

USED FOR

Diffused, coriander can be a powerful and uplifting mood enhancer. It relieves anxiety, insomnia, lethargy, and weariness. A few diluted drops, taken internally after a large meal, promote digestion.

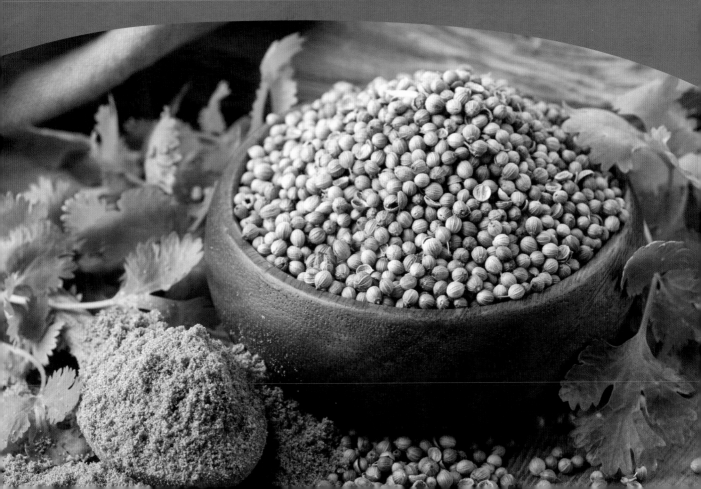

CYPRESS

BOTANICAL NAME: *CUPRESSUS SEMPERVIRENS*

Greeks say that cypress clears the mind during stressful times and comforts mourners. Cypress stanches bleeding (Hippocrates recommended it for hemorrhoids) and the Chinese chewed its small cones, rich in essential oils and astringents, to heal bleeding gums. The greenish essential oil is distilled from the tree's needles or twigs and sometimes from its cones.

THERAPEUTIC PROPERTIES

Antiseptic, astringent, deodorant; relieves rheumatic pain, relaxes muscle spasms and cramping, stops bleeding, constricts blood vessels.

USED FOR

Cypress's specialty is treating circulation problems, such as low blood pressure, poor circulation, varicose veins, and hemorrhoids. Because it helps heal broken capillaries and also discourages fluid retention, it is a favored essential oil at menopause. For these uses, add 8 drops to every ounce of cream or lotion and apply gently to the afflicted region a couple of times a day. You can also alleviate laryngitis, spasmodic coughing, and lung congestion just by putting a drop on your pillow. Because of its astringent, antiseptic, and deodorant properties, dilute about 6 drops of cypress essential oil in vinegar or aloe vera for an oily complexion or to reduce excessive sweating.

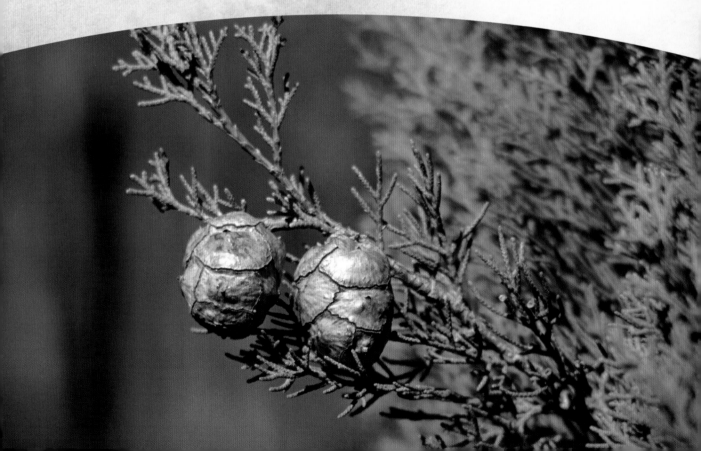

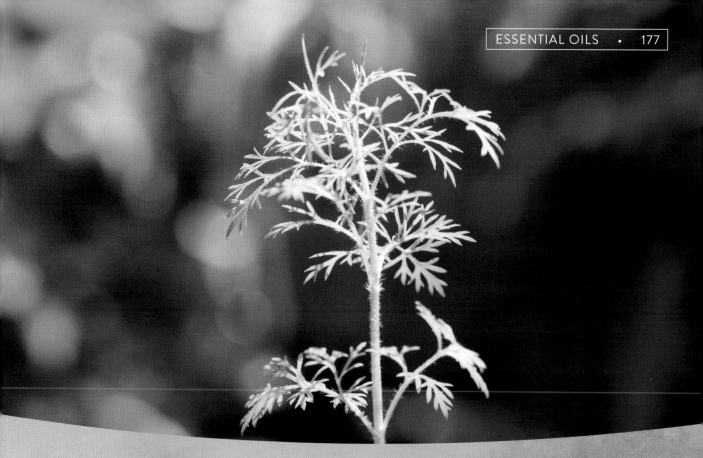

DAVANA

BOTANICAL NAME: *ARTEMISIA PALLENS*

Traditionally, the davana plant has been used in religious ceremonies in its native India, where it is offered to the god Shiva by Hindu devotees. But this flowering member of the daisy family has also been used in Indian folk medicine for hundreds of years to treat diabetes and high blood pressure. In fact, davana is offered to Shiva exactly for this reason: to show gratitude for the medicinal properties the plant possesses. In modern times, davana oil is especially prized for use in perfumes, because of its unique tendency to smell differently depending on the person wearing it. This results in a truly one-of-a-kind fragrance for perfume aficionados!

THERAPEUTIC PROPERTIES

Antimicrobial; helps to relieve coughs and congestion; may help to alleviate depression and anxiety; perfume additive.

USED FOR

Davana oil has been shown to rupture the protective cover of viruses, making it an effective remedy against colds and flu. It also fights bacterial infections in the body or on the skin, and can be used to disinfect surfaces in kitchens, bathrooms, and other rooms of your home. When used in aromatherapy, the soothing fragrance helps to lower blood pressure and may even help to relax the nervous system. The oil is used in the manufacture of perfumes, cosmetics, and some foods and beverages.

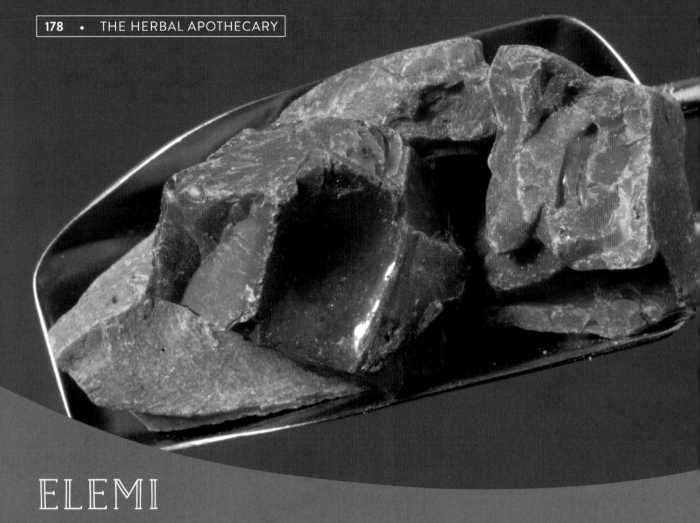

ELEMI

BOTANICAL NAME: *CANARIUM LUZONICUM*

Elemi is derived from a tree found in the tropical forests of the Philippines. It belongs to the same botanical family as frankincense and myrrh. Between January and June, when the leaves of the tree are budding, the gum resin is harvested from the trees. The essential oil is then steam extracted from the resin, producing a product with a peppery, lemony scent. By the 7th century, elemi oil was being used in religious ceremonies in China; but it was the explorer Magellan's discovery of the Philippines in 1521 that helped introduce the oil to Europe and the Middle East. By the 18th century, elemi had found a home among other therapeutic oils used in the West, where it was considered an essential medicinal ingredient.

THERAPEUTIC PROPERTIES

Antiseptic; analgesic; helps alleviate cold and flu symptoms; perfume additive.

USED FOR

Elemi's antiseptic properties help to protect against infections of many kinds, including bacterial, fungal, and viral. It helps to reduce pain caused by injuries, headaches, or arthritis. It helps to ease breathing and reduce congestion due to colds and coughs.

EUCALYPTUS

BOTANICAL NAME: *EUCALYPTUS GLOBULUS*

Eucalyptus or "gum" trees originated in Australia and Tasmania, but they are now found in subtropical regions all over the globe. Eucalyptus' thick, long, bluish-green leaves are distilled to provide essential oil. Blue gum eucalyptus, the most widely cultivated variety, provides most of the commercially available oil, although with more than 600 species, there are a variety of scents. Aromatherapists sometimes favor the more relaxing qualities and pleasant scent of the lemony *E. citriodora*. A very inexpensive oil, eucalyptus is used liberally to scent aftershaves and colognes and as an antiseptic in mouthwashes and household cleansers.

THERAPEUTIC PROPERTIES

Antibacterial, antiviral, deodorant; clears mucous from the lungs; as a liniment it relieves rheumatic, arthritic, and other types of pain.

USED FOR

It is the most popular essential oil steam for relieving sinus and lung congestion such as asthma. Inhale the steam, add one or two drops of oil to a compress, or put three or four drops in your bath. Especially appropriate for skin eruptions and oily complexions, it is also used for acne, herpes, and chicken pox. For a homemade preparation, mix eucalyptus essential oil with an equal amount of apple cider vinegar and dab on problem areas. This mix can also be used as an antiseptic on wounds, boils, and insect bites.

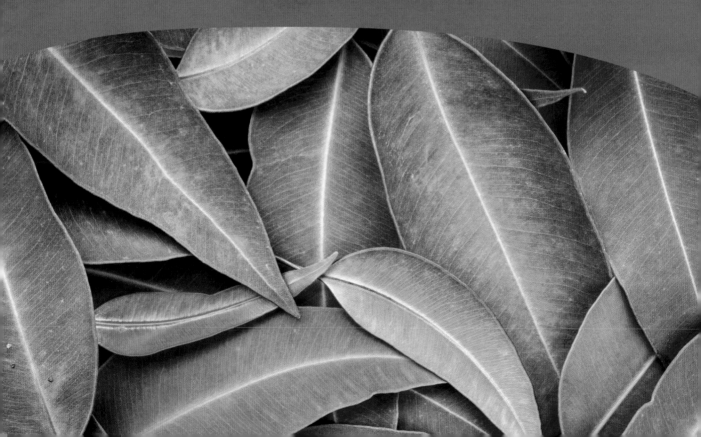

FENNEL

BOTANICAL NAME: *FOENICULUM VULGARE*

Known for its licorice-like flavor, fennel, a member of the carrot family, is native to the Mediterranean. But the flowering plant is now found all over the world, including Europe and the United States, and is coveted for both its taste and its therapeutic benefits. The herb was noted for its medicinal properties as far back as the 10th century, and even the poet Henry Wadsworth Longfellow wrote about fennel's "wondrous powers." Today, the herb is commonly used in foods, drinks, and cosmetics, but it is especially prized for its effectiveness at treating digestive issues.

THERAPEUTIC PROPERTIES

Antimicrobial; relieves digestive upset; may aid in weight loss.

USED FOR

Fennel oil can help to heal minor cuts and scrapes and prevent infection, and fights free radical damage in the body. The oil is especially useful for relieving digestive issues, including abdominal cramps, irritable bowel syndrome, gas, constipation, and diarrhea. Fennel oil may boost metabolism and suppress appetite, making it an excellent addition to a weight loss plan.

PRECAUTIONS

Heavy doses of fennel oil can have narcotic effects, causing hallucinations or convulsions. It is recommended that anyone with a history of seizures avoid using fennel oil.

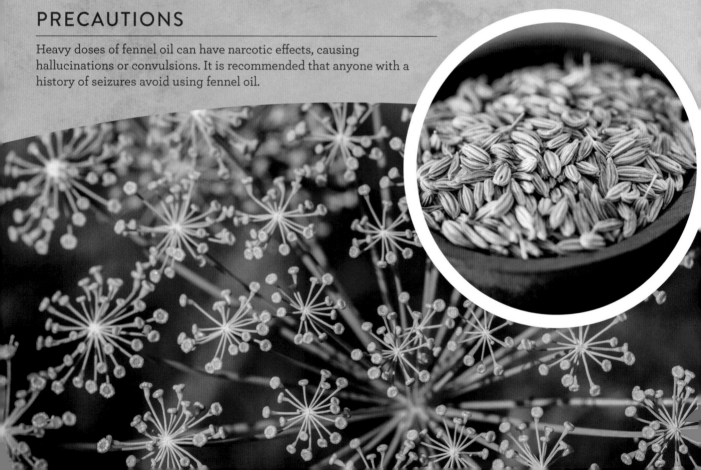

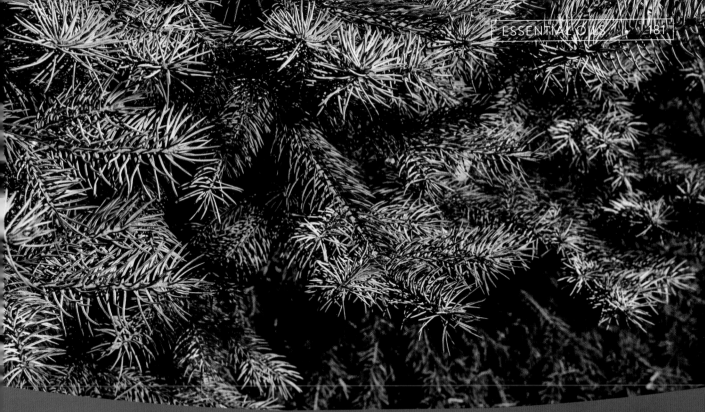

FIR

BOTANICAL NAME: *ABIES ALBA* AND OTHERS

For centuries, fir boughs were scattered over floors of churches and houses during winter, providing a clean, scented covering. Perhaps long ago, people realized that the uplifting fragrance helped overcome winter blues and encouraged feelings of contentment and joy.

Fir essential oil is distilled from the twigs or needles of many different conifers, yielding a rich variety of fragrances. The Canadian Balsam (*A. balsamea*) and Siberian firs (*A. siberica*) have an especially pleasant, forest-like scent, while the white fir (*A. concolor*) is excellent in massage blends. You may find other fir essential oils with similar uses and scent profiles, such as the Fraser (*A. fraseri*), Nordmann (*A. nordmanniana*), and Grand (*A. grandis*).

THERAPEUTIC PROPERTIES

Antibacterial, deodorant; relieves pain and coughing, clears mucous from the lungs, kills mold.

USED FOR

Fir essential oils soothe muscle and rheumatism pain and increase poor circulation when used in a massage oil or when added to a liniment or bath. They also help prevent bronchial and urinary infections and reduce coughing, including that caused by bronchitis and asthma. The best ways to utilize the essential oil are either through inhalation or via a chest rub. It is occasionally added to a salve or other skin preparation as an antiseptic for skin infections. An aromatherapy alarm clock from Japan uses the forest scent of pine or fir along with eucalyptus for its wake-up call.

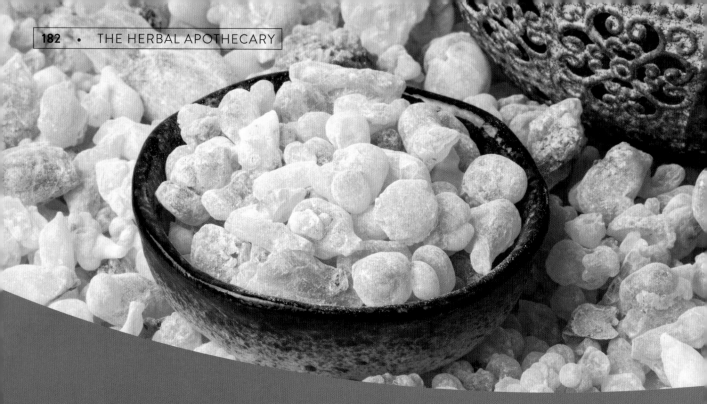

FRANKINCENSE

BOTANICAL NAME: *BOSWELLIA CARTERI*

The frankincense burned as church incense today is the same as that used by ancient peoples who inhabited the Middle East and North Africa. Eventually the use of frankincense spread throughout Europe and eastward into India, and it was burned as an offering to the gods of many cultures.

Aromatherapists and massage practitioners have observed that frankincense's fragrance can deepen breathing, aid relaxation, and cause the lungs to expand. Modern science backs up these observations by showing that, when burned, frankincense releases molecules of trahydrocannabinole, a psychoactive compound that may be responsible for uplifting the spirit. The pale yellow oil is steam distilled from hard "tears" of oleo gum resin.

THERAPEUTIC PROPERTIES

Antiseptic, anti-inflammatory, antifungal, astringent, sedative; clears lung congestion, decreases gas and indigestion, brings on menstruation.

USED FOR

Its antiseptic and skin-healing properties fight bacterial and fungal skin infections and boils. Since it's quite expensive, however, it is usually reserved for the most difficult cases, such as unsightly scars that remain after an infection has healed, and hard-to-heal wounds. For problem skin areas, use a couple drops of frankincense in an equal amount of vegetable oil. Frankincense is excellent on mature skin and acne. It is especially good when middle-aged women experience those conditions and also want to prevent wrinkles. Make a compress or massage oil with frankincense for breast cysts or for infection of the lungs, reproductive organs, or urinary tract. It also increases menstrual flow.

GALBANUM

BOTANICAL NAME: *FERULA GALBANIFLUA*

Originating on the slopes of mountain ranges in Iran, galbanum was used in ancient times for incense and perfume. In fact, the biblical book of Exodus mentions galbanum as a component in a sacred incense offering. But the flowering plant's healing and therapeutic properties are even more impressive than its scent. In fact, Hippocrates—known as the "Father of Modern Medicine"—made use of galbanum with his patients, and the herb was used medicinally in ancient Mesopotamia, India, and China. Often galbanum would be administered in pill form, making it one of the oldest "drugs" in the world.

THERAPEUTIC PROPERTIES

Antispasmodic; improves blood circulation; helps to diminish scars; decongestant; repels insects and parasites.

USED FOR

Galbanum has a relaxing effect on the muscles, and is often used by athletes to treat muscle cramps and pulls. Its ability to improve circulation, especially in the joints, helps to relieve pain from arthritis and rheumatism. Galbanum has been shown to speed up the growth of new cells in scarred areas, making it an ideal remedy for acne scars and stretch marks. When used in incense or sprays, the oil has been shown to repel insects and parasites, including mosquitoes, lice, and bed bugs.

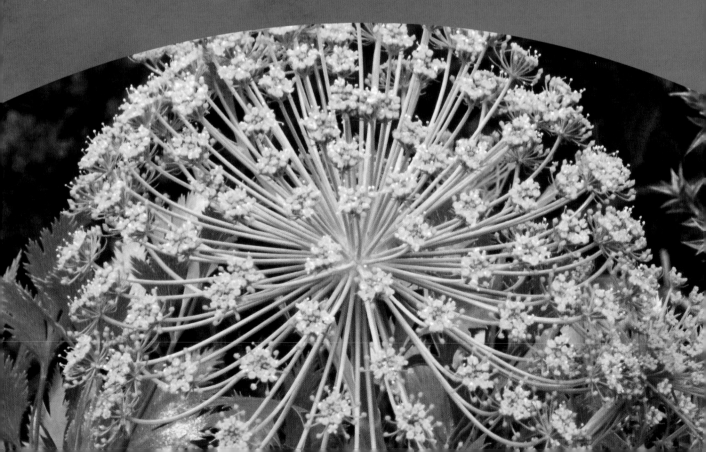

GERANIUM

BOTANICAL NAME: *PELARGONIUM GRAVEOLOENS*

A relative newcomer to the fragrance trade, geranium is a small, tender, South African perennial whose essential oil was not distilled until the nineteenth century. Since it is a veritable medicine cabinet with a lovely scent, it became an instant hit. It is also an insect repellent, and one that is certainly more aromatically pleasing than the commonly used citronella. The scent of geranium mixes well with almost any other essential oil. There are more than 600 varieties, including several with a rose-like fragrance.

THERAPEUTIC PROPERTIES

Antidepressant, antiseptic, astringent; stops bleeding; possibly gently stimulates the adrenals and normalizes hormones.

USED FOR

The essential oil treats a host of problems including inflammation, eczema, acne, burns, infected wounds, fungus (like ringworm), lice, shingles, and herpes. It also decreases scarring and stretch marks. Use it in the form of a salve, cream, lotion, or massage/body oil, whichever is most appropriate. It balances all complexion types and is said to delay wrinkling. Inhale this pleasant scent to treat PMS, menopause, fluid retention, and other hormone-related problems.

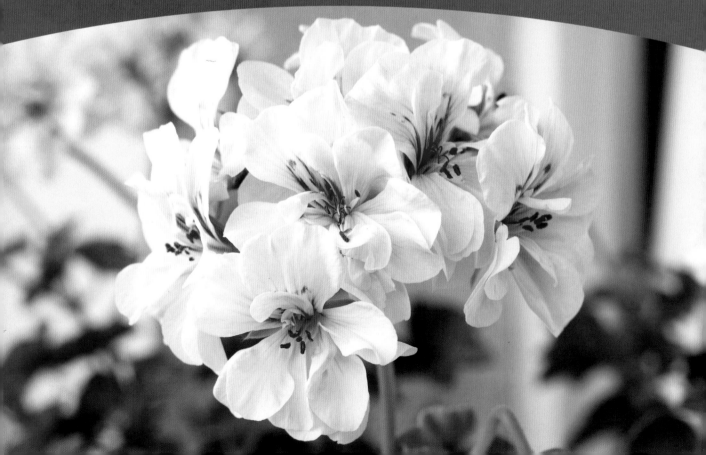

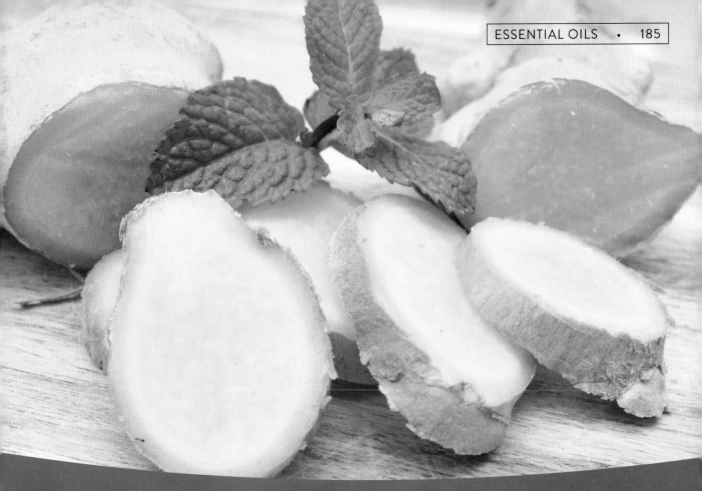

GINGER

BOTANICAL NAME: *ZINGIBER OFFICINALE*

You have certainly encountered ginger's succulent, spicy rhizome in the grocery store. Used fresh, or dried and powdered for a culinary spice, it flavors ginger ale, cakes, and cookies and is a major ingredient in curries and other Eastern cuisines. The Chinese scholar Confucius ate fresh ginger with every meal. Since it was one of the earliest herbs transported in the spice trade, it is now difficult to determine if ginger originated in India or China.

THERAPEUTIC PROPERTIES

Stimulates circulation, increases perspiration, relieves gas and pain, aids digestion.

USED FOR

Use a ginger compress wrapped around the neck or placed on the chest to ease sore throat or lung congestion. The smell of it alone will often open congested sinuses. If you experience nausea or motion sickness, inhale a drop placed on a hankie, eat a little candied ginger, or sip ginger ale, which contains a small amount of the essential oil. To relieve indigestion or menstrual cramps, rub a massage oil containing ginger into the skin on your abdomen or place a poultice made from the grated root on it. In a warming liniment, ginger essential oil treats poor circulation and sore or cramped muscles, since it decreases the substances in the body that make muscles cramp.

HELICHRYSUM

BOTANICAL NAME: *HELICHRYSUM ITALICUM*

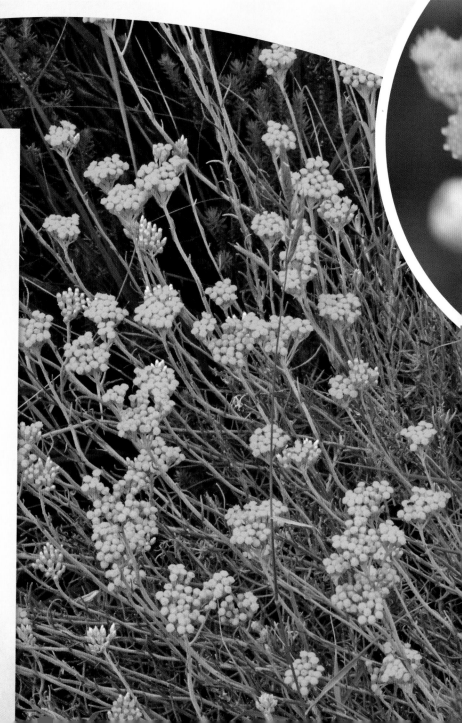

Helichrysum is a small perennial herb. The plant's medicinal and culinary uses go back to the days of ancient Greece. While there are a number of flowering species of helichrysum used in essential oil form, the most commonly available variety is *Helichrysum italicum*. The essential oil is obtained from its clusters of small, golden yellow blossoms.

Helichrysum's aroma is complex but nearly always described as sweet. Think caramelized sugar, honey, and nectar, wrapped in a floral bouquet. Its cloying fragrance is not for everyone, making its aromatherapy applications limited. No matter—this is an oil with amazing regenerative qualities when applied topically. Helichrysum is a skin care superstar: it's ideal for treating scars, blemishes, stretch marks, rashes, acne, and aging skin. It is even effective at treating sprains, muscle pain, and stiffness. Helichrysum promotes the regrowth of skin and the healing of wounds and cuts.

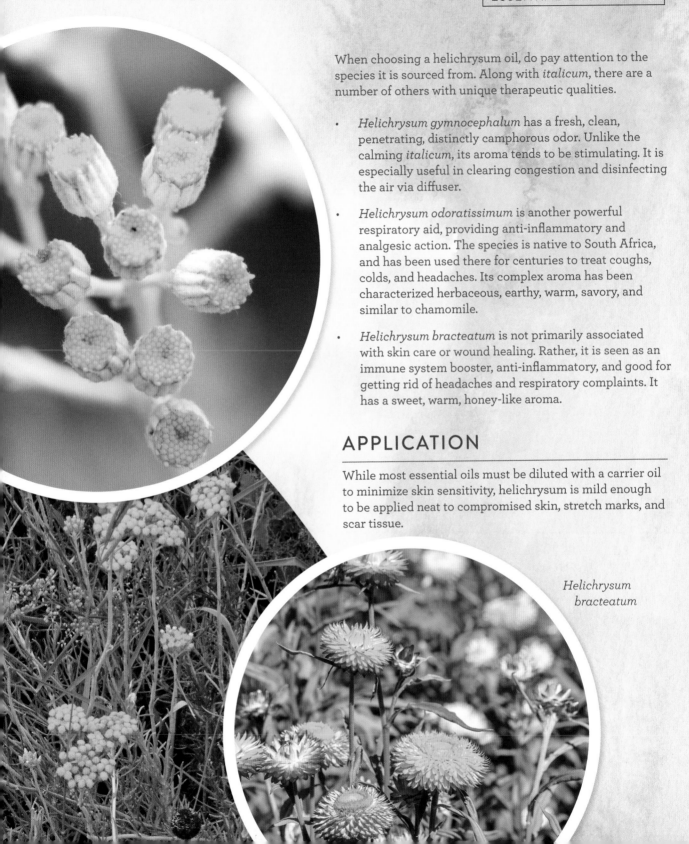

When choosing a helichrysum oil, do pay attention to the species it is sourced from. Along with *italicum*, there are a number of others with unique therapeutic qualities.

- *Helichrysum gymnocephalum* has a fresh, clean, penetrating, distinctly camphorous odor. Unlike the calming *italicum*, its aroma tends to be stimulating. It is especially useful in clearing congestion and disinfecting the air via diffuser.

- *Helichrysum odoratissimum* is another powerful respiratory aid, providing anti-inflammatory and analgesic action. The species is native to South Africa, and has been used there for centuries to treat coughs, colds, and headaches. Its complex aroma has been characterized herbaceous, earthy, warm, savory, and similar to chamomile.

- *Helichrysum bracteatum* is not primarily associated with skin care or wound healing. Rather, it is seen as an immune system booster, anti-inflammatory, and good for getting rid of headaches and respiratory complaints. It has a sweet, warm, honey-like aroma.

APPLICATION

While most essential oils must be diluted with a carrier oil to minimize skin sensitivity, helichrysum is mild enough to be applied neat to compromised skin, stretch marks, and scar tissue.

Helichrysum bracteatum

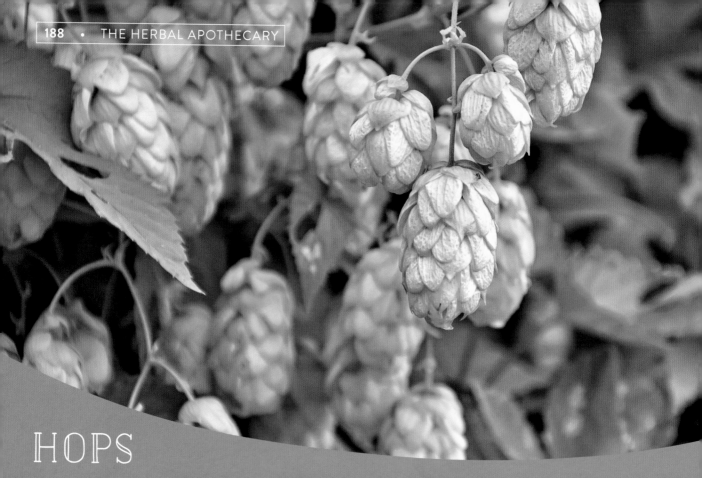

HOPS

BOTANICAL NAME: *HUMULUS LUPULUS*

If you only think of brewing beer when you think of hops, you may be missing out on some great essential oil benefits! The well-known libation ingredient is native to Europe, Asia, and North America, and the fragrant flowers of the plant attract butterflies. The essential oil is derived from these aromatic hops, and the spicy scent is used in perfumes and aromatherapy. Historically, the hops plant has been used as a sedative, and was often placed inside an insomnia sufferer's pillow—which was fittingly called a "hops pillow"—to promote better sleep. Nowadays, the oil can be added to a diffuser or to bath water to produce the same calming effects.

THERAPEUTIC PROPERTIES

Analgesic, anti-inflammatory; helps to relax nervous system.

USED FOR

Hops oil is most popularly used to reduce anxiety, relieve tension headaches, and promote better sleep. The oil has also been shown to relieve chronic pain and to soothe psoriasis and other skin irritations.

PRECAUTIONS

Because of its sedative properties, hops oil can exacerbate symptoms of depression. It is recommended that anyone suffering from depression avoid this essential oil.

HYSSOP

BOTANICAL NAME: *HYSSOPUS OFFICINALIS*

Hyssop is native to southern Europe and the Middle East, and has been used medicinally since antiquity due to its antiseptic, cough-relieving, and expectorant properties. It was also used for religious purposes in ancient Egypt, where priests would eat the herb during purification rituals. In the Middle Ages, hyssop was used to repel lice, to mask bad smells, and even to ward off plague. And Benedictine monks used the herb to create soups, sauces, and liqueurs. By 1631, the plant had made its way to North America with European settlers, and is now commonly grown throughout the northern United States and Canada. It has a bright medicinal smell that many people will associate with mouthwash.

THERAPEUTIC PROPERTIES

Antiseptic, antiviral, antispasmodic; helps stimulate digestive system; helpful for relieving respiratory ailments.

USED FOR

Hyssop has been shown to prevent infections when applied to wounds, and is effective against viral infections such as colds and flu. Its antispasmodic properties make it a great choice for calming coughs, and hyssop tea can soothe a sore throat. When used in steam inhalation, the oil helps to ease breathing and clear the respiratory tract. Hyssop has also been shown to stimulate the digestive system, and reduce discomfort due to indigestion or gas.

PRECAUTIONS

Hyssop oil contains a compound called pinocamphone, which can stimulate the nerves and cause seizures, especially in people with epilepsy. Those with epilepsy should avoid the oil.

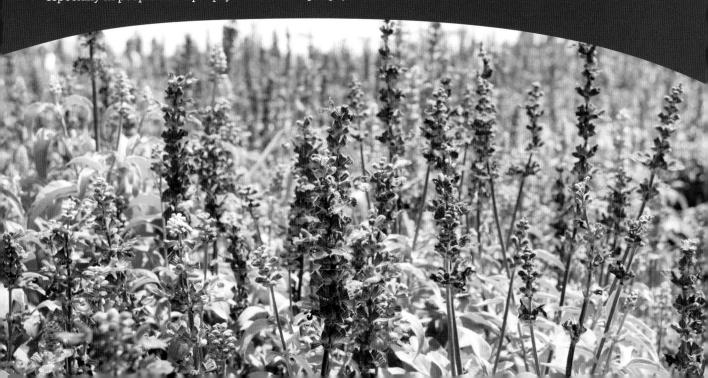

JASMINE

BOTANICAL NAME: *JASMINUM OFFICINALIS* AND *J. GRANDIFLORUM*

The small white flowers of this vinelike evergreen shrub, with their intriguing, complex scent, are intensely fragrant and found in most great perfumes. Jasmine is also known as "mistress of the night" and "moonlight of the grove" because its seductive scent reaches its peak late at night. Even the production of the essential oil is exotic. The flowers are gathered at night, when they produce the most oil, and laid on a layer of fat when using the enfleurage method. Try as chemists might to make it, the scent cannot be duplicated. Synthetic jasmine is so harsh, it demands a touch of the true essential oil to soften it.

THERAPEUTIC PROPERTIES

Antidepressant; relaxes nerves, relieves muscle spasms and cramping.

USED FOR

Jasmine sedates the nervous system, so it is good for jangled nerves, headaches, insomnia, and depression and for taking the emotional edge off PMS and menopause, although keep in mind its age-old reputation as an aphrodisiac! Studies at Toho University School of Medicine in Tokyo show that jasmine also enhances mental alertness and stimulates brain waves. It also eases muscle cramping, such as menstrual cramps. Cosmetically, the oil is wonderful for sensitive or mature skin. In its native India, jasmine flowers infused into sesame oil are applied to abscesses and sores that are difficult to heal. A similar preparation can be made by adding 2 drops of jasmine essential oil to 1 ounce vegetable oil.

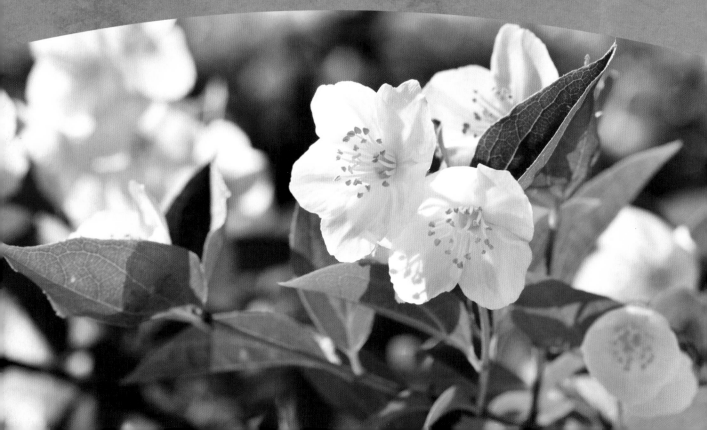

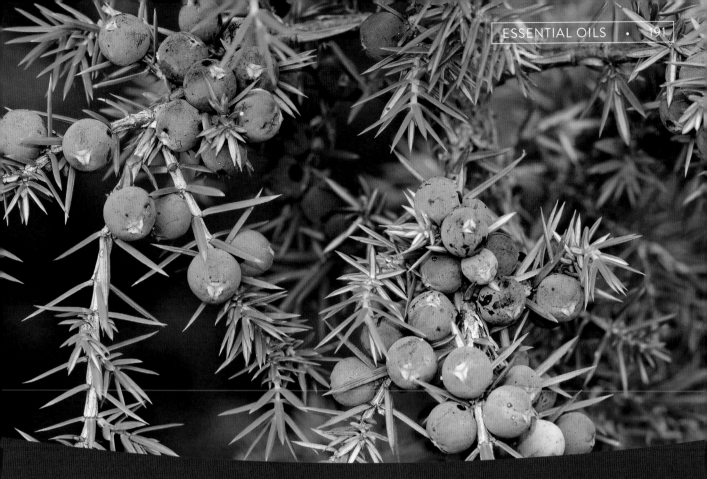

JUNIPER BERRIES

BOTANICAL NAME: *JUNIPERUS COMMUNIS*

Burning juniper branches was found to ward off contagious diseases, so medieval physicians chewed the berries while on duty and burned the branches in hospitals. In World War II, the French returned to burning juniper in hospitals as an antiseptic when their supply of drugs ran low. Fresh berries offer the highest quality oil, but needles, branches, and berries that have already been distilled to flavor gin are sometimes used. With many of the same properties as cedarwood, it also acts as a wool moth repellent.

THERAPEUTIC PROPERTIES

Antiseptic, astringent; relieves the aches of rheumatism, arthritis, and sore muscles; increases urination and circulation; encourages menstruation.

USED FOR

Juniper berry essential oil is used in massage oils, liniments, and baths to treat arthritic and rheumatic pain, varicose veins, hemorrhoids, fluid retention (especially before menstruation), and bladder infection. Inhale it in a steam to relieve bronchial congestion, infection, and bronchial spasms. Inhalation may also lift your spirits, as sniffing the oil seems to work as a pick-me-up and to counter general debility. Cosmetically it is suitable for acne complexions and eczema. Add approximately 6 drops per ounce to shampoos for greasy hair or dandruff.

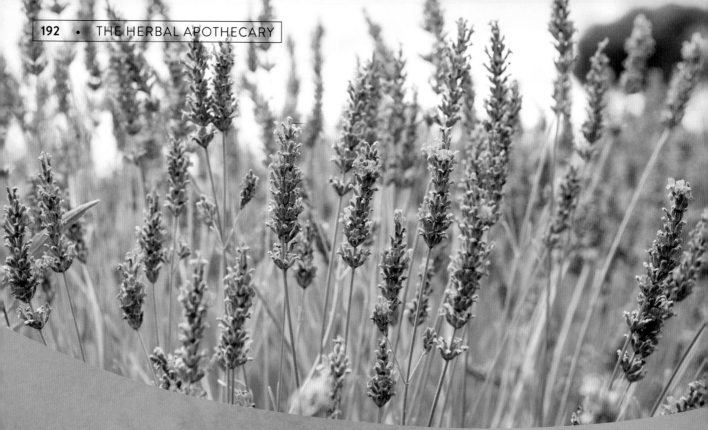

LAVENDER

BOTANICAL NAME: *LAVANDULA ANGUSTIFOLIA*

A well-loved Mediterranean herb, lavender has been associated with cleanliness since Romans first added it to their bathwater. In fact, the name comes from the Latin *lavandus*, meaning to wash. Today lavender remains a favorite for scenting clothing and closets, soaps, and even furniture polish. Lavender was traditionally inhaled to ease exhaustion, insomnia, irritability, and depression. Two related plants called spike (*L. latifolia*) and lavandin (*L. intermedia*) are produced in greater quantities; but they are more camphorous and harsher in scent, with inferior healing properties, although they are useful for disinfecting.

THERAPEUTIC PROPERTIES

Antiseptic, circulatory stimulant; relieves muscle spasms and cramping.

USED FOR

Lavender is among the safest and most widely used of all aromatherapy oils. It relieves muscle pain, migraines and other headaches, and inflammation. It is also one of the most antiseptic essential oils, treating many types of infection, including lung, sinus, and vaginal infections. Lavender is suitable for all skin types. Cosmetically, it appears to be a cell regenerator. It prevents scarring and stretch marks and reputedly slows the development of wrinkles. It is used on burns, sun-damaged skin, wounds, rashes, and, of course, skin infections. Of several fragrances tested by aromatherapy researchers, lavender was most effective at relaxing brain waves and reducing stress.

LEMON

BOTANICAL NAME: *CITRUS LIMONUM*

Most people would describe lemon as having a "clean" smelling fragrance. Aromatherapists use the tie-in with cleanliness to help people purge feelings of imperfection and impurity and to build up their confidence. Lemon essential oil is a major ingredient in commercial beverages, foods, and pharmaceuticals, although the cheaper lemongrass or even synthetic citral is often added to stretch it. It also is popular for its fresh aroma in cologne and many cosmetics, especially cleansing creams and lotions.

The flowers are occasionally distilled for their pleasant aroma, but cold pressing the peel produces the essential oil that you are most likely to find. Like other citruses, the oil keeps well for only about a year; so you can prolong its life by storing it in a cool place or even in the refrigerator.

THERAPEUTIC PROPERTIES

Antiseptic, antidepressant, antiviral; decreases indigestion, stops bleeding.

USED FOR

Studies show that the oil increases the activity of the immune system by stimulating the production of the white corpuscles that fight infection. Additionally, lemon essential oil counters a wide range of viral and bacterial infections. Massage it on the skin in a vegetable oil base to relieve congested lymph glands. Inhaled it has been shown to reduce blood pressure. Since it also reduces water retention and increases mineral absorption, it can be helpful in achieving weight loss. Incorporated into cosmetics, lemon is best used on oily complexions and to clean acne, blackheads, and other skin impurities.

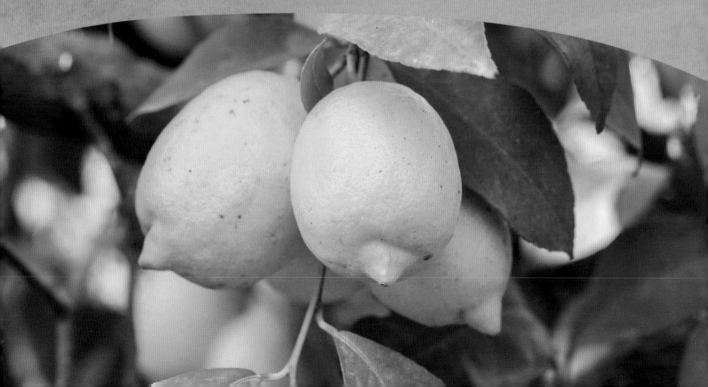

LEMONGRASS

BOTANICAL NAME: *CYMBOPOGON CITRATUS*

A relatively inexpensive essential oil, lemongrass is often the source of the lemon scent found in cosmetics and hair preparations. Its pleasant, clean fragrance is also incorporated into soaps, perfumes, and deodorants, and it flavors many canned and frozen foods. No wonder it is one of the ten best-selling essential oils in the world.

Along with related oils such as the lemon-rose scented palmarosa (*C. martini*) and citronella (*C. nardus*), it often adulterates more costly essential oils like melissa and lemon verbena to stretch quantities. Palmarosa is frequently used in skin preparations, while citronella is well known as an insect repellent and cleanser. The yellow to amber oil of these grasses is distilled from their partially dried leaves.

THERAPEUTIC PROPERTIES

Antiseptic, deodorant, astringent; relieves rheumatic and other pain, relaxes nerves.

USED FOR

Researchers also found this refreshing fragrance to reduce headaches and irritability and to prevent drowsiness. To make a foot bath, add about 3 drops of lemongrass oil to 2 or 3 quarts of warm water in a small tub. Stir well and keep your feet in the water for at least 20 minutes. You can also add a few drops to your bath. Lemongrass is an antiseptic suitable for use on various types of skin infections, usually as a wash or compress, and is especially effective on ringworm and infected sores. In fact, studies found that it is more effective against staph infection than either penicillin or streptomycin. When sprayed on a counter top, or along walls and floors, it discourages insect invasions and mold.

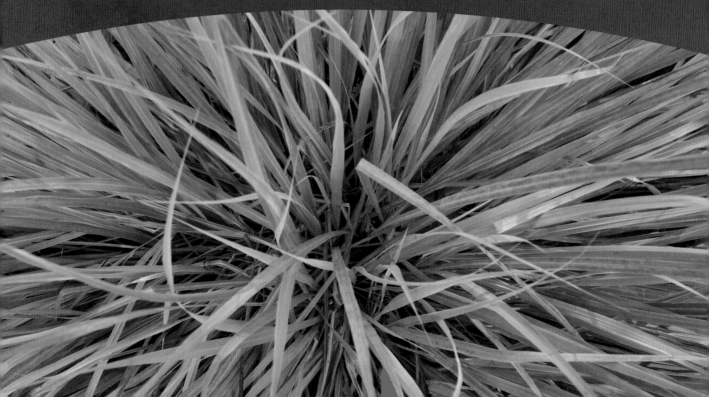

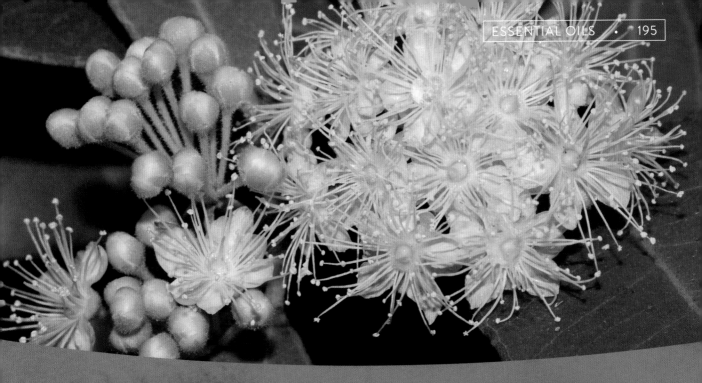

LEMON MYRTLE

BOTANICAL NAME: *BACKHOUSIA CITRIODORA*

Named after English botanist James Backhouse, *Backhousia citriodora* was once commonly known as lemon-scented myrtle. Eventually, the name was shortened to "lemon myrtle," to help the edible herb achieve more popularity in the culinary world. The lemony dried leaves are used in everything from sweet desserts to savory pastas, and are also popular in soaps, lotions, and bath products. The plant is native to Australia, where indigenous people have used it for medicine for hundreds of years due to its antimicrobial properties. Even today, the majority of lemon myrtle used for essential oil is grown only in Queensland and New South Wales, Australia.

THERAPEUTIC PROPERTIES

Antimicrobial, antifungal, anti-inflammatory; helps to relieve anxiety and stress; deodorizes; used in bath products.

USED FOR

Lemon myrtle's antimicrobial properties make it ideal for treating skin conditions such as acne and psoriasis, or preventing infections in minor cuts and scrapes. It can also ease itching and inflammation caused by insect bites and stings. It may help boost the immune system and keep colds and flu at bay. A few drops in bathwater help to relax the mind as well as the muscles. Lemon myrtle makes an excellent cleaner for your home, thanks to its antiseptic qualities and uplifting scent.

PRECAUTIONS

Because of its citric quality, lemon myrtle may make skin more susceptible to sunburn. If used topically, avoid direct exposure to sunlight for 48 hours.

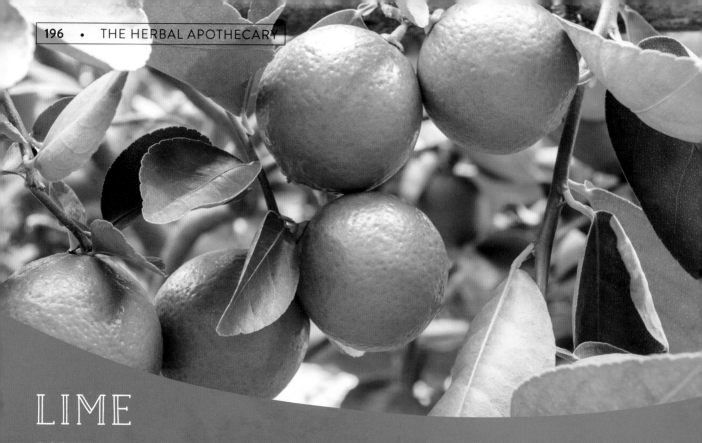

LIME

BOTANICAL NAME: *CITRUS AURANTIFOLIA*

Lime trees may be best known for providing the crucial ingredient in delicious key lime pies, but the tree is beneficial for more than just your taste buds. Lime has been used for therapeutic purposes since prehistoric times, when the leaves of the tree were used to treat bug bites and injuries. In the 19th century, British sailors would use the vitamin C rich fruit to prevent scurvy and skin problems. In fact, it is said that the sailor nickname "limey" came about because of the fruit's popularity with sailors! Today, lime oil is widely used in the food and beverage industry due to its refreshing, tart taste, but the same antioxidant properties that protected sailors still provide us with healthy benefits today.

THERAPEUTIC PROPERTIES

Antibacterial, antiviral, astringent; helps to stop bleeding from fresh wounds; excellent for use in aromatherapy.

USED FOR

Lime oil has been shown to protect against infections in minor cuts and scrapes, as well as ward off colds and flu. It works well to heal skin conditions such as psoriasis, rashes, and acne. Its astringent properties can help tone and tighten skin, keep gums healthy, and stop bleeding from minor injuries. Use a few drops in a diffuser for an uplifting, energizing scent.

PRECAUTIONS

As with other citrus-based oils, lime oil may make skin more susceptible to sunburn. If used topically, avoid direct exposure to sunlight for 48 hours.

LITSEA CUBEBA

BOTANICAL NAME: *LITSEA CUBEBA*

Also known as aromatic litsea and may chang, litsea cubeba is an evergreen tree native to Southeast Asia. The tree bears a fruit that resembles a pepper, giving it the nickname "mountain pepper." The essential oil—which has a lemony, citrusy scent similar to lemongrass—is extracted from these ripened and dried pepper-like fruits. The oil has traditionally been used in Chinese medicine to help with digestive issues, muscle aches, and asthma, and to relieve stress and anxiety. Although litsea cubeba is one of the least common essential oils on the market, its benefits should convince you to give it a try!

THERAPEUTIC PROPERTIES

Antibacterial, antiviral, antifungal, anti-inflammatory; helps reduce stress and anxiety; used to relieve digestive upset; insect repellant and home cleaner.

USED FOR

Effective in killing bacteria, viruses, and fungi, litsea cubeba aids a host of problems, including acne, athlete's foot, insect bites, and ringworm. The uplifting scent has been used for hundreds of years in aromatherapy to induce feelings of calm and reduce stress. A few drops added to a carrier oil and massaged into your stomach can reduce indigestion and stomach upset. The oil makes a great cleaner for your home, and the fresh-smelling scent helps keep bugs at bay.

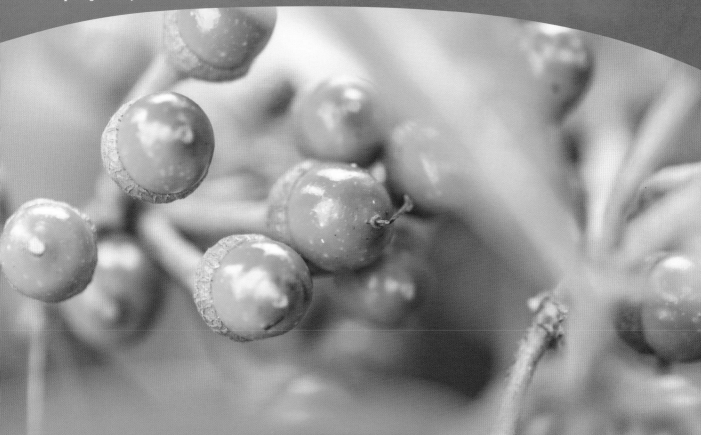

MARJORAM

BOTANICAL NAME: *ORIGANUM MARJORANA*

The greenish-yellow oil is distilled from the plant's flowering tops. Its taste and properties are milder than the closely related oregano, which is so strong and potentially toxic that it is seldom used in aromatherapy. The odor is sweet, herby, and pungent in concentration. When diluted, it mellows to an almost warm, spicy floral with a hint of camphor.

THERAPEUTIC PROPERTIES

Antioxidant; calms nerves, clears mucous from the lungs, relieves pain, improves digestion, brings on menstruation, lowers high blood pressure, stops bleeding.

USED FOR

A good sedative, marjoram eases stiff joints and muscle spasms, including tics, excessive coughing, menstrual cramps, and headaches (especially migraines). It also slightly lowers high blood pressure. Testing has shown it to be one of the most effective fragrances in relaxing brain waves. As a result, it makes an excellent calming massage oil, delightful when combined with the softer lavender. Add a few drops to your bath to counter stress or insomnia. Since it has specific properties that fight the viruses and bacteria responsible for colds, flu, or laryngitis, add a few drops of essential oil to either a chest balm or bath, or put 2 or 3 drops in a bowl of hot water and inhale the steam. In healing salves and creams, it also soothes burns, bruises, and inflammation. Marjoram is also an antioxidant that naturally preserves food.

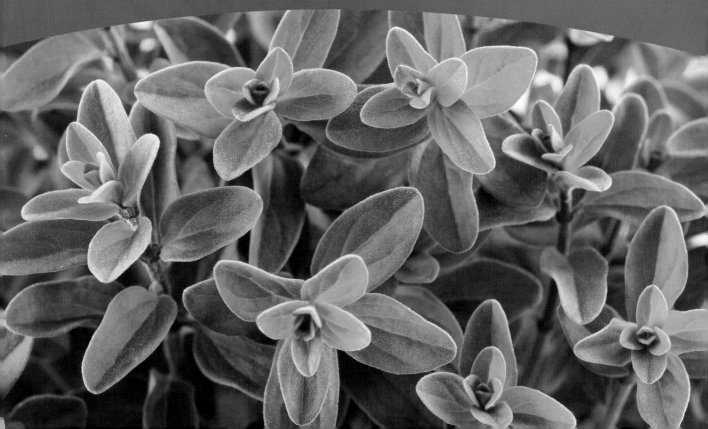

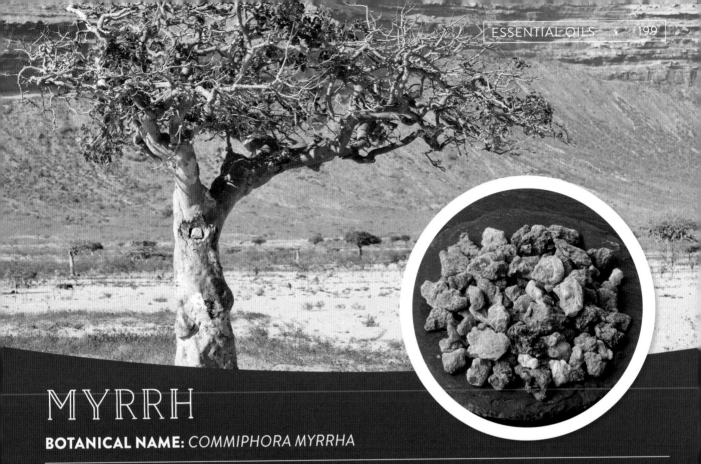

MYRRH

BOTANICAL NAME: *COMMIPHORA MYRRHA*

This small, scrubby, spiny tree from the Middle East and North East Africa is not very handsome, but it makes up for its looks with the precious gum it exudes. An important trade item for several thousand years, myrrh was a primary ingredient in ancient cosmetics and incenses. Believed to comfort sorrow, its name means "bitter tears." This may also refer to the bitter-tasting myrrh sap, which oozes in drops when the tree's bark is cut. Myrrh was added to wine by both the Greeks and Hebrews to heighten sensual awareness. The yellow to amber-colored oil is distilled from the gum and frequently added to toothpastes and gum preparations to help alleviate mouth ulcers, gum inflammation, and infection.

THERAPEUTIC PROPERTIES

Antiseptic, anti-inflammatory, antibacterial, antifungal, decongestant, astringent; heals wounds, brings on menstruation.

USED FOR

Myrrh is an expensive but effective treatment for chapped, cracked, or aged skin, eczema, bruises, infection, varicose veins, ringworm, and athlete's foot. Included in many ointments, it dries weepy wounds. It is a specific remedy for mouth and gum disease and is found in many oral preparations. It is very helpful applied on herpes sores and blisters: Add it to a lip balm, using about 25 drops per ounce. Lozenges or syrup containing myrrh treat coughs. As an additional bonus, it increases the activity of the immune system.

PRECAUTIONS

Due to a possible increase of thyroid activity, do not use myrrh if you have an overactive thyroid.

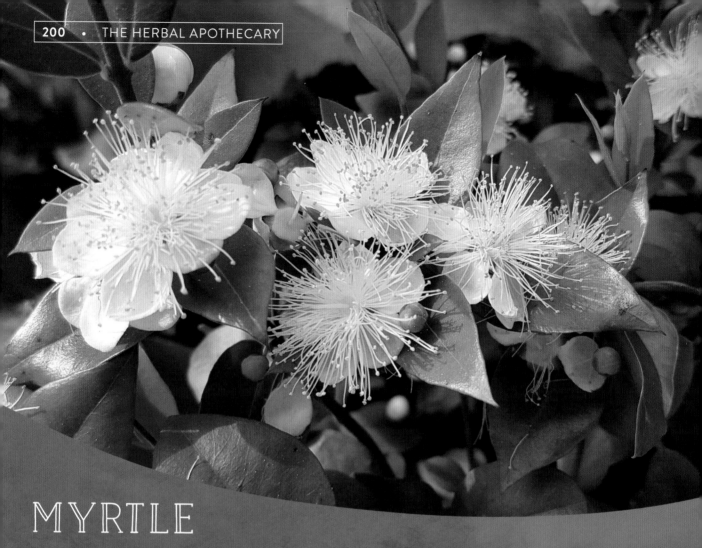

MYRTLE

BOTANICAL NAME: *MYRTUS COMMUNIS*

A flowering evergreen shrub, myrtle originated in Africa and southern Europe. According to Greek mythology, the plant was sacred to the goddesses Aphrodite and Demeter, and the plant is mentioned numerous times in ancient Greek and Roman writings. Myrtle has a long history of medicinal use, having been prescribed for fever and pain relief since at least 2500 BC. This may be due to its high concentration of salicylic acid, which is a compound related to aspirin and other modern-day pain relievers. Myrtle's scent is similar to eucalyptus oil, and, in fact, it comes from the same family as both eucalyptus and tea tree.

THERAPEUTIC PROPERTIES

Antimicrobial, antiseptic, anti-inflammatory; decongestant and expectorant; deodorant.

USED FOR

Myrtle oil can be applied to cuts and scrapes to prevent infection, or used to address skin conditions like acne. When used in a diffuser, the oil can help relieve congestion, coughs, and bronchial infections. Myrtle also makes an excellent deodorizer, either when used as incense or applied to the body like deodorant.

NEROLI

BOTANICAL NAME: *CITRUS AURANTIUM*

An Indochina native, the bitter orange produces the blossoms used for an oil known to aromatherapists and perfumers as neroli. Modern aromatherapists regard neroli as a treatment for depression. The blossoms may be distilled, made into a concrete by enfleurage, or extracted with solvents to create an absolute. A by-product of distillation, "orange flower water," is used in cooking and as a skin toner. Neroli is the main ingredient of the original eau de cologne, which was used both as a body fragrance and as a skin toner. Distilling the leaves and stems of the bitter orange produces an essential oil called petitgrain that is frequently used in men's cologne today and often adulterates the far more expensive neroli.

THERAPEUTIC PROPERTIES

Sedative; relieves muscle spasms and cramping, stimulates circulation.

USED FOR

Neroli's favored use is for circulation problems, especially hemorrhoids and high blood pressure. It makes a wonderfully fragrant and effective cosmetic for mature, dry, and sensitive skin and is also one of the best essential oils to add to a vaginal cream during menopause. It reputedly regenerates skin cells and has anti-aging properties. For the ultimate luxury, add it to your bath to ease tension from PMS, menopause, or life in general.

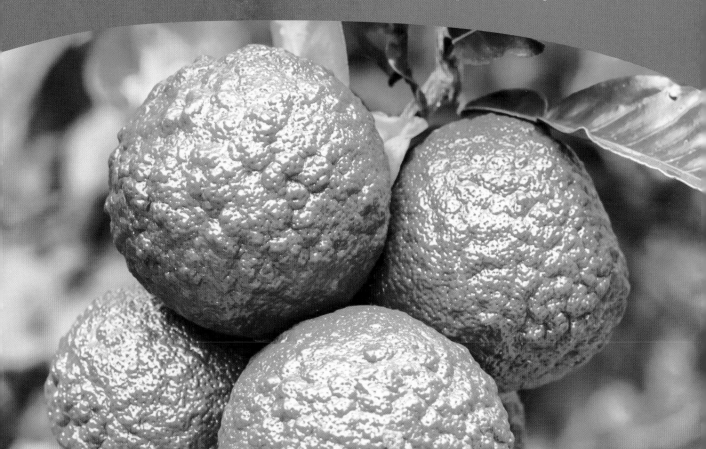

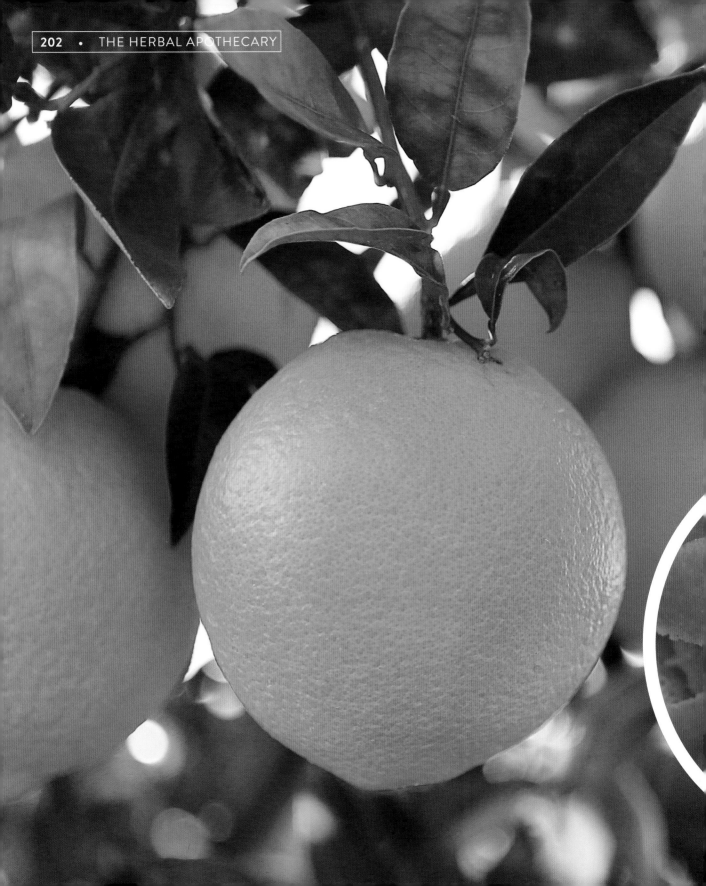

ORANGE

BOTANICAL NAME: *CITRUS SINENSIS*

Dispersed throughout the Mediterranean during the time of the crusades, the familiar sweet orange now comes from Sicily, Israel, Spain, and the U.S., each country's essential oil offering slightly different characteristics. They are rich in vitamins A, B, and C, flavonoids, and minerals. The Chinese, however, correctly warned in the *Chu-lu*—the first monograph describing the various citruses that was written in 1178—that they can increase lung congestion.

Oranges were considered symbols of fruitfulness, and the Greeks called them the "golden apple of the Hesperides." The god Zeus is said to have given an orange to his bride Hera at their wedding.

In 1290, Eleanor of Castile brought oranges to England, where they were grown as luxuries in greenhouses or "orangeries." In northern climates, only the very wealthy could afford oranges, and they were often given as extravagant gifts at Christmas time. In European courts they were stuck with cloves and carried as a pomander to dispel disagreeable odors and emotions such as depression and nervousness, as well as to bring more cheer into dreary winter days. The essential oil is cold pressed from the peel and lasts only about a year, so keep it cool and away from direct sunlight.

Orange's greatest claim to aromatherapy fame is its ability to affect moods and to lower high blood pressure. In fact, just sniffing it lowers blood pressure a couple points. It is also a good adjunct treatment for irregular heartbeat. Research at International Flavors and Fragrances, Inc., in New Jersey found that orange also reduces anxiety. You don't even need to buy the essential oil; simply peel an orange and inhale its aroma. Although not as antibiotic as lemon, it still has some value in fighting flu, colds, and breaking up congested lymph, especially when added to massage oil. The aroma of oranges is a favorite of children, and they will usually be more enthusiastic about an aromatherapy treatment when it is included. Also use the massage oil to ease a bout of indigestion or overcome a light case of insomnia or depression. Cosmetically it is good for oily complexions, although essential oils with more sophisticated fragrances are preferred.

PRECAUTIONS

The oil is only slightly photosensitizing, but still go easy in baths or any skin preparations since it can burn the skin—just 4 drops in a bathtub can be enough to irritate and redden sensitive skin. Related oils such as that of tangerine or mandarin are milder and safer choices for pregnant women and very young children.

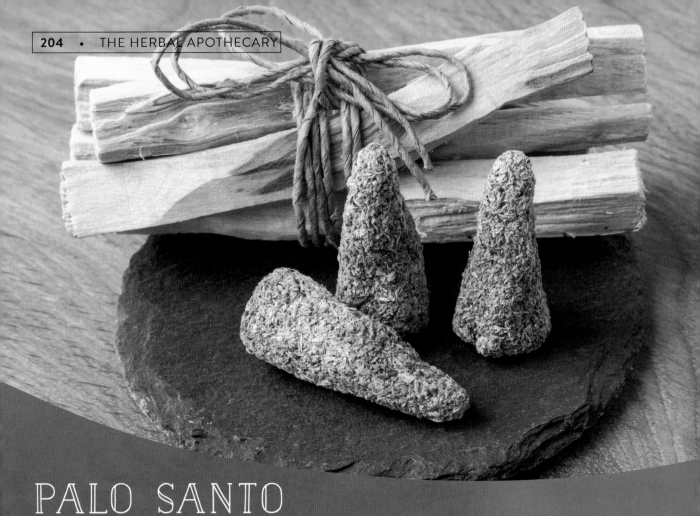

PALO SANTO

BOTANICAL NAME: *BURSERA GRAVEOLENS*

Palo santo, Spanish for "holy wood," is a tree native to Mexico, Central and South America, and the Galapagos Islands. The tree is from the same botanical family as frankincense and myrrh, which are also known for their beneficial essential oils. The oil from the palo santo tree has been used for centuries in folk medicine, as a way to relieve stomachaches and pain from arthritis, and was often burned by medicine men as a way to drive out "bad energy." Today, palo santo is seen as a promising aid for fighting inflammation and boosting immunity. Interestingly, the oil is distilled from fallen branches and dead trees, as palo santo wood develops a unique chemistry once it is dead.

THERAPEUTIC PROPERTIES

Antibacterial, anti-inflammatory; fights colds and flu; bug repellant; excellent household cleaner.

USED FOR

Palo santo's anti-inflammatory properties help to boost the immune system during times of stress or illness, and provide relief from headaches. Add a few drops to a bath to help fight colds and flu. The oil can be combined with water and sprayed on skin or clothes as a natural bug repellant. Its sweet scent and antibacterial effect make it a great choice for disinfecting and deodorizing your home.

PARSLEY SEED

BOTANICAL NAME: *PETROSELINUM SATIVUM*

Most of us are familiar with parsley as a leafy garnish on restaurant plates, but the Mediterranean herb has been prized for thousands of years for its medicinal benefits, as well as its culinary value. In fact, parsley is one of the oldest spices—and possibly medicines—known to man! Ancient Egyptians and Greeks were familiar with the plant, and the epic poet Homer even mentioned it in the *Odyssey*. Early Greek and Roman physicians found the herb useful for treating kidney and bladder disorders, digestive issues, gallstones, and dysentery. Oil can be extracted from the entire plant, but the seeds contain the highest concentration of this amazing substance.

THERAPEUTIC PROPERTIES

Antimicrobial, diuretic; aids digestion.

USED FOR

Parsley can prevent infections thanks to its antimicrobial properties. As a diuretic, it helps to detoxify the body of unwanted water, salt, and uric acid. This can not only lower blood pressure, but can relieve the symptoms of gout and arthritis, as well. One of parsley's oldest uses was aiding digestive issues, and this is still a great way to use it today: it stimulates digestion, while relieving constipation, indigestion, and gas.

PRECAUTIONS

Parsley seed oil should not be used by pregnant women as it can cause miscarriage.

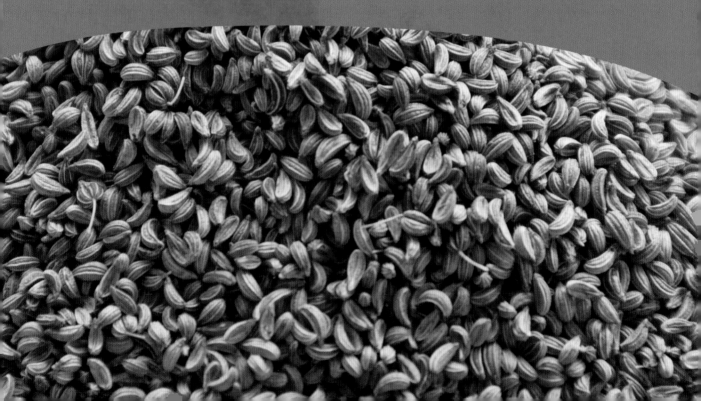

PATCHOULI

BOTANICAL NAME: *POGOSTEMON CABLIN*

To some people the scent of patchouli is exotic, sensual, and luxurious, but to others it's too forceful and repellent. It is so overpowering that most cosmetics forgo its virtues in favor of other essential oils that are more universally appealing. The leaves of this pretty Malaysian bush carry little indication of their potential, since the scent is only developed through oxidation. The leaves must be fermented and aged before being distilled. Even then, the translucent yellow oil smells harsh. As it ages, it develops patchouli's distinctive scent. Patchouli also has a reputation as an aphrodisiac, a notion that probably originated in India, where it is used as an anointing oil in Tantric sexual practices. All attempts to make a synthetic patchouli have failed.

THERAPEUTIC PROPERTIES

Antidepressant, anti-inflammatory, antiseptic, antiviral, antifungal; reduces fluid retention.

USED FOR

Cosmetically, the essential oil is a cell rejuvenator and antiseptic that treats a number of skin problems, including eczema and inflamed, cracked, and mature skin. As an antifungal, it counters athlete's foot. The aroma helps to relieve headaches, unless the patient doesn't like it!

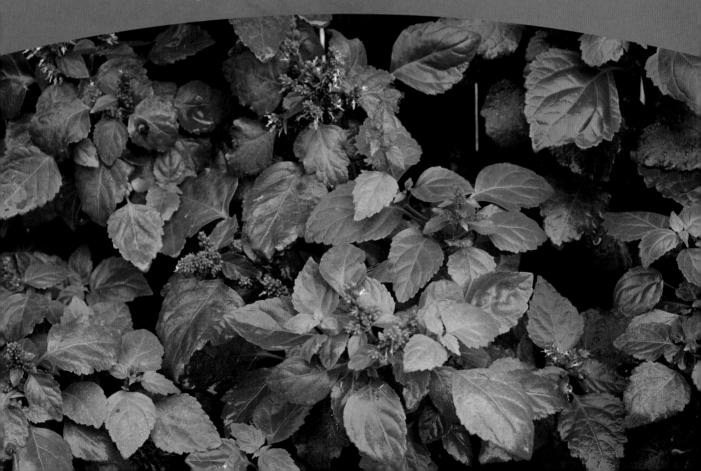

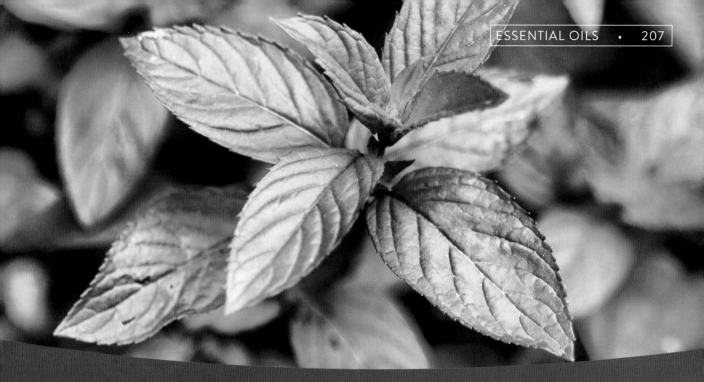

PEPPERMINT

BOTANICAL NAME: *MENTHA PIPERITA*

The most widely used of all aromatic oils, peppermint makes a grand and obvious appearance in all sorts of edible and nonedible products, including beverages, ice cream, sauces and jellies, liqueurs, medicines, dental preparations, cleaners, cosmetics, tobacco, desserts, and gums.

After the *British Medical Journal* noted in 1879 that smelling menthol (the main component in peppermint) relieves headaches and nerve pain, menthol cones that evaporate into the air became all the rage. Taking center stage in several controversies, herbalists have long argued for or against the assertion by the ancient Greek physician Galen that peppermint is an aphrodisiac. But everyone, including modern scientists, agrees that it is a strong mental and physical stimulant that can help one concentrate and stay awake and alert.

THERAPEUTIC PROPERTIES

Anti-inflammatory; relieves pain, muscle spasms, and cramping; relaxes the nerves, kills viral infections, decreases gas and indigestion, clears lung congestion, reduces fever.

USED FOR

Peppermint helps the digestion of heavy foods and relieves flatulence and intestinal cramping, actually relaxing the digestive muscles so they operate more efficiently. A massage over the abdomen with an oil containing peppermint can greatly aid intestinal spasms, indigestion, nausea, and irritable bowel syndrome. Peppermint essential oil is included in most liniments, where it warms by increasing blood flow, relieving muscle spasms and arthritis. Peppermint relieves the itching of ringworm, herpes simplex, scabies, and poison oak. It also clears sinus and lung congestion when inhaled directly. It also destroys many bacteria and viruses. Peppermint is not drying, as one might assume; rather, it stimulates the skin's oil production, so use it blended with other oils to treat dry complexions.

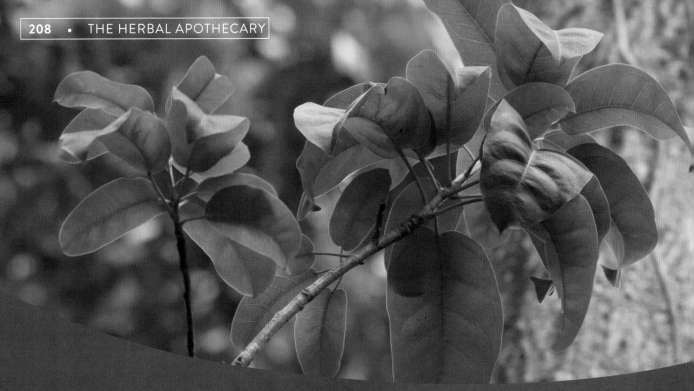

PERU BALSAM

BOTANICAL NAME: *MYROXYLON PEREIRAE*

With a lovely scent of vanilla and spice, Peru balsam is a favorite for use in aromatherapy. The oil comes from a tree in Central and South America, where a legend tells of a wounded Aztec princess who was healed by miraculous balsam resin. The traditional methods of oil extraction are quite interesting: balsam collectors, known as "balsameros," climb the 65-foot-high trunks of the trees and cut the trunks until the resin flows. Cloths are applied to absorb the balsam resin, and they are then combined with bark, pressed, and purified. The purified balsam is then distilled to produce the essential oil.

THERAPEUTIC PROPERTIES

Antioxidant, antiseptic, antibacterial; reduces stress and anxiety; helps eliminate dandruff; useful in dental hygiene.

USED FOR

Helps to eliminate free radicals and prevent infections. The oil has also been shown to repel mites, such as scabies. Peru balsam's calming scent has long been used in aromatherapy to relieve stress and anxiety. A few drops mixed with water and rinsed through the hair can eliminate dead skin cells on the scalp and prevent dandruff. The pleasant scent and taste makes the oil a popular additive to toothpaste and mouthwash.

PRECAUTIONS

Peru balsam is known to be a highly allergenic substance for some people. Always perform a patch test before using the essential oil.

PLAI

BOTANICAL NAME: *ZINGIBER CASSUMUNAR*

Native to Thailand, plai is a species of plant in the same family as ginger. Although it is relatively new to the essential oil scene, it has long been used by Thai massage therapists thanks to its ability to relieve discomfort and inflammation. But unlike ginger's warming effect, plai has a pleasant cooling effect that makes it especially soothing for aches and pains. The oil has a very high concentration of a substance called Terpinen-4-ol, which is the same ingredient that gives tea tree oil its antimicrobial properties—making plai an excellent addition to your healing essential oil arsenal.

THERAPEUTIC PROPERTIES

Anti-inflammatory, antimicrobial; helps ease respiratory problems; antispasmodic.

USED FOR

Plai's anti-inflammatory properties make it especially effective for treating aches and pains associated with muscle pulls and strains. It can be used to prevent infection and treat skin conditions such as acne. When used in a diffuser, plai has been shown to be helpful for asthma, bronchitis, and colds and flu. Its antispasmodic properties help to ease menstrual pain and irritable bowel syndrome.

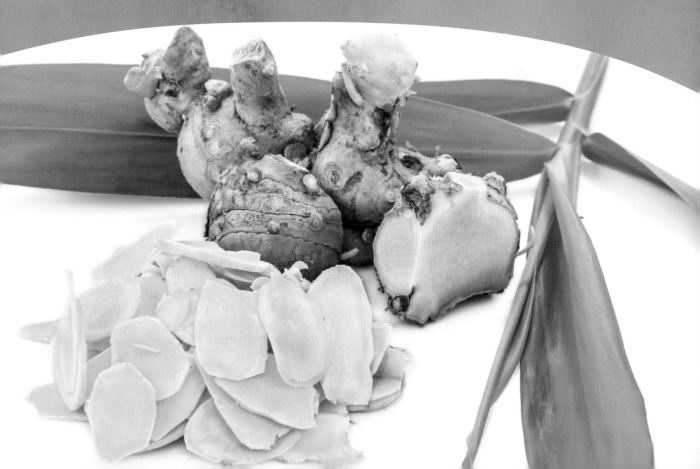

POPLAR

BOTANICAL NAME: *POPULUS BALSAMIFERA*

There are about 35 different trees in the *Populus* genus that are native to North America, and this large group is loosely divided into cottonwoods, aspens, and balsam poplars. Distilling the sticky, resinous, flowering buds of the balsam poplar is one way to produce the essential oil. While it is one of the rarer and lesser-known oils on the market, the buds of the poplar have been used by Native American medicine men for hundreds of years thanks to the medicinal properties of the buds. In fact, when Europeans first arrived in North America, the native people shared their healing balm with them, which the visitors dubbed "balm of Gilead" after the "healing balm of Gilead" referenced in the Bible.

THERAPEUTIC PROPERTIES

Antiseptic, anti-inflammatory; can help heal scars; analgesic.

USED FOR

The oil helps to heal many skin conditions and injuries, including cuts, bruises, acne, and scars. It has been shown to be an effective remedy for relieving the pain of sore muscles, arthritis, and injuries.

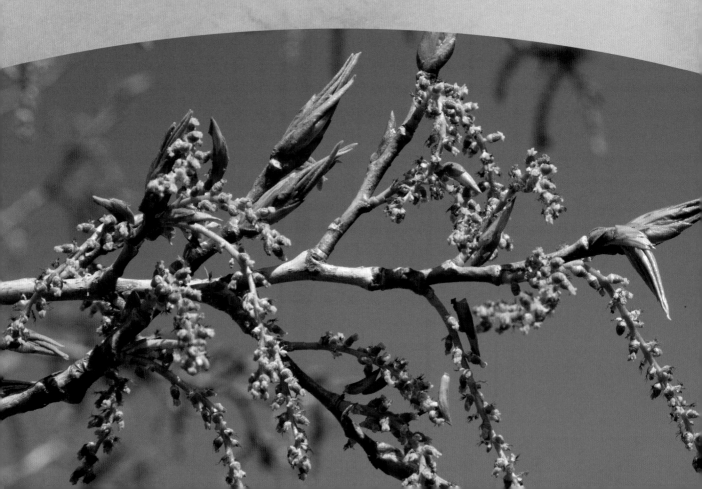

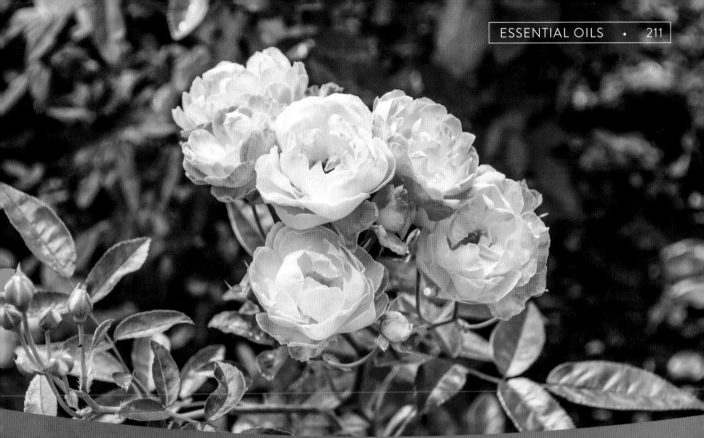

ROSE

BOTANICAL NAME: *ROSA DAMASCENA, R. GALLICA,* AND OTHERS

Originally from Asia Minor, the plant was brought by Turkish merchants to Bulgaria, where the most valued oil is now produced. It is gentle and nontoxic but extremely costly, because so little can be made during distillation and because the bushes need so much care. The oil is distilled or solvent-extracted from blossoms; but, as it is difficult to separate from water, the oil must be distilled at least twice, resulting in two products. The first is called attar of roses; the by-product is called rose water. The unadulterated oil congeals when it cools, but can be liquefied again by the warmth of the hand. It has been an age-old favorite essential oil in facial creams because, in addition to its incredible fragrance, it is reputed to fend off aging. It is also used in costly perfumes.

THERAPEUTIC PROPERTIES

Antidepressant, antiseptic, anti-inflammatory, astringent, antibacterial, antiviral; increases menstruation, calms nervous tension.

USED FOR

A cell rejuvenator and powerful antiseptic, rose essential oil soothes and heals skin conditions, including cuts and burns. It helps a variety of female disorders, possibly by balancing hormones. A massage oil helps various types of female problems, including menstrual cramps, PMS symptoms, and moodiness during menopause. Many women report that simply smelling rose's fragrance is enough to do the trick. Sniffing the oil or using a massage oil containing rose has even been suggested to help reverse impotency.

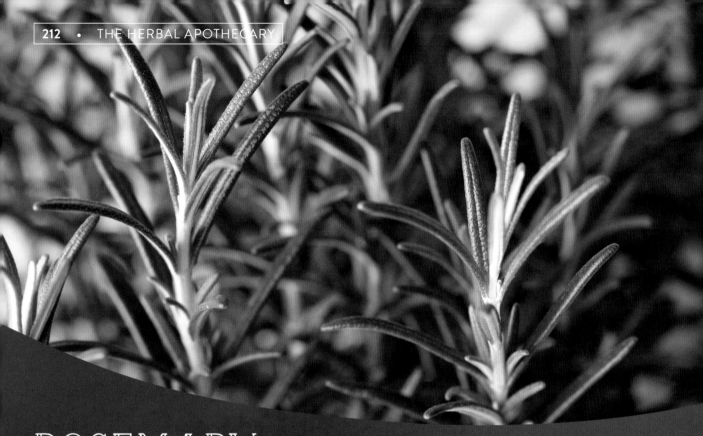

ROSEMARY

BOTANICAL NAME: *ROSMARINUS OFFICINALIS*

This Mediterranean native with tiny, pale blue flowers that bloom in late winter loves growing by the ocean—its latin name *rosmarinus* means "dew of the sea." It is cultivated worldwide, although France, Spain, and Tunisia are the main producers of the essential oil.

THERAPEUTIC PROPERTIES

Antiseptic, astringent, antioxidant; relieves rheumatic and muscle pain, relaxes nerves, improves digestion and appetite, increases sweating.

USED FOR

As an ingredient in a massage oil, compress, or bath, rosemary essential oil is excellent for increasing poor circulation and easing muscle and rheumatism pain. It is especially penetrating when used in a liniment. It is very antiseptic, so inhaling the essential oil or adding it to a vapor balm that is rubbed on the chest and throat relieves lung congestion and sore throat. It is a stimulant to the nervous system and increases energy. Cosmetically it encourages dry, mature skin to produce more of its own natural oils. It also helps get rid of canker sores. Add it to shampoos—it is an age-old remedy for dandruff and hair loss.

PRECAUTIONS

It can be overly stimulating and may increase blood pressure.

ROSEWOOD

BOTANICAL NAME: *ANIBA ROSAEODORA*

Brazil is famous for its rosewood trees, which can grow to more than 130 feet tall and produce heavy, strong wood that is prized for use in building materials, furniture, and musical instruments. The wood also has a high oil concentration, which produces an essential oil with a lovely rose scent, making it a favorite for perfumes and bath products. But the oil has many health benefits that go beyond its uplifting scent. Be sure to research sources before buying: responsible and reputable rosewood oil distilleries plant new trees for any that are cut down. This is an important step to maintain the beautiful and useful rosewood, which is known as "the ivory of the forest" due to illegal harvesting.

THERAPEUTIC PROPERTIES

Antiseptic; insect repellant; excellent for use in aromatherapy.

USED FOR

Rosewood oil helps cuts and scrapes heal faster and prevents infection. Although less potent than some oils, it can help to relieve headaches, toothaches, and muscle pain. Rubbed on the skin, rosewood can repel mosquitoes. The oil can also be used to kill small insects like bed bugs, fleas, and ants. Its sweet, floral scent makes it a great choice for adding to bath water or a diffuser.

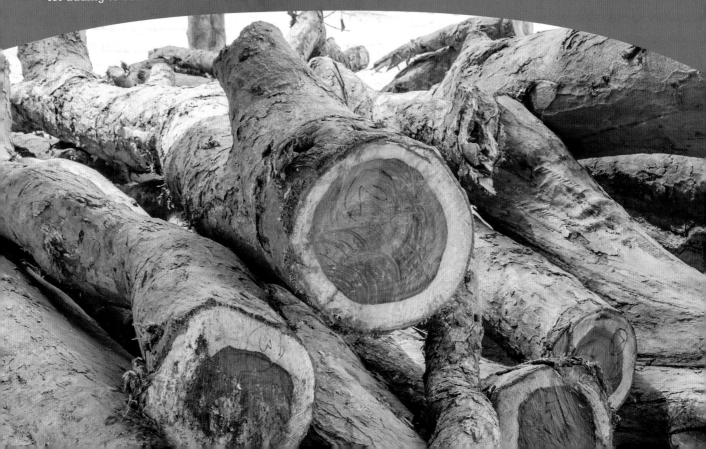

SAGE

BOTANICAL NAME: *SALVIA OFFICINALIS*

Native to the Mediterranean, sage has been known for its medicinal properties since ancient times, when the Greeks and Romans used it as a cure-all for everything from recovering memory loss to preventing plague. In fact, its very name is derived from the Latin *salvere*, which means "to feel healthy" or "heal." This herb is one of the oldest-known plants used not only in medicine, but also in food, and may conjure up memories of holiday tables laden with turkeys and sage stuffing. But the many uses of this ancient oil may persuade you to keep it on hand all year round!

THERAPEUTIC PROPERTIES

Antibacterial, antifungal, antioxidant, anti-inflammatory; helps relieve colds and coughs; eases digestion.

USED FOR

Sage is excellent at preventing infections, both internal and external. Its antioxidant and anti-inflammatory properties make it a valuable ingredient for skin care, as it provides an anti-aging effect and helps fade scars and marks. Sage oil provides relief from coughing and congestion due to colds or flu, and it promotes the production of bile, which helps the digestive system to run smoothly.

PRECAUTIONS

Sage oil is a stimulant, so should be avoided by those with epilepsy. The oil contains camphor, which is toxic in large amounts; always dilute before using, and avoid the oil during pregnancy.

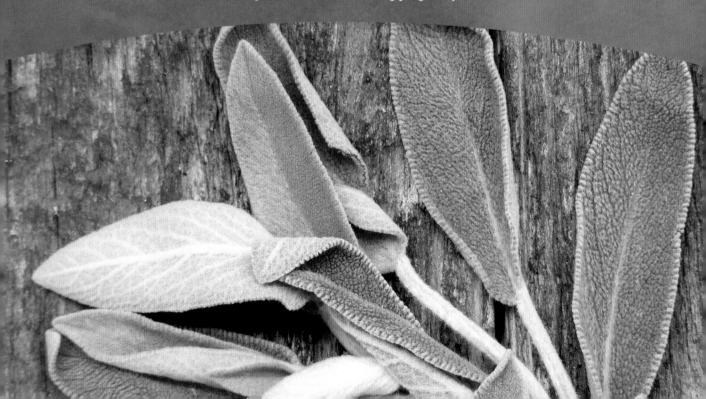

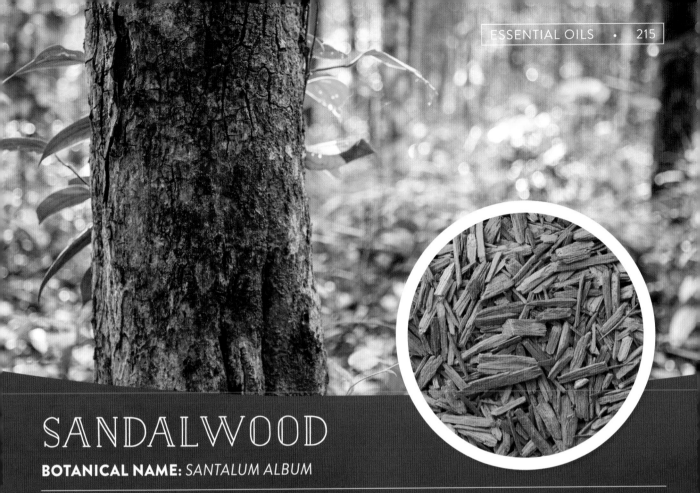

SANDALWOOD

BOTANICAL NAME: *SANTALUM ALBUM*

Sandalwood is distilled from the roots and heartwood of trees that take 50 to 80 years to reach full maturity. In an amazing and lengthy manufacturing process used since ancient times, the mature sandalwood trees are cut down, then left to be eaten by ants, which consume all but the fragrant heartwood and roots. The scent, called *chandana*, is used to induce a calm and meditative state. The lasting fragrance only improves with age. Temple gates and religious statues are carved from the wood because of the exquisite scent and because it is impermeable to termites and other insects. Mysore, India, produces the finest quality oil, and as an endangered species, sandalwood is regulated by the Indian government, which now grows the trees in cultivated plantations.

THERAPEUTIC PROPERTIES

Antidepressant, anti-inflammatory, antifungal, astringent, sedative, insecticide; relieves lung congestion and nausea.

USED FOR

The essential oil treats infections of the reproductive organs, especially in men, and helps relieve bladder infections. For either use, add 12 drops of essential oil for every ounce of vegetable oil and use as a massage oil over the infected area. This oil also counters inflammation, so it can be used on hemorrhoids. A syrup or chest balm containing sandalwood helps relieve persistent coughs and sore throat. One of sandalwood's most important uses is to sedate the nervous system, subduing nervousness, anxiety, insomnia, and to some degree, reducing nerve pain. Researchers have found it relaxes brain waves. Suitable for all complexion types, it is especially useful on rashes, inflammation, acne, and dry, dehydrated, or chapped skin.

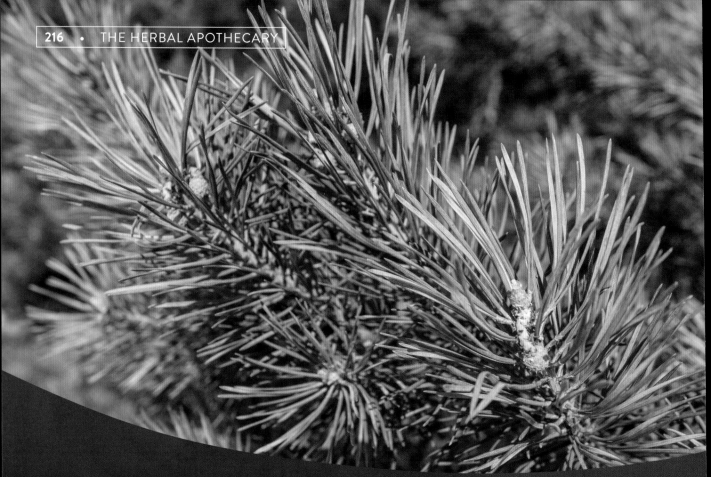

SCOTCH PINE

BOTANICAL NAME: *PINUS SYLVESTRIS*

You may already be familiar with the Scotch pine tree: it's one of the most common trees used for Christmas trees in the United States. The tree is native to Europe and Asia; in fact, it's the only pine tree native to northern Europe. The beneficial oil derived from the tree has been used since the time of Hippocrates, who took note of its healing effects on the respiratory system. And Native Americans would use mattresses stuffed with pine needles to repel fleas and lice. They were obviously on to something: the highest concentration of Scotch pine's essential oil is found in the fragrant needles.

THERAPEUTIC PROPERTIES

Antibacterial, anti-inflammatory, analgesic, decongestant, deodorizer; useful in aromatherapy.

USED FOR

Scotch pine oil is great for calming skin disorders like acne, eczema, psoriasis, or insect bites. Its anti-inflammatory and analgesic properties can help to reduce pain and swelling from arthritis or injuries. One of its most common uses is in cold and cough remedies: a few drops mixed with coconut oil and rubbed into the chest and neck can help open blocked nasal passages. Its familiar, uplifting scent and antibacterial properties make it a great choice to use as a household cleaner.

SPIKENARD

BOTANICAL NAME: *NARDOSTACHYS JATAMANSI*

Native to the Himalayas, spikenard is a flowering plant in the honeysuckle family. The roots and stems of the plant have been used since ancient times to create an aromatic oil, which is used for perfumes and medicine. Highly regarded in Indian Ayurvedic medicine, the oil is prized for its effects on depression, anxiety, and insomnia. Spikenard also has religious significance, and is referenced in both the Old and New Testaments of the Bible. Perhaps the most famous biblical reference is in the book of John, when Mary of Bethany spent a year's wages on spikenard ointment to anoint Jesus' feet. Luckily, today we can purchase this beneficial oil without breaking the bank.

THERAPEUTIC PROPERTIES

Antibacterial, anti-inflammatory, antiviral; aids respiratory issues.

USED FOR

Spikenard has been shown to help cuts and scrapes heal faster, and can be used to treat toenail fungus and athlete's foot. Its sedative properties can help those with insomnia fall asleep faster. The oil can be used as a natural laxative to relieve constipation. Spikenard's calming scent relaxes the mind as well as the body, and helps to quell the effects of depression and anxiety.

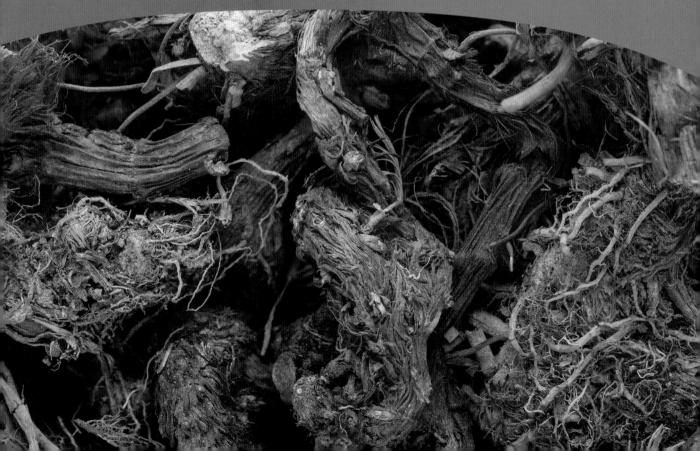

SPRUCE

BOTANICAL NAME: *PICEA MARIANA* (BLACK SPRUCE)

Thriving in the colder climate of the northern United States and Canada, several species of spruce trees produce essential oils, including the Norway and white spruce varieties. But the species most commonly used for its oil is the black spruce. Traditionally, Native Americans would use spruce mixed with honey to treat skin injuries, as well as using the tree in spiritual ceremonies. Meanwhile, Europeans used spruce to heal gum and stomach infections. Today, the essential oil, which is steam distilled from the needles and twigs of Canadian black spruce trees, is still used for these afflictions, and also has a long history of use in saunas and steam baths.

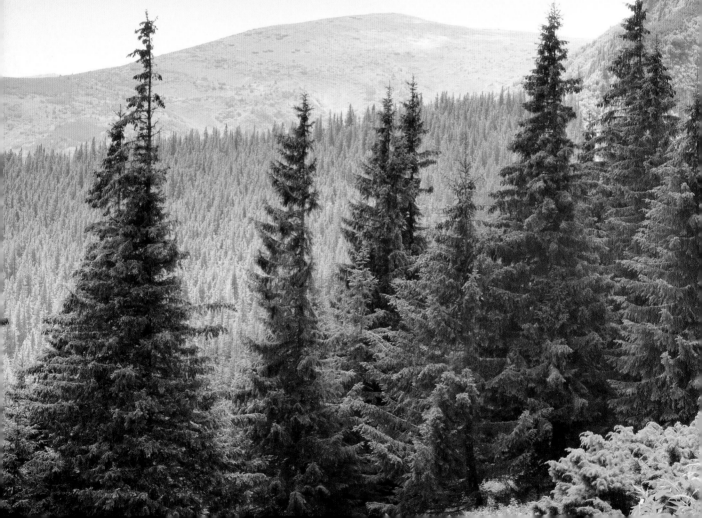

Black spruce essential oil comes from the tree's sharp, bluish-green needles and twigs. It has a refreshing, deep-forest scent, making it useful in aromatherapy for both energizing and calming effects. Via diffuser, it is used for relieving stress and mental fatigue, easing sadness, and providing spiritual uplift. Diluted in a carrier oil, it provides relief for muscle and joint pain, poor circulation, and flexibility issues.

Quite similar to black spruce, Norway spruce (Picea abies) essential oil has a crisp, green, uplifting scent, making it perfect for diffusion, as a cleaning agent for kitchens and bathrooms, as a health restorative, and as an addition to massage oil blends.

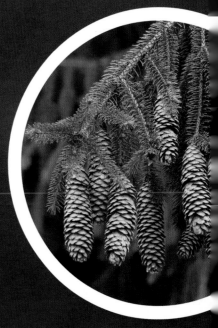

When diffused, the effects of white spruce (Picea glauca) have been described as grounding, centering, healing, uplifting, invigorating, and revitalizing. In fact, its rejuvenating effects on some people can be profound. It is also one of the best spruce oils to assist in breaking up mucus, easing asthma, bronchitis, and coughs, and providing all-around respiratory healing.

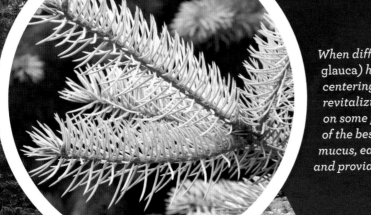

In general, the spruce essential oils can be used to speed the healing of minor cuts and scrapes, while preventing infection. A few drops added to a carrier oil and rubbed into muscles or joints can help soothe pain from injuries, strains, and arthritis. Spruce is an excellent oil to add to a steam bath to ease the symptoms of colds and flu. If these essential oils smell very familiar, that's because you've probably smelled them before in household cleaners, soaps, or air fresheners.

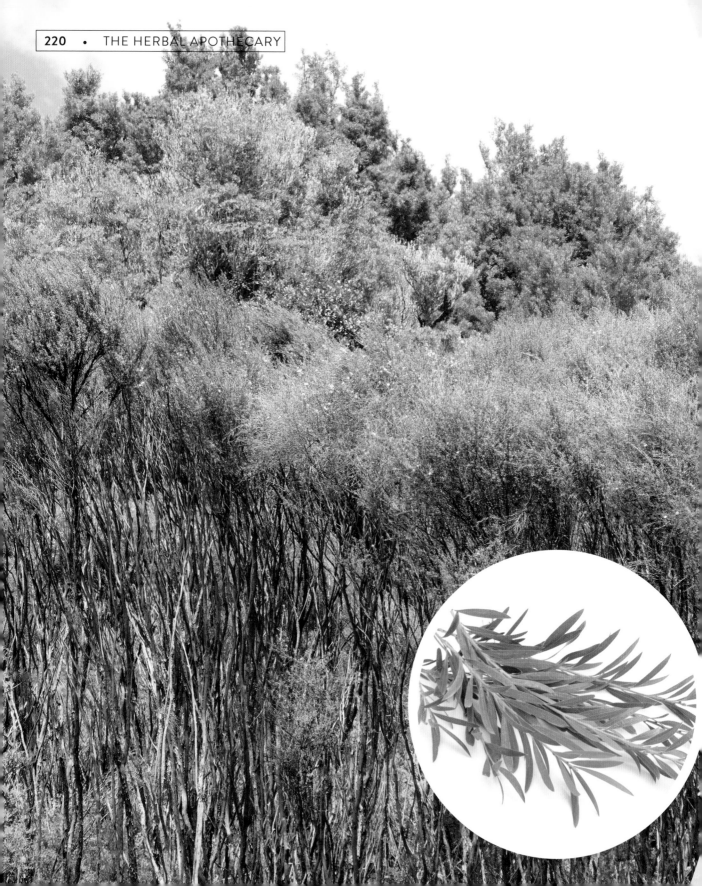

TEA TREE

BOTANICAL NAME: *MELALEUCA ALTERNIFOLIA*

On his first voyage to Australia, Captain Cook made a sharp-tasting tea from tea tree leaves and later used them in brewing beer. Eventually the leaves and then the essential oil were used to purify water. Australian soldiers and sailors used the essential oil as an all-purpose healing agent during World War II.

It's only recently, however, that essential oil companies have begun touting tea tree's healing properties. Medical journal articles support reports of its ability to heal mouth infections, and its primary use is in products for gum infection and canker sores, germicidal soaps, and deodorants. You will find several variations of tea tree, such as the harsher cajeput (*M. cajuputii*) and niaouli (*M. viridiflora*), favored for treating viral infections such as herpes. There is also a tea tree oil that is simply called MQV (*M. quinquenervia viridiflora*). Although it is more expensive, some aromatherapists prefer its softer, sweeter fragrance.

Tea tree essential oil is sometimes sold under its botanical name, Melaleuca.

A MEDICINE CABINET IN A BOTTLE

Tea tree is effective against bacteria, fungi, and viruses and stimulates the immune system. Use it in compresses, salves, massage oil, and washes to fight all sorts of infections, including herpes, shingles, chicken pox, candida, thrush, flu, cold, and those of the urinary tract. Studies show that the presence of blood and pus from infection only increase tea tree's antiseptic powers. It heals wounds, protects skin from radiation burns from cancer therapy, and encourages scar tissue to regenerate. Tea tree also treats diaper rash, acne, wounds, and insect bites. Adding just one drop to dish and diaper washing rinses gets rid of bacteria. It is one of the most nonirritating antiseptic oils, but this varies with the species, so a few people do find it slightly irritating.

MOLD DESTROYER

Add a teaspoon of tea tree oil, 10 drops of clove oil, and a cup of water to a spray bottle and shake thoroughly. Spray the mixture on moldy areas in the bathroom and kitchen. Leave it on for 10 or more minutes and then wipe it away. Tea tree oil can also be used as a mold preventative in toilets, tubs, and shower curtains.

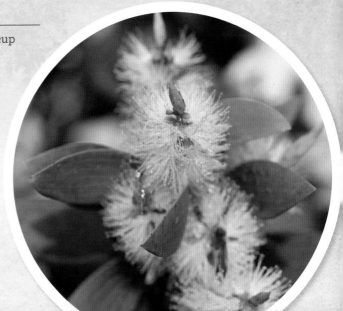

Tea tree's relative, cajeput, also has a broad range of applications. It is effective in fighting mold, bacteria, and viruses. It may be used topically in a carrier oil to alleviate joint pain, arthritis, and muscle cramps. It's also a great insect repellent.

THYME

BOTANICAL NAME: *THYMUS VULGARIS*

Most people consider this low-growing perennial evergreen no more than a culinary seasoning, yet its fragrance led Rudyard Kipling to write of "our close-bit thyme that smells like dawn in paradise."

Thyme was used in Muslim countries for fumigating houses; frankincense was added when people could afford it. The compound thymol, derived from thyme essential oil, is one of the strongest antiseptics known and has been isolated as an ingredient in drugstore gargles, mouthwashes, cough drops, and vapor chest balms. Some of the best-known products that contain thymol are Listerine mouthwash and Vicks VapoRub.

THERAPEUTIC PROPERTIES

Antiseptic, antibacterial, antifungal, antioxidant, astringent; destroys parasitic infections, helps dissipate muscle and rheumatic pain, stops coughing, decreases gas and indigestion, stimulates menstruation, clears lung congestion, stimulates the immune system and circulation.

USED FOR

Thyme essential oil is primarily used in a compress or sometimes in a salve or cream to fight serious infection. It is also useful for treating gum and mouth infections, such as thrush.

PRECAUTIONS

Thyme essential oil can irritate the skin and mucus membranes as well as raise blood pressure, so be sure to use it only in very low dilutions. Red thyme oil is even stronger than the white and is rarely used, except in a liniment for its increased heating effects. Essential oils of thyme are sometimes available in which the most potent components, thymol and carvacrol, are removed, although this decreases their antiseptic properties. Thyme essential oil should not be used with pregnant women or children. Thyme does destroy intestinal worms, but the essential oil should never be taken internally. Instead, use the herb itself in the form of a tea or tincture.

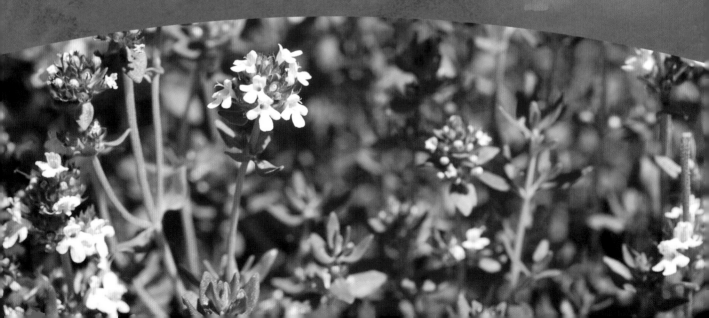

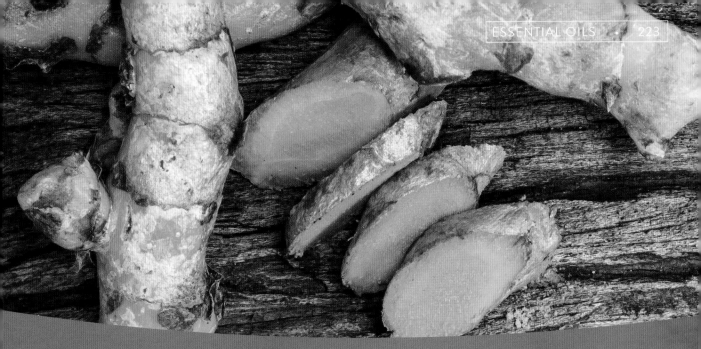

TURMERIC

BOTANICAL NAME: *CURCUMA LONGA*

A member of the ginger family, turmeric is native to Southeast Asia, where it is commonly used in cooking and for dyeing fabrics. But is has also been a staple in traditional medicine for thousands of years. The compound that gives the plant its distinctive yellow color, curcumin, also gives the essential oil powerful healing benefits. But curcumin isn't the only molecule in turmeric with healing properties: the plant is packed with such exotic-sounding substances as sesquiterpenes, borneol, and valeric acid, to name a few. They all work together to give turmeric its much-lauded anti-inflammatory and antioxidant qualities. And as an inexpensive and widely available essential oil, turmeric is a must-have for your medicine cabinet.

THERAPEUTIC PROPERTIES

Antioxidant, anti-inflammatory; helps to lower blood sugar and lowers blood pressure; supports the immune system.

USED FOR

Turmeric is especially prized for its anti-inflammatory properties, making it a great choice for soothing arthritis, muscle pain, headaches, and gastrointestinal inflammation. A few drops in a carrier oil applied to the skin can improve elasticity and reduce wrinkles, thanks to turmeric's antioxidant effects. When ingested in small quantities, turmeric oil helps to ward off infection and support the body's immune defenses. And research shows that turmeric can improve metabolic function in diabetics, as well as boost heart health.

PRECAUTIONS

Ingesting too much turmeric oil can cause stomach upset—use it in moderation. Because of its ability to lower blood pressure, avoid using turmeric if you are on blood pressure medication, as it can cause dangerously low blood pressure.

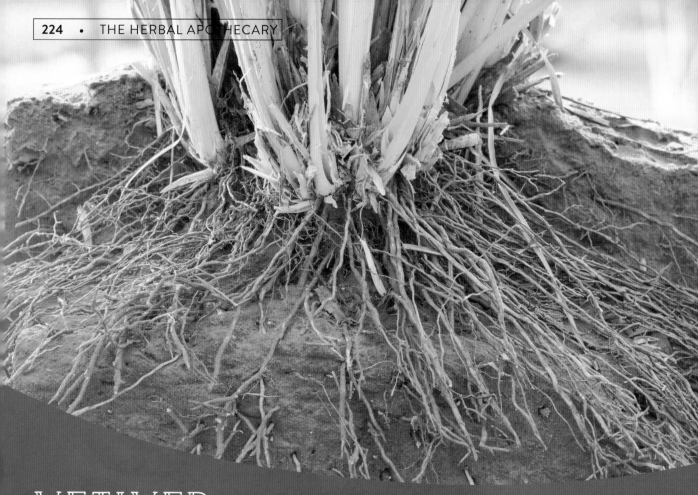

VETIVER

The complex, earthy essential oil is distilled from the roots of the plant.

BOTANICAL NAME: *CHRYSOPOGON ZIZANIODES*

Native to India, vetiver is a fragrant grass often grown as a barrier to protect crops from pests and weeds. Its lovely, musky, lemony scent has made it a favorite in the perfume industry. In fact, the scent of vetiver is included in 90 percent of perfumes and colognes sold in the West! But this grass is more than just a bug barrier and a pretty scent: vetiver has been used in traditional medicine in Asia and Africa for thousands of years. The essential oil is famous for its soothing, healing properties, and is known as "the oil of tranquility" in India and Sri Lanka.

THERAPEUTIC PROPERTIES

Antibacterial, anti-inflammatory; sedative; helps heal and fade scars.

USED FOR

Vetiver has been shown to stop the growth of bacteria and prevent infection, both when used topically and when ingested. The oil has a soothing and cooling effect, providing relief from aches and pains, and preventing overheating. Its sedative properties can help treat insomnia or anxiety. Vetiver has the ability to regenerate skin tissue, so try adding a few drops into a carrier oil or your favorite lotion and rubbing into scars and marks to help them fade.

YLANG YLANG

BOTANICAL NAME: *CANANGA ODORATA*

This fragrance is traditionally used to sharpen the senses and to temper depression, fear, anger, and jealousy. For these reasons, and also because of its reputation as an aphrodisiac, the flowers are spread on the beds of the newly married in Indonesia. Modern aromatherapists find the scent strongly sedating, easily sending the most reluctant sleeper off to dreamland. Science, on the other hand, regards ylang ylang more as a mental stimulant. Can it be both? Quite possibly it stimulates people's minds in one way while relaxing them in another.

THERAPEUTIC PROPERTIES

Antidepressant; stimulates circulation, relieves muscle spasms, lowers blood pressure, relaxes nerves.

USED FOR

Of all the essential oils, ylang ylang is one of the best at relaxing the mind and the body. Simply sniffing it can slightly lower blood pressure, although taking a bath with the oil or using it in a massage oil greatly enhances the relaxation experience. It can be helpful in cases of stress, shock, or anxiety. When used as a hair tonic, it balances oil production. Add about 6 drops to every ounce of hair conditioner.

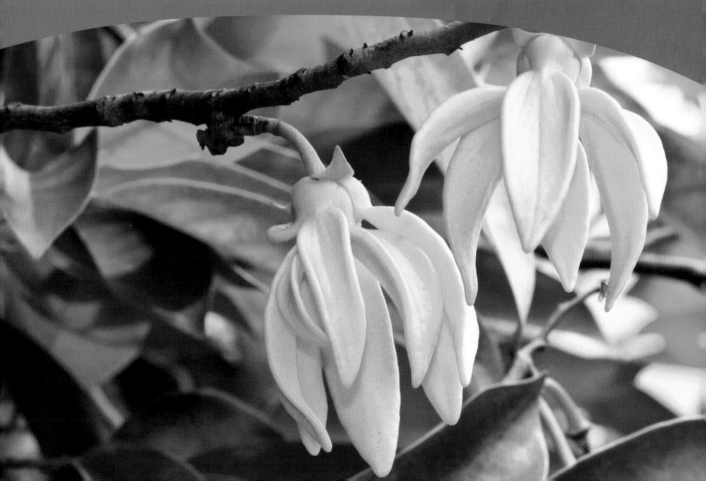

CARRIERS

Mixing your essential oil with a carrier is the most popular way of preparing topical aromatherapy products. It's also the simplest. There are several choices of carriers; the most common are vegetable oil, alcohol, water, and more rarely, vinegar. The carrier you choose will depend on how you plan to apply your treatment. For a massage or body oil, vegetable oil is the best choice. For a liniment, you may prefer alcohol as your base because it doesn't leave an oily residue. A room spray only needs a water base, while aloe vera juice is perfect for a complexion spray.

You can also dilute essential oils in ready-made products that use vegetable oils as their base, such as salves, creams, or lotions that you purchase at the store. This is a quick way to custom-make your own products. Select products that have little or no essential oils in them already to ensure that you do not end up with too much scent in the finished product. Many natural food stores sell unscented cream, lotion, and shampoo bases.

VEGETABLE OIL

Essential oils blend well into vegetable oils. Vegetable oils have other advantages, too: They are soothing to the skin, hold moisture in, and are easy to apply. Any high-quality vegetable oil such as almond, apricot kernel, fractionated coconut, hazelnut, jojoba, or grape seed can be a carrier oil. You don't necessarily need to use "cold-pressed" oil. In fact, you should avoid the heavily scented olive and peanut oils because they have their own odor, which may cover up the scent of the essential oils you are using.

Vegetable oils contain molecules that are too large to penetrate the skin as essential oil molecules do, but they slide smoothly over one another and over the skin, making them ideal for cosmetic products. Eventually, when you're more familiar with the properties of the various oils, you may vary the oil according to the application. But when starting out, use one of the carrier oils mentioned here. Store the carrier oils away from heat and light to ensure their freshness.

Vitamin E oil is an excellent antioxidant, and adding it to any aromatherapy blend will help extend the life of most vegetable oils. One or two capsules (200 to 400 IUs) per two-ounce bottle of carrier is enough. Just prick the end of the capsule with a pin and squeeze. To ensure freshness, make only enough of a blend to last for a couple months or keep it refrigerated. If you plan to keep a blend for a long time and are worried about rancidity, consider using jojoba oil. While more expensive than most, jojoba oil will never go rancid. If you're pinching pennies, use it as just a portion of your blend.

ALCOHOL

The same proportions suggested for diluting essential oils into vegetable oil will also work for alcohol. Although it is not used as often, alcohol is antiseptic and cooling and quickly evaporates, leaving no oily residue. You may choose between using a drinking alcohol, such as vodka, or a rubbing alcohol, which is poisonous. If you choose drinking alcohol, any type will work, but vodka is often used because it has no additional flavors or additives. An 80-proof vodka is 40 percent alcohol and 60 percent water. If you use rubbing alcohol (alcohol made from wood), be sure that it is not ingested. By itself, alcohol is far too drying to use on the skin or hair. Witch hazel, which is a blend of alcohol plus an extract of the bark and leaves of *hamamelis virginiana*, makes a good base for a mild astringent.

VINEGAR

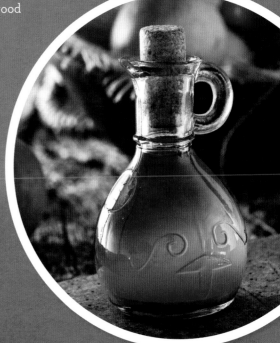

A few aromatherapy preparations incorporate vinegar. It is actually a better base for both skin and hair than alcohol, but it is not as popular due to its strong smell. The smell dissipates rather quickly, however, and you'll be pleased with the result if you try it. Vinegar is antiseptic, although not as antiseptic as alcohol. Its acidity helps restore the acid mantle or pH-balance to the skin and hair. For this purpose, apple cider vinegar is best, although many people prefer white vinegar because it has no color. Vinegar is water soluble, so you can dilute it with distilled water if you find its smell or sting too strong for the product you are making. Distilled water is used because it doesn't contain chlorine, salt, or city water additives and has none of the bacteria found in well water.

DILUTIONS

Some people find it easier to measure drops; others prefer measuring essential oils by the teaspoon. It depends on how much you need to measure at one time and the width of the container into which it's going. The size of a drop varies, depending on the size of the dropper opening and the temperature and viscosity (thickness) of the essential oil. Teaspoons are usually more convenient if you are preparing large quantities.

Most aromatherapy applications are a two-percent dilution. This means 2 drops of essential oil is added for every 100 drops of carrier oil—a safe and effective dilution for most aromatherapy applications. A one-percent dilution is suggested for children, pregnant women, and those who are weak from chronic illness. In some cases, you will want to use even less. Dilutions of three percent or more are used only for strong preparations such as liniments or for "spot" therapy, when you are only treating a tiny area instead of the entire body. Always remember that in aromatherapy, more is not necessarily better. In fact, too great a concentration may produce unwanted reactions. The following are standard dilutions:

- 1 percent dilution: 5–6 drops per ounce of carrier
- 2 percent dilution: 10–12 drops (about ⅛ teaspoon) per ounce of carrier
- 3 percent dilution: 15–18 drops (a little less than ¼ teaspoon) per ounce of carrier

BLENDING

For your very first aromatherapy blends, keep it simple. Use your favorite essential oils, but preferably no more than two to four at a time. Later, the many choices of oils will add to the excitement of creating your own blends.

Keep an aromatherapy notebook from the very beginning—you'll need exact records of how you made all your preparations. Jot down the ingredients, proportions, and processing procedures you used for each blend, as well as observations about how well it worked. Label your finished products with the ingredients, date, and special instructions, if any. You will be thankful for this information later when you come up with a formula everyone loves, and you want to duplicate it.

When considering blends, try to think about the characteristics of each oil, including what professional perfumers call personality, aroma notes, and odor intensity. Perfumers think of each oil as having its own unique personality, and they think of scent in terms of a musical scale: Fragrances have head or top notes, middle or heart notes, and base notes. The top notes are the odors that are smelled first but evaporate quickly, the heart is the scent that emerges after the first fifteen minutes, while the base note is the scent that lingers hours later.

Essential oils vary in odor intensity, which may or may not correspond to the evaporation rate of the aroma notes. Add much smaller amounts of strong essential oils, as it is extremely easy for an especially potent oil such as rosemary to completely overpower the soft scent of an oil such as sandalwood or cedar. When mixing small experimental quantities, one drop of a high intensity oil such as cinnamon can be way too much. Try adding just a smidgen of oil with the end of a toothpick. You can tell which oils have a high odor intensity, such as patchouli and cinnamon, just by smelling them. Use only about one drop of any of these oils to five drops of a more subtle essential oil, such as lavender. On the other hand, orange has such a low odor intensity, you will need about eight drops of it to blend evenly with four drops of lavender.

Here you have the makings of a formula: 8 drops orange, 4 drops lavender, and 1 drop clary sage. This formula presents a lesson in intensity and is arranged by notes. The scent leans toward the top and middle note regions. The orange brightens the top, evaporating relatively quickly, while the clary sage provides a sweetly sauntering base for comforting lavender.

There are many ways to alter the formula. For instance, add a drop of cinnamon instead of the clary sage for a scent that's a little more spicy and stimulating. If you want the woodsy smell of cedar, add several drops to balance the blend. Your options are endless.

Another way to expand a blend is to choose oils that have similar characteristics. It will make your blend seem more complicated and mysterious because no one can pinpoint exactly what the aroma is. Try combining peppermint and spearmint, lemon and bergamot, or cinnamon and ginger. Using oils that come from different parts of a plant tends to deepen and enrich the scent. For instance, add just the tiniest amount of turpentine-like juniper needles to a rich juniper berry to create a more detailed fullness.

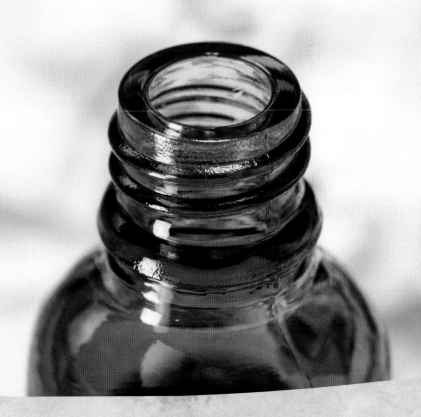

ESSENTIAL OIL APPLICATIONS

Making your own aromatherapy products has many advantages. You can be certain that your homemade products contain only the highest quality ingredients, yet they will likely cost a fraction of what you'd pay for them in the store. And using essential oils—rather than the whole herb—will eliminate complex procedures. Your finished product can usually be ready in a few minutes instead of hours.

VIA INHALATION

A pleasing and safe way to experience the benefits of essential oils is by simply breathing them in. This may be as simple as opening the bottle and taking a whiff. Steam inhalation is a great way to treat an upper respiratory problem. To create a steam inhalant, bring about 3 cups of water to a boil in a pan. Turn off the heat, and add 3-5 drops of essential oil to the water. Drape a towel over both your head and the pan to capture the steam, keeping your eyes closed and your head about 12 inches from the water. Take deep, relaxing breaths of the fragrant steam. You can also humidify and disinfect an entire room—just keep the mixture on a very low simmer. Essential oils can also be used in many humidifiers.

Diffusers are small electrical units that release water-based essential oil vapor into a room. Because they are unheated, the volatile compounds in the oils remain intact.

Nebulizers also pump essential oil vapor into the air, but do it without water. Generally, you place a few drops of essential oil in a hand-blown glass container and turn on a small compressor that's connected with a piece of tubing. The glass unit disperses a fine mist of micro-particles mixed with the stream of air produced by the pump. This method increases the surface area of the scent molecules. It's an extremely effective way to disinfect and energize the atmosphere. Diffusers and nebulizers can be used in a sick room for 10 to 15 minutes every hour to clear airborne bacteria that may spread infection.

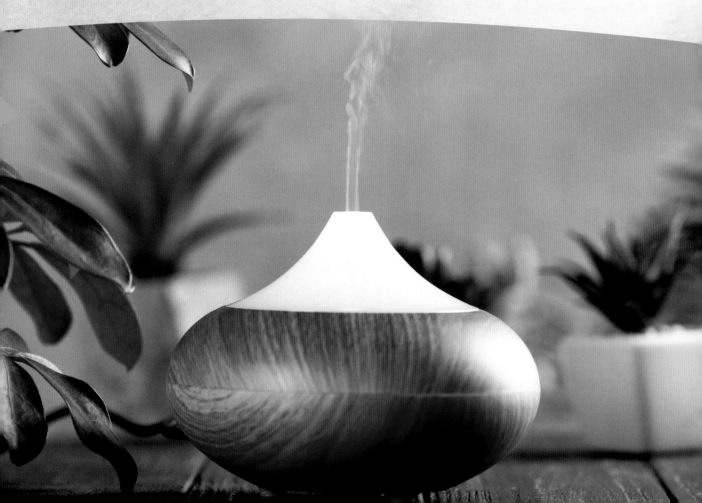

COMPRESS

An aromatherapy compress concentrates essential oils in a specific area of the body and keeps the area moist. It is one of the quickest and easiest therapeutic techniques to make. Add about 5 drops of an essential oil or a blend of oils to a cup of water. Use hot or cold water, whichever is best for the particular treatment: Cold water helps relieve itching, swelling, and inflammation, while hot water increases circulation and opens pores, helping to flush out blemishes. Fold a soft cloth and soak it in the water; then wring it out and apply it where needed. If you feel overheated, try a cold compress on your forehead. Cold is also usually the preferred temperature for relieving strained eyes. A cool compress can also help to get rid of a headache, although a few people find that heat works better for them. A hot compress against the back of the neck will relieve neck strain and tight muscles.

MASSAGE / BODY OIL

Massage oil consists of essential oils blended in a carrier oil. A small amount of healing essential oil can thus be evenly distributed over a large area of the body. Rubbing warms the body, relaxes muscles, relieves stress, encourages deep breathing, and helps the oils to penetrate deeply. All of these do their part in treating the whole person, rather than just focusing on a single symptom. To make either a massage or body oil, combine ½ teaspoon (50 drops) of essential oil with 4 ounces of any vegetable oil. A body oil made from essential oils is also a good alternative when the patient won't swallow a pill or drink tea. For example, if a child with a stomachache refuses to take any medicine, rub a therapeutic body oil on his or her stomach.

SALVE

Salves are made of herbal oils that are thickened with beeswax, so they form a healing and protective coating that adheres better to the skin. They are used on almost all skin problems, such as minor cuts, bruises, scrapes, diaper or heat rash, insect bites, eczema, psoriasis, and swelling. You can make any salve aromatherapeutic by stirring 24 drops of essential oil into 2 ounces of salve. This is fairly easy to do with a toothpick. The resulting salve will be a little runnier than usual, but it will stick to the skin perfectly well.

SCENTED CANDLE

Impregnated with essential oils, candles release the scent as they burn, creating whatever mood you want. You can make an aromatherapy candle from a purchased unscented candle by adding several drops of essential oil to the candle's wick. Wait 24 hours, until the wick absorbs the oil, before using the candle. You can make scented candles from scratch by adding oil to the melted wax or by saturating the wick just before pouring the candle. The wick method uses less oil, but many people like the scent of the candle.

TREATMENTS FOR COMMON AILMENTS

These simple aromatherapy treatments are for relatively minor problems that you would normally treat at home. The proportions have been carefully chosen to make the product both very therapeutic and pleasant to smell. Essential oil remedies are frequently administered as a massage or bath oil. That's because the safest way to use essential oils is externally and in a diluted state.

HELPFUL HINTS BEFORE YOU BEGIN

- In recipes that call for 12 drops of an essential oil, you might prefer using the equivalent measurement of $1/8$ teaspoon.

- If you plan to keep a preparation longer than six months, use the more expensive jojoba oil because it won't ever go rancid. Or add one or two capsules of vitamin E, which will preserve your recipe longer than other oils, but not as long as jojoba.

- When preparing recipes to be used by the elderly, the very young (less than 12 years of age), or anyone who is very ill or frail, be sure to cut the amount of essential oils in half, keeping the carrier (vegetable oil, water, alcohol, vinegar, etc.) the same. These people are so sensitive that they will react equally well to the smaller amount.

- Just want to try something out? Make a smaller amount by cutting the proportions in half. If the drops don't divide evenly, use the smaller number. Use a clean toothpick if you only want a smidgen of something, such as patchouli (yes, it's that powerful!).

ACNE AND OILY SKIN

Acne may not be a hazard to your health, but it does impair your looks. The problem typically is the result of clogged skin pores. When the pores and follicles (canals that contain hair shafts) are blocked, oil cannot be secreted and builds up. Bacteria feed on the oil and multiply. People with oily skin have a greater chance of developing acne, as do teenagers and anyone experiencing hormonal fluctuations. Although not medically proven, stress may also contribute to acne breakouts.

Luckily, quite an array of essential oils is available to help you deal with acne. That's because many oils help manage the specific underlying problems that cause acne: They balance hormones, reduce stress, improve the complexion, and regulate the skin's oil production. This makes aromatherapy the ideal treatment for blemishes, pimples, and other skin eruptions. Commercial acne remedies have long recognized this.

Essential oils for acne or an oily complexion include: cedarwood, clary sage, eucalyptus, frankincense, geranium, juniper berry, lavender, lemon, lemongrass, sandalwood, and tea tree.

FACIAL TONER FOR OILY COMPLEXIONS

- 12 drops lemongrass oil
- 6 drops juniper berry oil
- 2 drops ylang ylang oil
- 1 ounce witch hazel lotion
- 1 ounce aloe vera gel

Combine all of the ingredients in a glass bottle. Give the mixture a good shake and it's done! Apply at least once a day. If you find witch hazel too drying, vinegar is an excellent substitute. It is not as drying as the witch hazel lotion and helps to retain the skin's natural acid balance.

ZIT ZAP COMPRESS

- 4 drops cedarwood oil
- 2 drops eucalyptus oil
- 1 teaspoon Epsom salts
- ¼ cup water

Pour the boiling water over the Epsom salts. When the salts are dissolved and the water has cooled just enough to not burn the skin, add the essential oils. Soak a small absorbent cloth in the hot solution, then press the cloth against the blemishes for about one minute. Repeat several times by rewetting the cloth in the same solution.

INTENSIVE BLEMISH TREATMENT

Stir the water and essential oil into the herb powder to make a paste. Apply as a mask directly on the blemished area. Let the paste dry and keep it on your skin for at least 20 minutes, then rinse off. This routine can be done more than once a day, if you wish. The vitamin E can be obtained by poking open a vitamin capsule and squeezing out the oil. It is a good addition when obstinate sores need to heal or if there is any chance of scarring.

ASTHMA

The characteristic wheezing of asthma is made by the effort to push air through swollen, narrowed bronchial passages. During an asthma attack, stale air cannot be fully exhaled because the bronchioles are swollen and clogged with mucous, and thus less fresh air can be inhaled. The person gasps and labors for breath. Allergic reactions to food, stress, and airborne allergens are the common causes of asthma. Allergies trigger production of histamine, which dilates blood vessels and constricts airways. Asthma sufferers fight an ongoing battle with such low-level congestion, which is actually an attempt by unhappy lungs to rid themselves of irritations.

Many aromatherapy books warn against using essential oils to treat asthma. Some asthmatics are sensitive to fragrance and find that it triggers their attacks. While you certainly don't want to make the situation any worse, aromatherapy offers promising results when used judiciously.

The safest time for aromatherapy treatments is in between attacks. Use a chest rub made from essential oils that have decongestive and antihistamine properties, such as peppermint and ginger. German chamomile, which contains chamazulene, is thought to actually prevent the release of histamine. Frankincense, marjoram, and rose encourage deep breathing and allow lungs to expand. To reduce bronchial spasms, use the relaxants: chamomile, lavender, rose, geranium, and marjoram.

A lavender steam can be used by some asthmatics even during an attack. The steam opens airways, while lavender quickly relaxes lung spasms. This may halt the attack right in its tracks or at least make it less severe. As an added bonus, lavender also relaxes the mind, so it helps dissipate the panic you feel when you can't catch your breath. If you find that steaming only makes it more difficult to breathe, use an aromatherapy diffuser or a humidifier instead.

ASTHMA INHALATION RUB

- 6 drops lavender oil
- 4 drops geranium oil
- 1 drop marjoram oil
- 1 drop peppermint or ginger oil
- 1 ounce vegetable oil

Combine the ingredients. Rub on chest as needed, especially before bedtime. Since asthmatics can be extremely sensitive to scent, do a sniff test first. Test the formula by simply sniffing it to make sure there is no adverse reaction.

Essential oils are not powerful enough to heal an asthmatic condition all by themselves. Herbs that repair lung damage and improve breathing are also needed, along with avoiding whatever sparks the allergic reaction. If this means stress, then other aromatherapy techniques such as massage, relaxation techniques, and fragrant baths can help you de-stress your life.

Essential oils for asthma: chamomile, eucalyptus (don't use during an attack), frankincense (deepens breathing, allows lungs to expand), geranium, ginger, lavender, marjoram, peppermint, rose.

BLADDER INFECTION

Bladder infections are common, especially in women. So common, in fact, that you may already be familiar with the medical term cystitis to describe the inflammation that can result when bladder infections are unattended. Fortunately, several essential oils can come to the rescue. Juniper berry, sandalwood, chamomile, pine, tea tree, and bergamot are especially effective treatments. However, juniper berry is so strong that it could irritate the kidneys if the bladder infection has spread into them. If that is the case, stick to the other oils. In fact, if there is any chance that you have a kidney infection, be sure to seek a doctor's opinion, as it can have serious consequences.

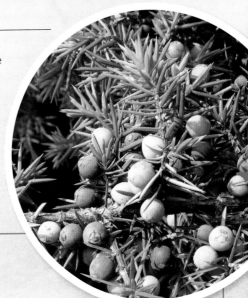

BLADDER INFECTION OIL

- 8 drops juniper berry or cypress oil
- 6 drops tea tree oil
- 6 drops bergamot oil
- 2 drops fennel oil
- 2 ounces vegetable oil

Combine the ingredients. Massage over the bladder area once daily. For a preventive treatment, add a tablespoon of this same oil to your bath.

BURNS AND SUNBURN

The first step in treating any minor burn or sunburn is to quickly immerse the afflicted area in cold water (about 50°F) containing a few drops of essential oil. Or you can apply a cold compress that has been soaked in the same water. If the person feels overheated or if the eyelids are sunburned, place the compress on the forehead.

Burned skin is tender to the touch, so spraying a remedy is preferable to dabbing it on. A spray also is extra cooling and is especially handy when sunburn covers a large area. For your burn wash, compress, or spray, lavender is an all-time favorite among aromatherapists. Lavender and aloe vera juice both promote new cell growth, reduce inflammation, stop infection, and decrease pain. Aloe has even been used successfully on radiation burns. There are several other essential oils that reduce the pain of burns and help them heal, so feel free to experiment. Use them in the same proportions suggested for lavender, except rose oil for which 1 drop equals 5 drops of other essential oils.

A small amount of vinegar helps to heal a minor burn and provides an additional cooling effect, but it is painful on an open wound. Reserve it for cases in which the skin is unbroken. In general, stick to treating minor, first-degree burns at home, and leave the care of deeper or more extensive burns to a doctor.

Essential oils for burns and sunburn include: chamomile, geranium, lavender, marjoram, peppermint (cooling in small amounts), rose, and tea tree.

EMERGENCY BURN WASH / COMPRESS

- 5 drops lavender oil
- 1 pint water, about 50°F

Add the essential oil to the water and stir well to disperse the oil. Immerse the burned area for several minutes, or take a soft cloth, soak it in the water, and apply it to the burn. Leave the compress on for several minutes, then soak again and reapply at least twice more.

SUNBURN SOOTHER

- 20 drops lavender oil
- 4 ounces aloe vera juice
- 200 IU vitamin E oil
- 1 tablespoon vinegar

Combine ingredients. Shake well before using. Keep this remedy in a spritzer bottle, and use as often as needed. If you keep the spray in the refrigerator, the coolness will provide extra relief. For the best healing, make sure you use aloe vera juice and not drugstore gel.

CONGESTION, SINUS AND LUNG

The most common cause of sinus and lung congestion is a cold or flu virus. Additionally, secondary bacterial infections that follow on the heels of colds and flus can be especially nasty, irritating the delicate lining in the respiratory tract. The mucous that causes the congestion is produced to protect that lining and wash away the infection.

For quick relief, thin out congestion by using the essential oils of eucalyptus, peppermint, and bergamot combined with steam. Remember how much easier it is to breath when you step into a steamy, hot shower? The steam opens up tightened bronchial passages, allowing the essential oils to penetrate and wipe out the viral or bacterial infection that is causing the problem.

Two of the best essential oils to eliminate infection are lavender and eucalyptus. In fact, studies prove that a two percent dilution of eucalyptus oil kills 70 percent of airborne staphylococcus bacteria. Anise, peppermint, and eucalyptus reduce coughing, perhaps by suppressing the brain's cough reflex. If congestion is severe, also use essential oils that loosen congestion. Cypress dries a persistently runny nose.

To create a therapeutic steam, add a few drops of essential oil to a pan of water that is simmering on the stove. You can also use a humidifier—some actually provide a compartment for essential oils. If you are at the office or traveling and steaming is impractical, try inhaling a tissue scented with the oils, or use a natural nasal inhaler.

VAPOR RUB

- 12 drops eucalyptus oil
- 5 drops peppermint oil
- 5 drops thyme oil
- 1 ounce olive oil

Combine ingredients in a glass bottle. Shake well to mix oils evenly. Gently massage into chest and throat. Use one to five times per day and especially just before bed.

GERM FIGHTER SPRAY

- 12 drops tea tree oil
- 6 drops eucalyptus oil
- 6 drops lemon oil
- 2 ounces distilled water

Combine the ingredients, and shake well to disperse the oils before each use. Dispense this formula from a spray bottle as needed on minor cuts, burns, or abrasions to prevent infection and speed healing. As an alternative to the distilled water, you can use a tincture made from an antiseptic herb such as Oregon grape root. If you do this, keep in mind that tinctures contain alcohol, which will make the essential oils disperse better and increase the antiseptic properties of the spray, but it will also sting more on an open wound. Apply immediately and then several times a day to keep the wound clean and encourage healing.

CUTS, SCRAPES, AND BRUISES

Simple cuts and scrapes can easily be treated with antiseptic essential oils. A mist of diluted oil is an excellent way to apply them. Herbal salves containing antiseptic essential oils are also effective in treating scrapes or wounds that aren't too deep. Need to protect your cut? Many of the resins and balsams such as benzoin, frankincense, and myrrh actually form a protective barrier over the wound that acts as an antiseptic "Band-Aid." In an emergency, don't forget that you can dab a little lavender or tea tree oil directly on a scrape as they are among the least irritating of oils.

Essential oils for cuts and scrapes include: benzoin, eucalyptus, frankincense, geranium, lavender, lemon, myrrh, rose, and tea tree.

DEPRESSION/ANXIETY

It's no secret that fragrance lifts and enhances one's mood. The aroma of many plants, such as the elegant orange blossom aroma of neroli or the closely related and less expensive petitgrain, as well as jasmine, sandalwood, and ylang ylang, relieve depression and anxiety. Modern aromatherapists agree with the 17th-century herbalist John Gerard, who recommended the use of clary sage to ease depression, paranoia, mental fatigue, and nervous disorders.

Fragrances are generally effective for people who have mild forms of depression that do not require drugs. And they can be especially helpful when the doctor is trying to wean patients off drugs. Aromatherapy can be used safely in conjunction with antidepressant medications because it will not interfere with the dosage or effect. If you are currently taking prescription drugs to deal with depression or anxiety, however, don't abruptly stop taking them or replace them with essential oils without your doctor's okay.

Massage and bath oils are probably the most relaxing forms of antidepressant aromatherapy. If you wish to make your environment more uplifting at home or at work, try using an aromatherapy room spray, or put the essential oils in an aromatherapy diffuser, potpourri cooker, or a pan of simmering water. You can make a constant companion of your favorite oil, or of a blend of oils by carrying them in a small vial. Then, when you need a lift, just take a whiff.

UPLIFTING FORMULA

- 6 drops bergamot oil
- 3 drops petitgrain oil
- 3 drops geranium oil
- 1 drop neroli
- 2 ounces vegetable oil

Combine all the ingredients. Use as a massage oil, add 1 or 2 teaspoons to your bath, or add 1 teaspoon to a foot bath. For an equally uplifting room or facial spritzer, substitute the same amount of water for the vegetable oil in this formula. Put the water formula in a spray bottle, and spritz or sniff throughout the day as needed.

DERMATITIS, PSORIASIS, AND ECZEMA

Dermatitis is an inflammation of the skin that causes itching, redness, and skin lesions. It's difficult even for dermatologists to uncover the source of this bothersome skin problem. Some obvious causes, though, are contact with an irritant such as poison oak or ivy, harsh chemicals, or anything to which one is allergic. Stress also seems to be a contributing factor in many types of dermatitis. Essential oils that counter stress, soothe inflammation and itching, soften roughness, and are both antiseptic and drying are used to treat these skin conditions.

One type of dermatitis is eczema, a word that describes a series of symptoms rather than a disease. Eczema is characterized by crusty, oozing skin that itches and may feel like it burns. Psoriasis is a dermatitis with red lesions covered by silver-like scales that flake off. This condition can be hereditary, but its cause is unknown. It has an annoying tendency to come and go for no apparent reason.

One of the best vehicles for essential oils in these cases is an herbal salve that already contains a base of skin healing herbs such as comfrey and calendula. You can use a store-bought herbal salve or one that you make yourself. Stir in 15 drops (or less) of essential oils per ounce of salve. Since salves come in a two-ounce jar, that means adding no more than 30 drops; use less if the salve already contains some essential oils. Secondary skin infections, which often occur with eczema, need to be treated with antiseptic essential oils, such as those suggested for acne.

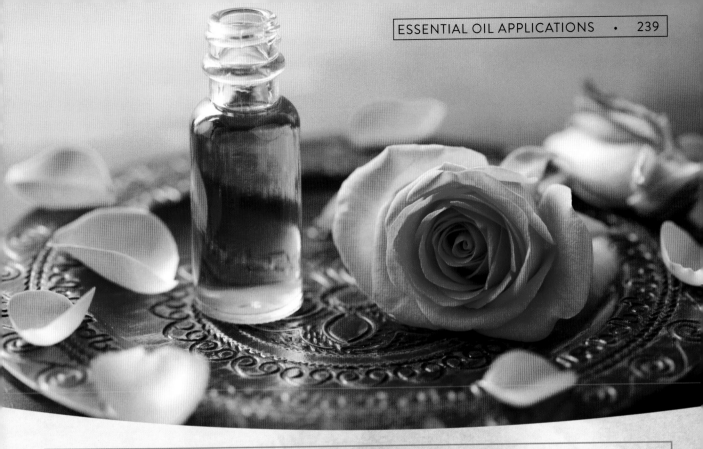

DERMATITIS SKIN CARE

- 8 drops tea tree oil
- 8 drops chamomile oil
- 1 teaspoon Oregon grape tincture
- 2 ounces healing salve

With a toothpick, stir the tincture and essential oils into the salve. This will make the salve semi-liquid. You can purchase the tincture at a natural food store. Apply one to four times a day.

DRY COMPLEXION SCRUB

- 6 drops lavender oil
- 2 drops peppermint oil
- 1 tablespoon dried elder flowers, lavender, or chamomile (optional)
- 2 tablespoons oatmeal
- 1 tablespoon cornmeal

Grind dry ingredients in a blender or electric coffee grinder. (Drugstores sell colloidal oatmeal, which needs no grinding.) Add the essential oils, and stir to distribute. Store in a closed container, and use instead of soap for cleansing your face. For clean skin, moisten 1 teaspoon with enough water to make a paste, dampen your face with a little water, then gently apply scrub. Rinse with warm water. Use this daily instead of soap.

ANTI-AGING COMPLEXION CREAM

- 15 drops geranium oil
- 3 drops rose oil
- 2 drops frankincense or neroli oil
- 2 ounces complexion cream

Stir the essential oils into the cream. Use daily.

DIAPER RASH

Aromatherapy baby oil and powder can help protect your little one from diaper rash. The oil repels moisture, and the powder absorbs moisture and prevents chafing. Use one or the other with every diaper change, or more often if needed. Baby oil is also good for the skin. Make your own baby powder from plain old corn starch and essential oils.

Essential oils for diaper rash: chamomile, lavender, sandalwood, tea tree

AROMATHERAPY BABY OIL

- 6 drops lavender oil
- 2 drops chamomile oil
- 2 ounces vegetable oil

Combine the ingredients. Use after each diaper change and as an all-over massage oil. The same amount of lavender and chamomile can also be stirred into a basic herbal salve with a toothpick and used on the diaper area.

FRAGRANT BABY POWDER

- 20 drops (¼ teaspoon) lavender oil
- 5 drops mandarin or tangerine oil
- ½ pound corn starch

Put the corn starch in a plastic zip-lock bag and drop in the essential oils. Tightly close the bag, and toss back and forth to distribute the oil, breaking up any clumps by pressing them with your fingers through the bag. Let stand at least four days to distribute the essential oil. Spice, salt, or Parmesan cheese shakers with large holes in their lids make good powder applicators. Powder after each diaper change or bath.

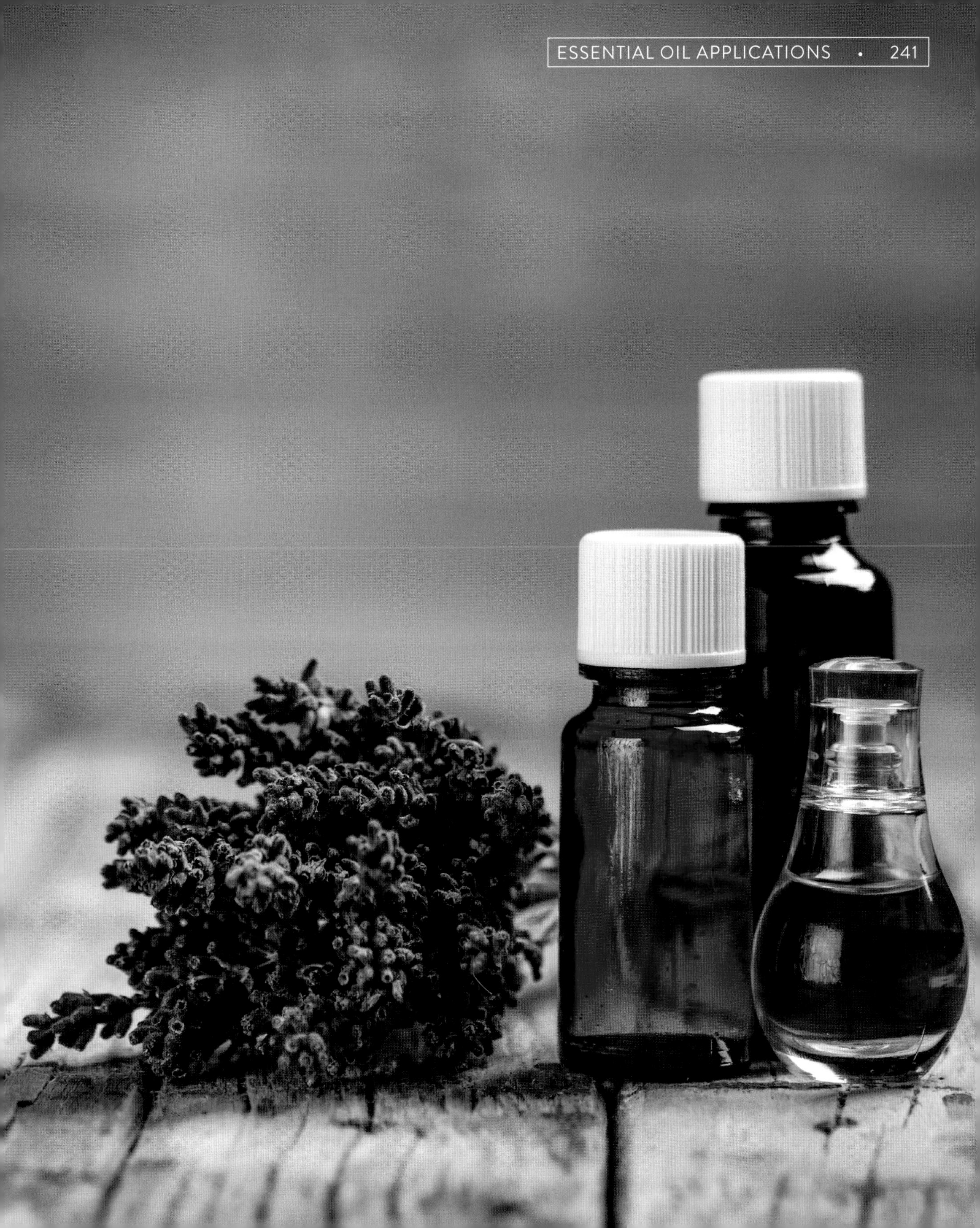

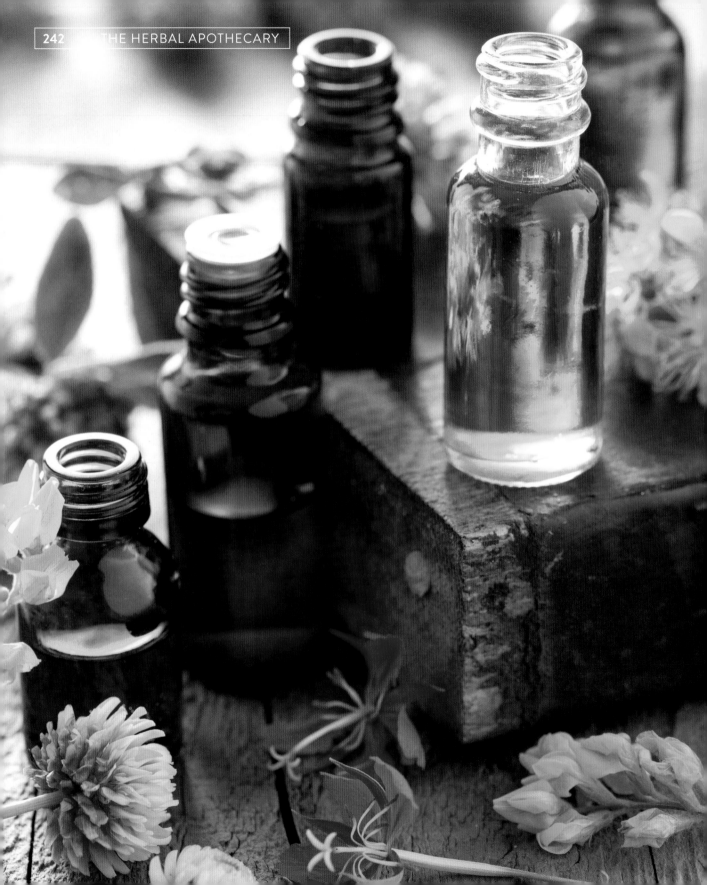

EARACHE

An earache is most likely due to an infection. While this is not the sort of condition to treat exclusively with aromatherapy, an aromatherapy massage oil rubbed on the outside of the ear is an excellent adjunct to other treatments. Dilute an antiseptic essential oil like lavender or tea tree in olive oil. Lavender has the added benefit of helping to reduce inflammation. Gently rub this around the outside of the ear and down along the lymph nodes on the side of the neck. Do not put it in the ear itself. Instead, make a warm compress using these same oils and place it directly over the ear. Always treat both ears, even if only one hurts, and continue treating them for a couple days after the pain is gone.

Essential oils for earache: lavender, tea tree.

AROMATHERAPY EAR RUB

- 3 drops lavender oil
- 3 drops tea tree oil
- 1 tablespoon vegetable oil

Combine ingredients. Rub this oil around the ear and down the side of the neck. For children, remember to use half this dilution (no more than 3 drops total of essential oil to 1 tablespoon carrier oil). Rub on two to four times a day, especially before bed.

FATIGUE

Just as some aromas calm you down, others will perk you up. Researchers found that this is especially true of eucalyptus and pine. The spicy aromas of clove, basil, black pepper, and cinnamon—and to a lesser degree patchouli, lemongrass, and sage—are other aromatherapy stimulants that reduce drowsiness, irritability, and headaches. Several large Tokyo companies circulate lemon, cypress, and peppermint through their air-conditioning and heating systems to keep employees alert. These stimulating essential oils have been shown to prevent the sharp drop in attention that typically hits after working for thirty minutes. Clove, cinnamon, lemon, cardamom, fennel, and angelica act as stimulants. Using aromatherapy stimulants is healthier for you than ingesting stimulants such as coffee because the scents provide energy without causing an adrenaline rush that strains the adrenal glands.

Essential oils for energy: cinnamon, clove, cypress, eucalyptus, fir, ginger, lemon, lemongrass, peppermint, rosemary.

PICK-ME-UP COMBO

- 8 drops lemon oil
- 2 drops eucalyptus oil
- 2 drops peppermint oil
- 1 drop cinnamon leaf oil
- 1 drop cardamom oil (expensive, so optional)
- 2 ounces vegetable oil

Combine the ingredients. Use as a massage oil, add 2 teaspoons to your bath, or add 1 teaspoon to a footbath. Without the vegetable oil, this combination can be used in an aromatherapy diffuser, simmering pan of water, or a potpourri cooker, or it can be added to 2 ounces of water for an air spray. The cardamom oil is optional, but, oh, does it enhance this massage oil! Use it as often as you like.

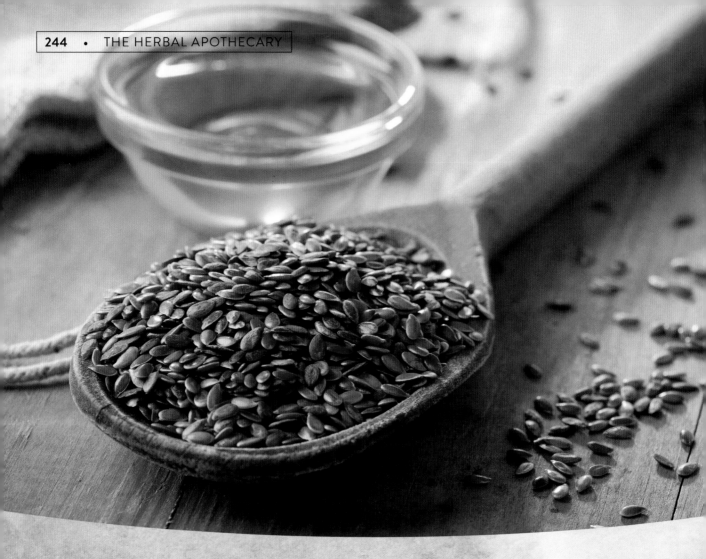

HEADACHES

Aromatherapy really proves its worth with headaches. Peppermint, eucalyptus, and lavender are especially helpful in reducing headache pain. A tincture of lavender called "Palsy Drops" was recognized by the British Pharmacopoeia for more than 200 years and used by physicians to relieve muscle spasms, nervousness, and headaches until the 1940s, when herbs and aroma preparations fell out of favor and chemicals became more popular.

In a 1994 U.S. study by H. Gobel, the essential oils of peppermint and eucalyptus relaxed both the mind and muscles of headache sufferers when the oils were diluted in alcohol and rubbed on their foreheads. Essential oils can be used to make a compress to place on your forehead whenever a headache hits.

Most people find that their headaches respond best to a cold compress, but you can use a warm or hot compress—or alternate the two—for the result that works best. You can also place a second compress at the back of the neck. When you do not have time for compresses, dab a small drop of lavender, eucalyptus, or peppermint oil on each temple. For some people, a hot bath only makes their head pound more. However, if bathing does ease your pain, add a few drops of relaxing lavender or chamomile to your bath water.

HEADACHE-BE-GONE COMPRESS

- 5 drops lavender or eucalyptus oil
- 1 cup cold water

Add essential oil to water, and swish a soft cloth in it. Wring out the cloth, lie down, and close your eyes. Place the cloth over your forehead and eyes. Use throughout the day, as often as you can.

MIGRAINE HEADACHE HAND SOAK

- 5 drops lavender oil
- 5 drops ginger oil
- 1 quart hot water, about 110°F

Add essential oils to the hot water, and soak hands for at least 3 minutes. This therapy can be done repeatedly.

RESTFUL HEADACHE PILLOW

- 12 drops lavender oil
- 12 drops marjoram oil
- 1 cup flax seeds
- Small piece of silk cloth

Add essential oils to flax seeds (found at any natural food store) in a glass jar and let them sit for a week until the oils are absorbed. Fold and stitch the cloth (an old scarf works fine) into a bag and add the scented flax seeds. Sew up the opening. Lie down, and lay this "pillow" over your eyes when you feel a headache coming on. Store the pillow in a glass jar to preserve the scent. If the scent starts to dissipate, you can add more essential oil directly through the cloth as needed.

Migraine headaches can be especially painful. Raising the temperature of the hands a few degrees by soaking them in warm water seems to short-circuit a vascular headache such as a migraine by regulating circulation. Adding a couple drops of essential oil to the water increases the effect. Migraines often respond best to a blend of ginger and lavender.

Cluster headaches can also be quite severe and require special treatment. In addition to the headache compress, try a cream made from capsaicin, the active compound in cayenne peppers. Spread it on your forehead, temples, or any other area where you experience pain, but not too close to the eyes. Capsaicin blocks a neurotransmitter called substance P (which stands for pain), stopping pain impulses from registering in the brain. The cream works best as a preventative, keeping the headache from forming in the first place. Available for sale in drug and natural food stores, it needs to be applied four to five times a day for about four weeks to do much good, yet it is well worth the trouble.

Essential oils for headaches include: chamomile, cinnamon, clove, eucalyptus, ginger, jasmine, lavender, lemongrass, marjoram, patchouli, and peppermint.

HIVES

Hives are rashlike, itchy skin bumps that are most often seen in children, but anyone can get them. They are often caused by a food allergy, although it may be difficult to diagnose at first because the reaction can occur hours or even a day after eating the culprit food. While it's a good idea to eliminate the allergen and build up the immune system, the immediate need is to stop the itching.

The essential oil of chamomile is an excellent first choice to treat hives, but if it's too expensive or you don't have any on hand, you can turn to an essential oil that decreases inflammation, such as lavender. The fragrance of either lavender or chamomile oil can also be very calming to someone who feels that they are going to go mad from the itching.

First wash off the skin. If the itching is not sufficiently relieved, apply the Hives Paste. A child who normally objects to having a poultice smeared on his or her skin will often accept this poultice because it so effectively stops the itching.

HIVES SKIN WASH

- 5 drops chamomile or 10 drops lavender oil
- 2 drops peppermint oil
- 3 tablespoons baking soda
- 2 cups water (or use peppermint tea instead)

Combine the ingredients. If you are making a tea to use as the base instead of water, pour 2 ½ cups of boiling water over 4 teaspoons of dried peppermint leaves, and steep 15 minutes. Strain out the herb. Add the remaining ingredients. Use a soft cloth or a skin sponge to apply on irritated skin until itching is alleviated. Chamomile is the best choice for this recipe, but it is expensive, so 10 drops of lavender essential oil can be substituted, if necessary.

HIVES PASTE

- ¼ cup of the Hives Skin Wash
- 3 tablespoons bentonite clay

Stir the ingredients into a paste, and wait about five minutes for it to thicken. Apply to irritated skin with your fingers or a wooden tongue depressor. Let dry on skin, and leave for at least 45 minutes before washing off. Reapply for another 30 minutes if the area is still itching.

IMMUNE SYSTEM, WEAKENED

Many essential oils have a remarkable ability to both support the immune system and increase one's rate of healing. Some of these same essential oils are also powerful antiseptics. One way these oils fight infection is to stimulate the production of white corpuscles, which are part of the body's immune defense. Still other essential oils encourage new cell growth to promote faster healing. As an extra bonus, the regenerative properties of these essential oils improve the condition and tone of the skin. All can be used in conjunction with herbal remedies designed to improve immunity. Relaxation achieved through a massage or bath lowers stress, improves sleep, and thus stimulates the immune system.

One important way to assist your immune system is with a lymphatic massage that uses essential oils. Lymph nodes are located around the body, particularly in the throat, groin, breasts, and under the arms. They are like filtering centers for cleansing the blood. The lymphatic system moves cellular fluid through the system, cleansing the body of waste produced by the body's metabolic functions. Lemon, rosemary, and grapefruit are especially good at stimulating movement and supporting the cleansing action. A lymphatic massage involves deep strokes that work from the extremities toward the heart. You can even do this on yourself. Rub the oil up your arms to the lymph nodes in your armpits. From the center of your chest, rub again toward the armpit, and then down your neck. Massage your legs from your feet up to the groin.

Essential oils for the immune system: bergamot, grapefruit, lavender, lemon, myrrh, rosemary, tea tree, thyme.

LYMPH MASSAGE OIL

- 6 drops lemon oil
- 6 drops grapefruit oil
- 3 drops rosemary oil
- 2 drops bay laurel (if available)
- 2 ounces vegetable oil

Combine ingredients. You can use this for any type of massage, but it is particularly effective when used in a lymphatic massage as described above.

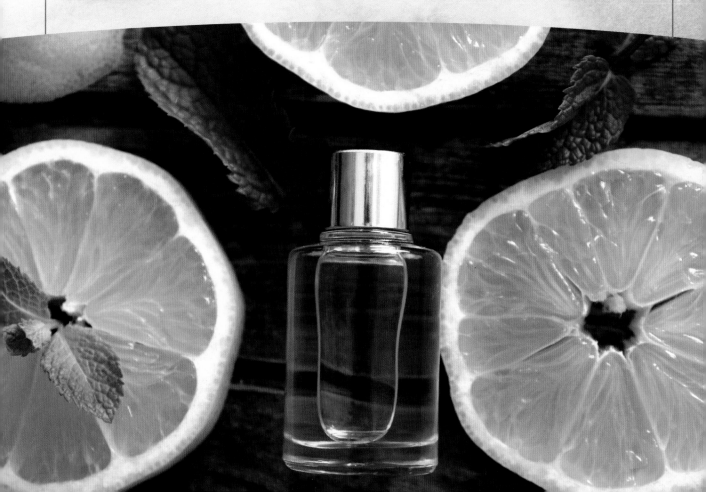

INDIGESTION / NAUSEA

Digestive woes such as belching, stomach pains, and intestinal gas are easily remedied with aromatherapy. A massage oil rubbed on the stomach is especially good for fussy children or anyone who refuses to swallow medicine.

Don't overlook the role that stress plays in impairing digestion. It can restrict the flow of digestive juices and constrict muscles in the digestive tract. No wonder so many people get a queasy stomach when encountering stressful situations. Tension is also thought to contribute to digestive complaints such as colitis and ulcers and most other digestive tract problems.

Aromatics start working at the first stage of digestion, when they signal the brain that food is coming. The response is almost immediate: Digestive juices are released in the mouth, stomach, and small intestine, preparing the way for proper assimilation. To aid digestion, add spices such as anise, basil, caraway, coriander, and fennel to your cooking, or drink a cup of peppermint, thyme, lemon balm, or chamomile tea. Even though many herb books describe these herbs as digestive stimulants, researchers found that most of them actually relax intestinal muscles and relieve cramping. This slower pace gives food more time to be adequately digested and, therefore, prevents gas. Thus, the same essential oils that improve poor appetite also relieve intestinal gas. These include peppermint, ginger, fennel, coriander, and dill.

TUMMY OIL

- 2 drops lemongrass oil
- 1 drop fennel oil
- 2 drops chamomile oil
- 2 ounces vegetable oil

Combine the ingredients and massage over the abdominal area. This all-purpose formula will thwart indigestion, including nausea, gas, appetite loss, and motion sickness, as well as help improve appetite and digestion. You can also add 1 to 2 teaspoons to bathwater. Use as needed. Feel free to alter this formula by choosing other oils on the list, but be careful of hot oils like thyme, peppermint, and black pepper, especially in a bath since they can burn the skin.

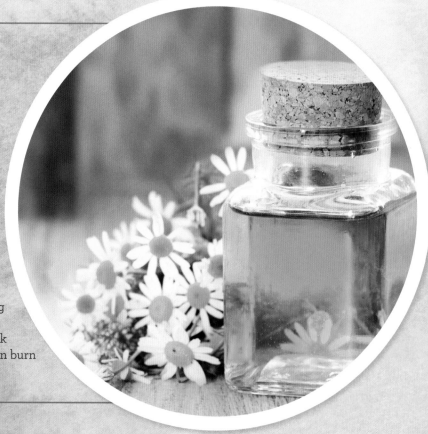

INSECT BITES

For mosquito or other insect bites that don't demand much attention, a simple dab of essential oil of lavender or tea tree provides relief from itching. Chamomile and lavender essential oils reduce swelling and inflammation, and diminish itching or other allergic response. Bentonite clay poultices are of great help for more painful stings or bites. As the clay dries, it pulls toxins to the skin's surface to keep them from spreading, and it pulls out pus or stingers imbedded in the skin. Adding essential oil to clay keeps the clay reconstituted, preserved, and ready for an emergency. If an allergic reaction, such as excessive itching, swelling and inflammation, or difficulty breathing, occurs following a bite, call a doctor immediately.

BUG-OFF REPELLENT

- 12 drops citronella oil
- 12 drops eucalyptus oil
- 6 drops cedarwood oil
- 6 drops geranium oil
- 1 ounce rubbing alcohol or vodka

Mix ingredients together, and dab on exposed skin. This recipe contains a lot of essential oil and is highly concentrated, so don't use it like a massage oil. Rubbing alcohol is poisonous if drunk, so if you use it, be sure to mark the container accordingly. Pat on as needed. Since it won't harm fabrics (except silk), use some of it on your clothes so that you won't apply too much to your skin or absorb too much through the skin.

BITE AND STING POULTICE

- 12 drops lavender oil
- 5 drops chamomile oil
- 1 tablespoon bentonite clay
- 2 teaspoons distilled water

Put clay in the container to be stored. Add the water slowly, stirring more in as the clay absorbs them. Add essential oils, stirring to distribute them evenly. The resulting mixture should be a thick paste. If necessary, add more distilled water to achieve this consistency. Store the paste in a container with a tight lid to slow dehydration. It should last several months, but if the mixture starts to dry out, add a little distilled water to reconstitute it. Use as much and as often as needed.

JOINT PAIN

A liniment heats the skin and underlying muscles and joints to relieve pain. The base of a liniment may be either rubbing alcohol or an edible alcohol such as vodka. If you do use rubbing alcohol, remember that it is toxic to drink, so label it accordingly. Alcohol is cooling and quickly evaporates, leaving no oily residue. Occasionally, though, a person will prefer using a vegetable oil base, making the liniment more like a concentrated massage oil. Oil heats up faster and will stay on the skin longer, making it better for massages.

Essential oils such as cinnamon, peppermint, and clove give a liniment its heating action. Skin-heating preparations like Tiger Balm and White Flower Oil contain peppermint and/or camphor, which stimulate both hot and cold reactions in nerve endings in the skin. The brain registers these sensations at the same time. The contrast between the two messages makes a liniment seem much hotter than it really is.

The most effective liniments also contain muscle-relaxing and inflammation-reducing essential oils such as rosemary, marjoram, and lavender. They penetrate into the skin to work directly on the muscle.

For arthritis, rheumatism, and other inflammatory conditions, use chamomile, marjoram, birch, and ginger in a massage oil. These same oils can also be added to a pain-relieving bath. For arthritic hands or feet, try a daily hand or foot bath.

NERVE PAIN OIL

- 4 drops chamomile oil
- 3 drops marjoram oil
- 3 drops helichrysum oil
- 2 drops lavender oil
- 1 ounce vegetable oil or St. John's wort oil

Combine the ingredients. Apply as needed throughout the day for pain relief. This formula is even more effective if St. John's wort oil is used instead of plain vegetable oil. Buy it at a natural food store.

LINIMENT

- 8 drops eucalyptus oil
- 8 drops peppermint oil
- 8 drops rosemary oil
- 4 drops cinnamon leaf oil
- 4 drops juniper berry oil
- 4 drops marjoram oil
- 2 ounces alcohol (either rubbing or vodka)

Mix ingredients. Shake or stir a few times daily for three days to disperse the essential oils in the alcohol. This formula is stronger than a typical massage oil, so don't use it over a large area of the body. Instead, concentrate on painful joints. It will also work well as a warm-up liniment before exercising or heavy physical work to help prevent muscles from cramping or becoming stiff. If preferred, the alcohol in this recipe can be replaced with a vegetable oil. Use several times a day as needed.

Essential oils for joint pain include: birch, chamomile, clove, cypress, fir, ginger, juniper berry, marjoram, peppermint, and rosemary.

MUSCLE CRAMPS

Muscles can hurt after a vigorous day of exercise or work, especially if you aren't exercising on a regular basis and then really go for it. Activities that you repeat daily can also tighten muscles and cause them to cramp. This cramp relief oil formula is excellent for lower back or shoulder pain, tight muscles from working at a computer, or the aftereffects of physical exercise. Even menstrual cramps, which are really little more than the cramping of the uterine muscle, respond well to this remedy. By the way, this same recipe can be used as a first-aid treatment along with ice on sprains and bruises. The sooner it is applied, the better. It reduces the swelling and pain and promotes faster healing.

CRAMP RELIEF OIL

- 12 drops lavender oil
- 6 drops marjoram oil
- 4 drops chamomile oil
- 4 drops ginger oil
- 2 ounces vegetable oil or St. John's wort oil

Combine ingredients. Apply throughout the day as often as needed over the cramping area. This formula is also excellent for the lower back pain that sometimes accompanies menstrual cramps. It works well when made with plain vegetable oil, but if you can, use an herbal oil made from St. John's wort oil instead, as it is excellent for sore muscles. You can buy a ready-made version at natural food stores.

NAUSEA/MOTION SICKNESS

That queasy feeling in the stomach that signals nausea can be caused by quite a few different problems. Topping the list are motion sickness, food poisoning, the flu, headaches, emotional upset, anxiety, medications, and pregnancy. Peppermint and ginger ease both nausea and motion sickness. Chamomile and fennel relax the stomach and soothe burning irritation and inflammation. Basil overcomes nausea from chemotherapy or radiation treatments (even when conventional drugs have little effect). Lemongrass is used in Brazil, the Caribbean, and much of southeast Asia to relieve nervous digestion. Sometimes the smell alone of such essential oils as peppermint, ginger, or basil is enough to quell nausea. If not, use them in a massage oil where they will enter the bloodstream.

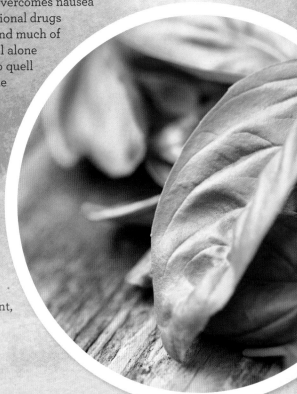

Prefer the taste of peppermint? It comes in a close second in preventing motion sickness and works equally well for general stomach upsets. While essential oils are far too potent to ingest, you can take the extract of peppermint that is sold at the grocery store in the baking section. Used mostly to flavor candy, this product is a diluted and water soluble form of the essential oil. A couple drops of peppermint extract in a glass of water makes a handy first aid remedy. If you are prone to motion sickness, carry a small vial of the extract with you on your next airplane flight, boat ride, or any form of travel.

Essential oils for nausea and motion sickness: ginger, peppermint, sandalwood.

STOMACH SOOTHER

- 1–3 drops peppermint extract (not in essential oil form!)
- ½–1 cup water (preferably warm)

Add the extract to the water. Sip to ease nausea or stomach upset, and repeat after 20–30 minutes if you haven't experienced relief.

PREMENSTRUAL SYNDROME (PMS)

Premenstrual syndrome, better known as PMS, is a collection of many different symptoms that typically begin several days or even a week before menstruation. The host of symptoms include water retention, breast swelling and tenderness, depression, irritability, mood swings, and headaches. Not all women who get PMS experience all of these symptoms, but any one of them can greatly alter one's life while going through it. In many ways, aromatherapy is ideal to treat PMS. Taking time out to lounge in an aromatic bath or getting a massage with a fragrant oil helps most women tremendously. For depression and mood swings associated with PMS, nothing can beat clary sage. The essential oils of neroli, rose, and jasmine may be expensive, but their heavenly fragrances help dispel moodiness and irritability.

For the excessive bloating and swollen breasts of PMS, use the essential oils of juniper berry, patchouli, grapefruit, and carrot seed. Another good oil for this is birch, which is also a natural pain reliever. Use juniper berry if you experience water retention. If headache is among your PMS symptoms, try an inhalation of lavender or marjoram. For best results with any PMS or menstruation remedy, begin using it a couple of days before you experience any symptoms.

Essential oils for PMS: chamomile, clary sage, geranium, jasmine, marjoram, neroli, rose.

MOOD OIL

- 9 drops geranium oil
- 6 drops chamomile oil
- 3 drops clary sage oil
- 3 drops angelica oil (optional)
- 2 drops marjoram oil
- 2 ounces vegetable oil

Combine the ingredients. The angelica oil is heavenly, but optional, as it may be hard to find. Use daily as a massage oil or add 1 to 2 teaspoons to a bath. To make it more elegant and effective, add 1 or 2 drops of neroli, rose, or jasmine. Without the vegetable oil, you can use this in a diffuser or simply carry around a vial of it to smell as needed.

BLOATING AND HEADACHE RELIEF OIL

- 6 drops lavender oil
- 3 drops juniper berry oil
- 2 drops birch oil
- 1 drop patchouli oil (optional)

Combine ingredients. Use as a massage oil or add 1 to 2 teaspoons to your bath or 1 teaspoon to a foot bath. Don't use the patchouli if you don't like the smell; it can easily overwhelm a formula.

SORE THROAT/LARYNGITIS

A bacterial infection or lots of singing, talking, or yelling can cause a sore throat. At times, the throat can be so inflamed and painful that it becomes difficult to swallow. If the inflammation is in the voice box, you can easily come down with laryngitis, in which your voice is reduced to a hoarse whisper or it even may become impossible to talk at all. For centuries, European singers have known the secret to preserving their voices with aromatherapy and herbal remedies. Their most popular sore throat and laryngitis cure is to gargle with a marjoram herb tea that has been sweetened with honey. You can use the essential oil of marjoram to make a similar remedy. As both an antiseptic and anti-inflammatory, it is a good choice. Other essential oils or herb teas to use as a gargle are sage, hyssop, and thyme, all of which kill bacterial infections.

Any of these essential oils can easily be gargled or sprayed into the throat. This brings the antibacterial and soothing essential oils into direct contact with the bacteria responsible for causing a sore throat or laryngitis. In an emergency, a few drops of essential oil diluted in two ounces of water may also be used. Both lavender and eucalyptus work so well in an aromatherapy steam to recover your voice that you must remind yourself to not overstress it until your throat fully recovers. And don't forget the old standard of a hot drink made with fresh lemon juice and honey.

Essential oils for sore throat: bergamot, eucalyptus, lavender, lemon, marjoram, sage, sandalwood, tea tree, thyme.

THROAT SPRAY OR GARGLE

- 4 drops marjoram oil
- ½ cup warm water
- ½ teaspoon salt

Combine ingredients. Shake well to dissolve the salt and disperse the oils before spraying or gargling. Gargle every half hour at first and then several times a day.

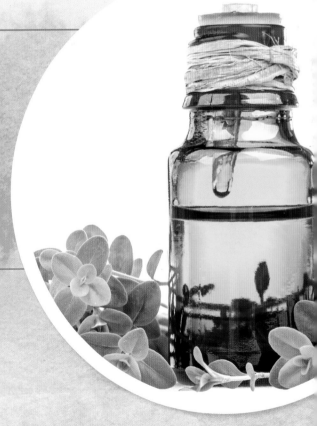

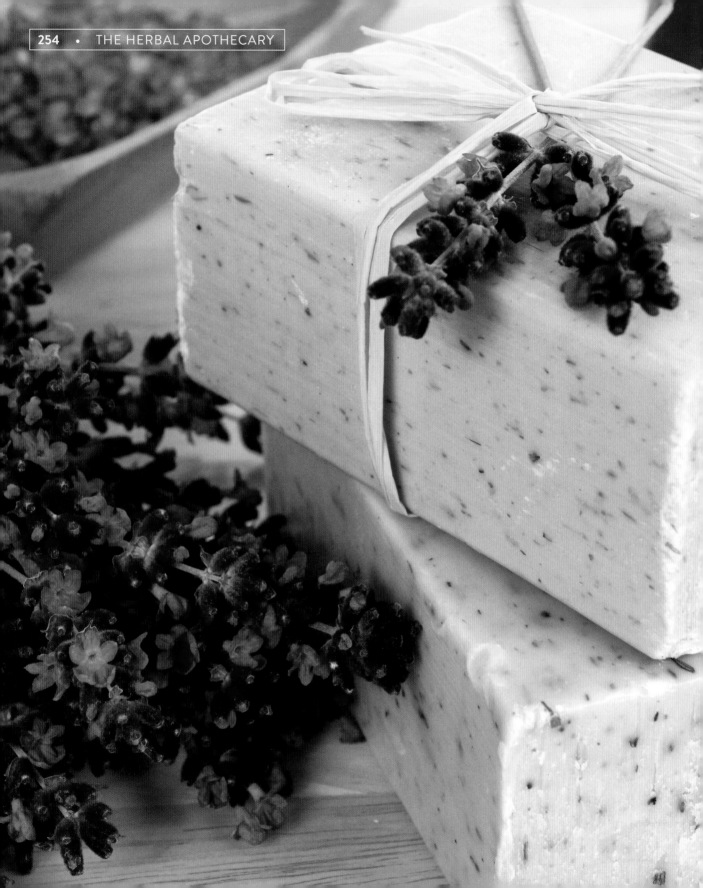

SOAPS AND CLEANING PRODUCTS

LAVENDER-SCENTED LIQUID SOAP

- 1 cup liquid bubble bath base
- ¾ cup distilled water
- ¼ teaspoon lavender essential oil
- 8-10 drops purple soap coloring

Combine bubble bath base, distilled water, essential oil, and coloring in a 2-cup measuring cup. Stir well. Insert funnel into a 16-ounce clear bottle with a tight-fitting cap. Pour in mixture.

LAVENDER SOAP

- 1 bar unscented white soap
- 15 drops lavender essential oil
- 5 drops rose essential oil
- 8-10 drops violet or purple soap coloring
- ¼ cup hot distilled water
- ¼ cup dried lavender buds or blossoms

Grate soap into medium bowl with a cheese grater. Add essential oils and soap coloring. Add the hot water and stir vigorously to distribute color evenly. Mixture will be the consistency of wet dough. Working quickly, knead in the lavender buds before the soap firms up. Form soap into 3 small balls or oval bars. Set aside on plastic wrap to dry at room temperature 24 hours.

ORANGE BLOSSOM LIQUID SOAP

- Grated peel of 1 lemon
- Grated peel of 1 orange
- 1 cup liquid bubble bath base
- ¼ teaspoon orange blossom essential oil

Combine lemon peel, orange peel and 1 cup water in small saucepan. Simmer 5 minutes. Remove from heat. Set aside to steep 1 hour. Insert funnel into a 16-ounce clear bottle with a tight-fitting cap. Place a small coffee filter in funnel. Pour lemon/orange mixture into bottle. Discard the filter and add the bubble bath base and essential oil. Seal bottle tightly and shake well.

ALMOND AND TANGERINE GLYCERIN FACIAL SOAP

- Sunflower oil or jojoba oil
- 12 ounces clear or white glycerin soap base
- ½ cup ground raw almonds
- 1 tablespoon honey
- 15 drops tangerine or orange essential oil

Lightly grease 6 muffin cups with sunflower oil; set aside.

Slice soap base into slivers. Place in microwave-safe bowl. Cover loosely with plastic wrap. Microwave on high in 30-second intervals, stirring the soap in between intervals, until the soap is liquid. Stir in almonds, honey, and tangerine oil.

Quickly pour mixture into muffin cups, filling about ¾ full. Set aside to firm up, about 1 hour. Run a small sharp knife around the inside edge of the muffin cups to release soap.

LEMONGRASS SOAP

- ½ gallon cardboard milk or orange juice carton, empty, rinsed, and dried
- ½ pound white vegetable soap compound
- 2 teaspoons finely minced dried or fresh lemongrass stalk
- 2-3 drops lemongrass essential oil or cosmetic bath salt or soap fragrance

Measure 2 inches up from bottom of milk carton. Using serrated knife or scissors, cut off bottom of carton and reserve.

Break or cut soap compound into 1-inch cubes. Place into 1-quart microwave safe glass measuring cup. Microwave on high in 30-second intervals or less, stirring the soap in between intervals, until the compound melts. Remove from microwave and stir in the lemongrass and essential oil (stir gently to avoid creating bubbles).

Pour the mixture into the carton and let cool 10-15 minutes. Use a toothpick or bamboo skewer to distribute lemongrass in compound, if needed. Place mold in refrigerator for 1 hour. Turn the soap out and cut into cubes.